NUTRITION 97/98

Ninth Edition

W9-ARS-103

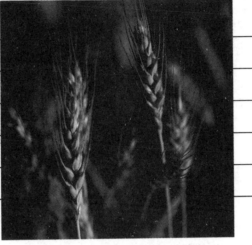

Editor

Charlotte C. Cook-Fuller
Towson State University

Charlotte Cook-Fuller has a Ph.D. in community health education and graduate and undergraduate degrees in nutrition. She has worked for several years in public health services and has also been involved with the federally funded WIC (Women, Infants, and Children) program. Now as a professor, she teaches nutrition within both professional and consumer contexts, as well as courses for health education students. She has coauthored a nutrition curriculum for grades K–12 and is currently involved in a multidisciplinary effort to provide strategies to public school teachers for teaching about global issues such as hunger.

Editorial Consultant

Stephen Barrett, M.D.
Editor, *Nutrition Forum*

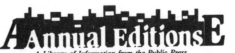

Annual Editions
A Library of Information from the Public Press
Dushkin/McGraw·Hill
Sluice Dock, Guilford, Connecticut 06437

Visit us on the Internet—http://www.dushkin.com

The Annual Editions Series

ANNUAL EDITIONS is a series of over 65 volumes designed to provide the reader with convenient, low-cost access to a wide range of current, carefully selected articles from some of the most important magazines, newspapers, and journals published today. ANNUAL EDITIONS are updated on an annual basis through a continuous monitoring of over 300 periodical sources. All ANNUAL EDITIONS have a number of features that are designed to make them particularly useful, including topic guides, annotated tables of contents, unit overviews, and indexes. For the teacher using ANNUAL EDITIONS in the classroom, an Instructor's Resource Guide with test questions is available for each volume.

VOLUMES AVAILABLE

Abnormal Psychology
Adolescent Psychology
Africa
Aging
American Foreign Policy
American Government
American History, Pre-Civil War
American History, Post-Civil War
American Public Policy
Anthropology
Archaeology
Biopsychology
Business Ethics
Child Growth and Development
China
Comparative Politics
Computers in Education
Computers in Society
Criminal Justice
Criminology
Developing World
Deviant Behavior
Drugs, Society, and Behavior
Dying, Death, and Bereavement

Early Childhood Education
Economics
Educating Exceptional Children
Education
Educational Psychology
Environment
Geography
Global Issues
Health
Human Development
Human Resources
Human Sexuality
India and South Asia
International Business
Japan and the Pacific Rim
Latin America
Life Management
Macroeconomics
Management
Marketing
Marriage and Family
Mass Media
Microeconomics

Middle East and the
   Islamic World
Multicultural Education
Nutrition
Personal Growth and Behavior
Physical Anthropology
Psychology
Public Administration
Race and Ethnic Relations
Russia, the Eurasian Republics,
   and Central/Eastern Europe
Social Problems
Social Psychology
Sociology
State and Local Government
Urban Society
Western Civilization,
   Pre-Reformation
Western Civilization,
   Post-Reformation
Western Europe
World History, Pre-Modern
World History, Modern
World Politics

Cataloging in Publication Data
Main entry under title: Annual editions: Nutrition. 1997/98.
   1. Nutrition—Periodicals. 2. Diet—Periodicals. I. Cook-Fuller, Charlotte C., *comp.* II.
Title: Nutrition.
   ISBN 0–697–37331–2   613.2′.05   91–641611

Ninth Edition

Cover image © 1996 PhotoDisc, Inc.

Printed in the United States of America

Editors/Advisory Board

Staff

To the Reader

In publishing ANNUAL EDITIONS we recognize the enormous role played by the magazines, newspapers, and journals of the *public press* in providing current, first-rate educational information in a broad spectrum of interest areas. Many of these articles are appropriate for students, researchers, and professionals seeking accurate, current material to help bridge the gap between principles and theories and the real world. These articles, however, become more useful for study when those of lasting value are carefully *collected, organized, indexed,* and *reproduced* in a *low-cost format,* which provides easy and permanent access when the material is needed. That is the role played by ANNUAL EDITIONS. Under the direction of each volume's *academic editor,* who is an expert in the subject area, and with the guidance of an *Advisory Board,* each year we seek to provide in each ANNUAL EDITION a current, well-balanced, carefully selected collection of the best of the public press for your study and enjoyment. We think that you will find this volume useful, and we hope that you will take a moment to let us know what you think.

You may agree with Pudd'nhead Wilson (a character created by Mark Twain), who said, "The only way to keep your health is to eat what you don't want, drink what you don't like, and do what you'd rather not." Nutritionists would argue that you cannot achieve or maintain good health on a diet of soft drinks and vending machine foods. But you might be surprised to learn that many of your favorite foods can fit into a good diet. In making food choices, remember that variety and moderation are two key words that will assist you in achieving positive health outcomes and avoiding the negative results of excesses or deficiencies.

An array of resources is available to help you make decisions, including popular publications, the news media, scientific journals, and people from many educational backgrounds. Your dilemma is to select reliable sources that will supply factual information based on science rather than exaggerations based on bias. It is important to avoid overreacting to nutrition- and food-related news items or promotional materials, especially if they sound sensational or have shock value. The exaggeration and the myth are what much of the public grasps and, in large measure, reacts to. My challenge to you is to use *Annual Editions: Nutrition 97/98,* preferably with a standard nutrition text, as an invitation to learning. Become a discriminating learner. Compare what you hear and read to the accepted body of knowledge. If this volume provides you with useful information, challenges your thinking, broadens your understanding, or motivates you to take some useful action, it will have fulfilled its purpose.

While this entire volume is essentially one of current events and current thinking, the first unit focuses on trends that give a preview of the future and that relate to characteristics of today's food consumer, the food industry, and views of foods and food components. The next three units are devoted to nutrients, diet and disease, and weight control. All are topics which directly relate to our health, and the dynamic state of knowledge on these subjects requires each of us to be constantly learning and adjusting. Units on food safety and health claims follow—areas in which consumers are especially vulnerable to media and promotional hype and misinformation. The last unit addresses hunger and malnutrition as a social and political issue as well as one requiring scientific knowledge for solution. Originally, this unit was intended as a forum for global concerns, but it has become abundantly clear that hunger is also a national issue.

Although the units in this book are distinct, many of the articles have broader significance. The topic guide will help you to find other articles on a given subject. You will also find that many of the articles contain at least some element of controversy, the origin of which may be incomplete knowledge, questionable policy, pseudoscience, or competing needs. Sometimes these are difficult issues to resolve, and frequently any resolution creates further dilemmas. But creatively solving problems is our challenge. We take the world as it is and use it as the foundation for tomorrow's discoveries and solutions.

Annual Editions: Nutrition 97/98 is an anthology, and any anthology can be improved, including this one. You can influence the content of future editions by returning the postage-paid article rating form on the last page of this book with your comments and suggestions.

Charlotte C. Cook-Fuller

Charlotte C. Cook-Fuller
Editor

Contents

UNIT 1

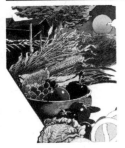

Trends Today and Tomorrow

Eleven articles examine the eating patterns of people today. Some of the topics considered include nutrients in our diet, eating trends, food labeling, self-service outlets, and the impact of biotechnology.

The concepts in bold italics are developed in the article. For further expansion please refer to the Topic Guide, the Glossary, and the Index.

Overview   46

UNIT 2

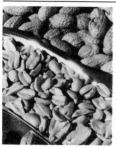

Nutrients

Ten articles discuss the importance of nutrients and fiber in our diet. Topics include dietary standards, carbohydrates, fiber, vitamins, supplements, and minerals.

UNIT 3

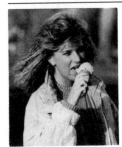

Through the Life Span: Diet and Disease

Seven articles examine our health as it is affected by diet throughout our lives. Some topics include the links between diet and disease, cholesterol, and eating habits.

The concepts in bold italics are developed in the article. For further expansion please refer to the Topic Guide, the Glossary, and the Index.

UNIT 4

Fat and Weight Control

Seven articles examine weight
management. Topics include
the relationship between dieting
and exercise, the effects of
various diet plans, and the
relationship between being
overweight and fit.

Overview   114

The concepts in bold italics are developed in the article. For further expansion please refer to the Topic Guide, the Glossary, and the Index.

UNIT 5

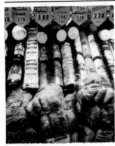

Food Safety

Eight articles discuss the safety of food. Topics include food-borne illness, pesticide residues, naturally occurring toxins, and food preservatives.

The concepts in bold italics are developed in the article. For further expansion please refer to the Topic Guide, the Glossary, and the Index.

UNIT 6

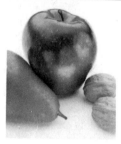

Health Claims

Eleven articles examine some of the health claims made by today's "specialists." Topics include quacks, fad diets, and nutrition myths and misinformation.

The concepts in bold italics are developed in the article. For further expansion please refer to the Topic Guide, the Glossary, and the Index.

UNIT 7

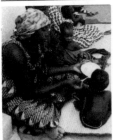

Hunger and Global Issues

Five articles discuss the world's food supply. Topics include global malnutrition, communicable diseases, and famine.

Topic Guide

This topic guide suggests how the selections in this book relate to topics of traditional concern to students and professionals involved with the study of nutrition. It is useful for locating articles that relate to each other for reading and research. The guide is arranged alphabetically according to topic. Articles may, of course, treat topics that do not appear in the topic guide. In turn, entries in the topic guide do not necessarily constitute a comprehensive listing of all the contents of each selection.

TOPIC AREA	TREATED IN	TOPIC AREA	TREATED IN
Additives	41. New Scientific Review Reaffirms Safety of MSG	Dieting	25. Teens at Risk 32. Dieting and Weight Loss Increase Osteoporosis Risk 33. Losing Weight Safely
Alcohol	11. Alcohol: Spirit of Health?		
Antioxidants	5. Phytochemicals 17. Trials of Beta-Carotene 18. Vitamin E	Diet/Disease	5. Phytochemicals 6. Taking Soy to Heart 27. Is Butter Really Better for Me?
Athletes	25. Teens at Risk 51. Supplements Are Unnecessary to Enhance Athletic Performance	Eating Disorders	25. Teens at Risk
		Elderly	26. Boning Up on Osteoporosis 31. New Study Finds Higher Weight Protects Elderly 32. Dieting and Weight Loss Increase Osteoporosis Risk 57. Federal Food Assistance Programs
Attitudes/ Knowledge	1. Consumer Nutrition and Food Safety Trends 1996 9. Genetic Engineering 24. Kids Just Want to Have Fun 25. Teens at Risk		
Biotechnology	9. Genetic Engineering 10. Genetically Altered States	Fats/Substitutes	7. Taking the Fat Out of Food 8. Fast Food: Fatter than Ever 14. Facts about Fats 27. Is Butter Really Better for Me?
Cancer	5. Phytochemicals 11. Alcohol: Spirit of Health? 14. Facts about Fats 17. Trials of Beta-Carotene	Fiber	21. Fiber 41. New Scientific Review Reaffirms Safety of MSG 53. Herbal Roulette
Children	24. Kids Just Want to Have Fun 28. Vegetarian Diets 35. New Paradigm of Trust 57. Federal Food Assistance Programs	Food and Drug Administration (FDA)	7. Taking the Fat Out of Food 9. Genetic Engineering 10. Genetically Altered States
Controversies	7. Taking the Fat Out of Food 9. Genetic Engineering 19. Vitamin C 27. Is Butter Really Better for Me? 30. New Study Questions Weight Guidelines 42. After the Glow 53. Herbal Roulette 55. Averting a Global Food Crisis 59. Modern Farming Yields Bountiful Fields of Dreams	Food-borne Illness	36. Foodborne Illness: Role of Home Food Handling Practices 37. New Risks in Ground Beef Revealed 38. Botulinum Toxin 39. Mad Cow Madness 42. After the Glow
		Food Safety	9. Genetic Engineering 10. Genetically Altered States 37. New Risks in Ground Beef Revealed 38. Botulinum Toxin 39. Mad Cow Madness 40. How Much Are Pesticides Hurting Your Health? 41. New Scientific Review Reaffirms Safety of MSG 42. After the Glow 43. Naturally Occurring Toxins
Coronary/Heart Disease	5. Phytochemicals 6. Taking Soy to Heart 11. Alcohol: Spirit of Health? 14. Facts about Fats 18. Vitamin E 27. Is Butter Really Better for Me?		
Cultural Influence	22. Nutritional Implications of Ethnic and Cultural Diversity	Food Supply	55. Averting a Global Food Crisis 56. Nibbling at Famine's Edge 59. Modern Farming Yields Bountiful Fields of Dreams

TOPIC AREA	TREATED IN	TOPIC AREA	TREATED IN
Guidelines/ Recommendations	2. 1995 Dietary Guidelines 3. Food Pyramid 4. Not-So-Great Mediterranean Diet Pyramid 5. Phytochemicals 8. Fast Food: Fatter than Ever 12. Should You Be Eating More Protein— or Less? 16. Vitamin A 20. Special Report: Iron Overkill 21. Fiber 24. Kids Just Want to Have Fun 26. Boning Up on Osteoporosis 28. Vegetarian Diets 30. New Study Questions Weight Guidelines 31. New Study Finds Higher Weight Protects Elderly 36. Foodborne Illness: Role of Home Food Handling Practices 37. New Risks in Ground Beef Revealed 38. Botulinum Toxin	Recommended Daily Allowances (RDA)	16. Vitamin A 19. Vitamin C
		Risk/Benefit	7. Taking the Fat Out of Food 9. Genetic Engineering 10. Genetically Altered States 11. Alcohol: Spirit of Health? 15. Food for Thought about Dietary Supplements 16. Vitamin A 17. Trials of Beta-Carotene 18. Vitamin E 19. Vitamin C 27. Is Butter Really Better for Me? 28. Vegetarian Diets 31. New Study Finds Higher Weight Protects Elderly 34. Surgery for Obesity 41. New Scientific Review Reaffirms Safety of MSG 42. After the Glow 43. Naturally Occurring Toxins 49. Vitamin Pushers and Food Quacks 53. Herbal Roulette
Herbals	53. Herbal Roulette 54. Herbal Warning		
Hunger/ Malnutrition	55. Averting a Global Food Crisis 56. Nibbling at Famine's Edge 57. Federal Food Assistance Programs 58. Thunder in the Distance	Sugar/Sugar Substitutes	13. What's Wrong with Sugar?
Labeling	33. Losing Weight Safely 50. Supplement Bill Passes	Supplements	15. Food for Thought about Dietary Supplements 16. Vitamin A 17. Trials of Beta-Carotene 18. Vitamin E 19. Vitamin C 49. Vitamin Pushers and Food Quacks 50. Supplement Bill Passes 51. Supplements Are Unnecessary to Enhance Athletic Performance 52. Nutrition Shortcut in a Can? 53. Herbal Roulette 54. Herbal Warning
Minerals	20. Special Report: Iron Overkill 25. Teens at Risk 26. Boning Up on Osteoporosis		
Myths/ Misinformation	13. What's Wrong with Sugar? 15. Food for Thought about Dietary Supplements 44. How Quackery Sells 47. Food for Thought 48. Why Do Those #&*?@! "Experts" Keep Changing Their Minds? 49. Vitamin Pushers and Food Quacks 51. Supplements Are Unnecessary to Enhance Athletic Performance		
		Teenagers	25. Teens at Risk
		Vegetarians	28. Vegetarian Diets
Obesity	25. Teens at Risk 29. Obesity: No Miracle Cure Yet	Vitamins	15. Food for Thought about Dietary Supplements 16. Vitamin A 17. Trials of Beta-Carotene 18. Vitamin E 19. Vitamin C 49. Vitamin Pushers and Food Quacks
Pesticides	40. How Much Are Pesticides Hurting Your Health?		
Phytochemicals	5. Phytochemicals	Weight/Weight Control	14. Facts about Fats 29. Obesity: No Miracle Cure Yet 30. New Study Questions Weight Guidelines 31. New Study Finds Higher Weight Protects Elderly 32. Dieting and Weight Loss Increase Osteoporosis Risk 33. Losing Weight Safely 34. Surgery for Obesity 35. New Paradigm of Trust
Policy Decisions	2. 1995 Dietary Guidelines 50. Supplement Bill Passes		
Pregnancy	16. Vitamin A 25. Teens at Risk		
Protein	12. Should You Be Eating More Protein— or Less? 28. Vegetarian Diets 51. Supplements Are Unnecessary to Enhance Athletic Performance		

Trends Today and Tomorrow

It is change, continuing change, inevitable change, that is the dominant factor in society today. No sensible decision can be made any longer without taking into account not only the world as it is, but the world as it will be.
—Isaac Asimov

The average consumer is a phantom, constantly reshaping and reemerging under the influences of the food industry, the media, activist organizations, and whatever health messages are currently most persuasive. Years ago, for the sake of heart health, we were persuaded to switch from butter and lard to vegetable oil and margarine. Later, we obediently avoided tropical oils. Now we are told to beware of the trans fatty acids produced in the manufacture of solid margarines. Indeed, for the last half-century, Americans have been bombarded by health and nutrition messages and admonitions at an increasingly rapid rate, many of which have been misleading and contradictory. It is no wonder that consumers have become more and more confused and have grown disenchanted with conventional sources of advice. In a recent poll, half of the respondents reported being unhappy with conflicting information, and 81 percent said they would rather get information *after* nutrition and health professionals have reached consensus. As more and more people access the Internet, this problem may be exacerbated rather than alleviated.

All of this does not mean that Americans are unconcerned or disinterested in their dietary habits. The first article identifies several trends and issues of interest and concern to consumers, more than a third of whom indicate they are doing all they can to achieve a healthy diet. Americans say their priority issues for today are weight, dietary fat, and children's nutrition. That fat is of concern can be verified by the reduction of daily fat calories as a portion of meals from 40 percent in the 1970s to 34 percent in 1994. Paradoxically, total caloric intakes have increased during the same time period, causing many of us to gain eight pounds or more. Consumers also report that taste and time are high-priority issues. McDonald's McLean Deluxe burger, considered unpalatable by the public, has finally disappeared from the market, and it is reported that this chain will stop selling salads as well. In another development that contradicts good eating habits, many restaurants and fast-food chains report a move toward larger serving sizes. That we now spend 44 percent of our food budgets outside the home, double the

percentage since 1955, speaks to our willingness to go along with, even to promote, these trends.

New, lower-fat products are constantly entering the market. Fat replacers, which make many of these new items possible, are a hot news topic today, especially the recent controversial addition of Olestra, discussed in "Taking the Fat Out of Food." Even as snack chips made with Olestra are being market-tested in three states, the Center for Science in the Public Interest (CSPI) has accelerated its negative campaign. Limited approval from the FDA requires Proctor & Gamble to monitor Olestra's effects and undergo a review within the next 30 months. Meanwhile, an announcement of a newer product called Z-Trim has already been made. If we want our lower fat in other ways, we might check out the low-calorie, low-fat ostrich meat now being ranch-raised in several western states or the two new lower-fat Girl Scout cookies. A low-cholesterol egg yolk product, already being used in food products, may soon reach the shelves as a stand-alone egg product as well.

Today's consumer is sophisticated and desirous of information about diets and food. Responses have come from government agencies and the food industry as well as professionals and voluntary associations. The revised Recommended Dietary Allowance (RDAs) are not yet published, but the 1995 Dietary Guidelines are now available and are discussed in the second article in this unit. Issued jointly by the U.S. Departments of Agriculture and Health and Human Services, their purpose is to provide advice to healthy Americans about the relationship between food choices and health. This edition has been changed to reflect a clear linkage to the Food Pyramid and the Nutrition Facts Label and emphasizes the advantages of fruits, vegetables, and grain products. A review of these guidelines is mandatory every five years, and publication of a new edition follows a lengthy process of literature review; solicitation of written comments from health professionals, trade organizations, and the public; and public hearings.

Perhaps an issue of greater significance than fat replacements is the controversy over whether to use butter or margarine, since the physiological effects of the trans fatty acids produced in hydrogenation may also be unhealthy. Does that mean, then, that the saturated fat in butter is less dangerous to health than margarine? The key issue is the *amount* of fat.

Another trend worthy of note is the increased interest in food chemicals other than nutrients. Called phytochemicals, they represent an expanded knowledge of the chemical composition of normal foods and their potential for promoting good health and preventing diseases such as cancer and heart disease. More and more frequently we read about the possible advantages of isoflavones, saponins, flavinoids, phytoestrogens, and many others. The promises are great but are mostly unproven, making the balance between developing this new market and maintaining public health and safety a challenge. The best current wisdom dictates eating a wide variety of foods with emphasis on fruits, vegetables, and whole grains rather than on supplements or manufactured foods. Two articles on phytochemicals and soy products discuss these issues.

In "Genetic Engineering: Fast Forwarding to Future Goals," John Henkel relates the use of genetic engineering or biotechnology to produce modified, but familiar, foods. Reports indicate that the first genetically altered food, the Flavr Savr tomato, a vine-ripened fruit that has a prolonged shelf life, is well accepted. Other possibilities may be even more exciting in the future: disease- or insect-resistant crops, potatoes that absorb less fat, plants that resist freezing. Some see gene splicing as simply shortening the time required by older, more cumbersome plant

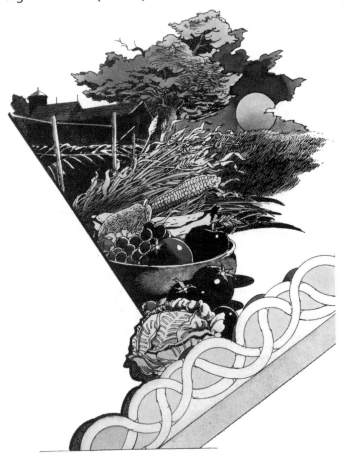

breeding programs. Others have worries about safety and ethical issues and public acceptance. The article "Genetically Altered States" reports that one of the concerns, the possibility of transferring a gene that will initiate allergies, has occurred. Fortunately, the industry involved responded in a proactive and highly responsible fashion.

Finally, an article on alcohol discusses the evidence regarding its benefits in protecting against heart disease and other conditions. As always, this is a case of "some will win and some will lose." Small deviations in the amount of alcohol consumed can spell the difference between benefit and risk.

In other news, a maroon-colored carrot, called Beta Sweet, is reported ready to enter the market by the end of this year. Originally bred to match the football colors at Texas A&M University, it was found to have six times the beta carotene of other carrots. Barbie dolls are promoting milk drinking by clutching a milk carton and wearing cow-print clothes. Coca-Cola is to have a newly contoured can, something else for those of us who must have change. And, of course, the big news includes the price wars being waged by the top three cereal companies, a response to a sluggish market. Thus we end another year.

Cultural change clearly is occurring in our lifetimes. An orange was a treat in the toe of my mother's Christmas stocking. As a child I had fresh oranges and orange juice in cans. For my daughters, frozen orange juice was commonplace. My grandchildren enjoy drinking it from sealed cartons and fortified with calcium, although all of the previous options remain. Which of the new food experiences being planned for us will we like, and which will retreat into oblivion? Perhaps all we can say with certainty is that there will be change.

Looking Ahead: Challenge Questions

What current consumer trends and trends in the food industry will and will not support healthier lifestyles?

Based on Figure 1 in the article "Consumer Nutrition and Food Safety Trends 1996," identify specific organizations that fit each category. Which ones do you believe to be operating responsibly to assist the consumer?

Discuss the implications of promoting genetically engineered foods as they relate to health and ethical issues.

Compare the 1995 Dietary Guidelines to an earlier version. In what ways does the newest edition better represent good dietary practice? What further suggestions do you have for alteration?

What would be a knowledgeable consumer response to all of the information about phytochemicals and the availability of highly fortified foods?

Does change always equal progress? Why or why not? Give examples from the nutrition field.

Consumer Nutrition and Food Safety Trends 1996

An Update

Nine consumer nutrition and food safety trends, identified in 1995, have been revisited and updated to reflect the status of current consumer influencer activities. Major forces that influence the consumer nutrition environment have been closely scrutinized. Significant activities that have occurred in the last half of 1995 are put into perspective to anticipate what lies ahead for consumers in 1996.

KATHLEEN E. MCMAHON, Ph.D., R.D.

Kathleen E. McMahon, Ph.D., R.D., is Vice President, Nutrition and Scientific Communications, at Edelman Public Relations Worldwide. She has more than 10 years of consumer nutrition issues management and communications experience in the food industry. In addition, Dr. McMahon, a member of the American Institute of Nutrition, served on the Board of Directors of the Society for Nutrition Education from 1990 to 1993. Correspondence can be directed to Dr. McMahon at Edelman Public Relations, 200 East Randolph Drive, 63rd Floor, Chicago, IL 60601.

An approach to predicting and monitoring major consumer nutrition trends, based upon the activities of major consumer influencer groups, was extensively outlined previously.[1] This 1996 update analyzes recent key consumer influencer activities from the end of 1995 to gain insight into the nutrition and food safety issues consumers will face in 1996.

WHERE CONSUMERS ARE HEADING IN 1996

According to The American Dietetic Association (ADA) 1995 Nutrition Trends Survey,[2] only 35% of Americans are doing all they can to achieve a healthy diet, down from 44% in 1991 and 39% in 1993. Consumers' perceived obstacles continue to be taste, time, and confusion. Consumers report that the biggest source of their nutrition information is television (42%), followed by magazines (39%) and newspapers (19%). However, 49% of consumers found the increasing level of news reports somewhat or very confusing. They found much of it negative and difficult to apply to their diets and lifestyle. This represents a challenge for each of the influencer groups to realize and

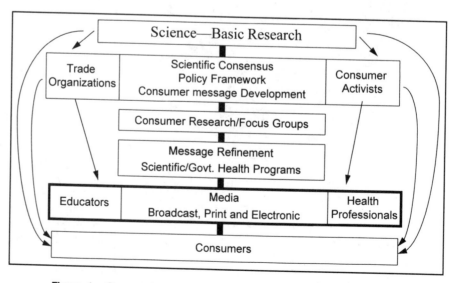

Figure 1. Communication flow from key influencers to consumers.

From *Nutrition Today*, January/February 1996, pp. 19-23. © 1996 by Williams & Wilkins. Reprinted by permission.

take responsibility for the impact their actions and media communications have on consumer attitudes and behavior.

SNAPSHOT OF THE NUTRITION INFLUENCER ENVIRONMENT

Current consumer nutrition influencers' activities serve as the basis for predicting what consumers will be exposed to and what will drive their concerns and understanding (or misunderstanding) of nutrition and health in 1996. The major influencer groups include the media; consumer product and food service industry; regulatory and legislative arena; scientific and academic community; food, nutrition and education professional organizations; and consumer advocacy groups.[1] The complexity in which these groups interact to reach the consumer is displayed in Figure 1. Communications with consumers are coming from all influencer sources. It is no wonder that consumers are confused by the seemingly conflicting information that reaches them on complex nutrition issues.

> **"Publishing science by press release" fails to place complex findings in a context useful for consumers.**

For example, the phenomenon of "publishing science by press release" is only beginning. Scientists, universities, and professional societies trying to gain visibility for their articles and journals are going directly to the general media. This process has one major flaw: complex nutrition scientific information needs to be placed in a practical, useful context for consumers. As a matter of fact, the ADA 1995 Nutrition Trends Survey uncovered a strong consumer preference, 81%, to hear findings on new research only after there has been general acceptance among nutrition and health professionals.[2]

The most recent information source gaining ground is the electronic media. Increased access to

the Internet represents opportunities for nutrition information exchange as well as raising issues about the accuracy and sources of the information that reaches consumers. In November 1995, it was reported that over 24 million consumers have access to the Internet in the United States and Canada. This area will experience rapid growth and will warrant serious attention from influencer groups in 1996.

> **Access to the Internet creates opportunities while raising concerns about accuracy and sources of information reaching consumers.**

Using consumer-driven research for nutrition message and program development is on the cutting edge with regulators, the public health community, and health professionals. Focus groups are being used for testing the US Department of Agriculture (USDA) Dietary Guidelines, Dietary Guidelines Alliance message development, and development of strategies for Centers for Disease Control and Prevention (CDC)'s Nutrition and Physical Activity Communication Team (NuPACT) healthy eating and physical activity campaign. The focus groups' discussions have provided unexpected insights into consumers' perceived needs and understanding of dietary recommendations. The issue for nutrition educators and communicators then becomes how to juggle "what consumers want" with "what educators need to teach." The challenge is to deliver what consumers *think* they need while motivating them to take action.

> **Communicators must balance "what consumers want to know" with "what educators want to teach."**

Meanwhile, the 1996 consumer nutrition environment will be affected by advances in basic research findings in areas as dietary components and cancer, antioxidants, phytochemicals, and molecular genetics. Health professional initiatives and new/existing partnerships among influencer groups will continue to have an impact on consumers. Finally, during 1996, whatever issues Center for Science in the Public Interest (CSPI) targets will always loom on the horizon.

UPDATE 1996: NINE ISSUES REVISITED ON CENTER STAGE

Nine key consumer nutrition and food safety issues identified in 1995 (Table 1) have been revisited to reflect current consumer influencer activities that will shape what consumers will be exposed to in 1996 (Table 2):

1. Weight Maintenance—Physical Activity Leads Calorie Intake. The key question currently under debate in the scientific community is: What is a "healthy weight?" The

**Table 1
Nine Nutrition and Food Safety Issues of 1995**

1. Weight control/weight management Calorie intake and physical activity gain prominence
2. Healthy eating—What is it?
3. Fat stays first
4. Food safety maintains its position
5. Building blocks for kids' nutrition
6. The dawn of "nutraceuticals"
7. Calcium to take center stage
8. Biotechnology gains momentum
9. Tailor-made for rugged individualists

**Table 2
Nine Nutrition and Food Safety Issues Take Center Stage Revisions for 1996**

1. Weight maintenance—Physical activity leads calorie intake
2. Healthy eating—What is it?
3. Fat stays first
4. Building blocks for kids' nutrition
5. Antioxidants and phytochemicals in light of "the dawn of nutraceuticals"
6. Food safety stays important
7. Calcium yet to take center stage
8. Advances in genetics drive potential for individualized dietary recommendations
9. Biotechnology lags behind

1995 Dietary Guidelines Advisory Committee[4] recommends that the "maintain healthy weight" guideline be changed to "Balance the food you eat with physical activity; maintain or improve your weight." The new weight tables do not allow for weight gain with age, a departure from earlier recommendations. In September 1995, headlines such as "Even moderate weight gain can be deadly"[5] suggested to consumers that maintaining a "healthy weight" is even more difficult than the 1995 Dietary Guidelines suggest. For example, media coverage sent the message that unless you are 5 feet, 5 inches tall and weigh 110 pounds, you *must* lose weight. Meanwhile, as the guidelines are in the process of changing, most health professionals continue to recommend against taking drastic measures and encourage consumers to simply make gradual changes over time.

Actually, the physical activity side of the energy input = energy output equation will be the major focus in the weight issue. Although 1995 recommendations from CDC and the American College of Sports Medicine call for moderate levels of physical activity,[3] no official government policy standards are in place that are comparable to the Dietary Guidelines for Americans or the Food Guide Pyramid. The policy recommendations generated at the December 1995 National Institutes of Health (NIH) Consensus Development Conference for physical activity and its role in cardiovascular health are a step toward official recommendations for consumers.

The Report of the Dietary Guidelines Advisory Committee on the Dietary Guidelines for Americans, 1995,[4] brings an increased focus on weight maintenance and, specifically, physical activity (as a key component of weight maintenance). This is a major change in emphasis that will certainly keep this issue in front of consumers in 1996.

With regard to energy intake, calorie counting will be coming back. In 1995, media coverage has focused on the "exposé" that fat-free foods are not the panacea to lowering calorie intake and losing weight. It has been reported that consumers perceive the term "fat free" as "calorie free" and a license to overeat. This has brought a renewed interest in calorie intake and calorie content, as well as fat content, of the foods we eat. Health professionals will place greater emphasis on communicating concepts of appropriate serving sizes and portion control as it relates to energy intake.

Finally, consumers continue to hope for a magic bullet. That hope was fueled again with media coverage of a hormone that reportedly can take weight off without having to change diet or physical activity levels.

2. Healthy Eating—What Is It?

Food patterns from other cultures—Mediterranean, vegetarian, Asian—continue to gain consumer interest as approaches to healthful eating. The publication of the revised Dietary Guidelines for Americans in 1995 has triggered the health and regulatory professionals to revamp the Food Guide Pyramid, to make it more consumer friendly and more ethnically diverse. To evaluate the healthfulness of American diets, the USDA has developed a Healthy Eating Index. The Index takes into account 10 dietary components identified in current dietary recommendations (*ie*, Food Guide Pyramid food

> **Consumers are attracted to cultural food patterns as a basis for healthful living.**

groups, macro- and micronutrients, and even variety of foods) to assess overall diet quality. The Index demonstrates that Americans have much room for improvement—the average score was 63.9 out of a possible 100.[6]

It is interesting to note that USDA Dietary Guidelines focus group results demonstrate that consumers don't really understand how the principle of moderation applies to healthful food choices. Consumers want practical tips and specific dos and don'ts. Essentially, they want to be told what food choices are "good" and "bad." And, they want the food they eat to taste good. This represents quite a challenge to health professionals who are trying to teach how all foods can be incorporated into healthful diets.

3. Fat Stays First with Consumers.

At 65%, the highest level to date, fat remains the number one nutrition concern of consumers, according to the 1995 Food Marketing Institute Trends Survey.[7] In the Food Marketing Institute/Prevention 1995 Shopping for Health Survey,[8] fat content is the primary reason for not purchasing certain foods; 77% of shoppers stopped buying food products because of the amount of fat listed on the nutrition label. The release of the Surgeon General's Second Report on Diet and Health in early 1996 is bound to direct more attention to dietary fat issues. In 1988, when it was first released, it set a precedent for dietary recommendations in the United States.

The research on physiological, behavioral, and cognitive factors on the role dietary fats and fat-modified foods play in satiety and weight maintenance has only begun and will certainly impact dietary advice in the near future.

4. Building Blocks for Kids' Nutrition.

There appear to be two important issues that have not been resolved in the influencer communities. First, is the dietary recommendation that less than 30% calories come from fat an appropriate dietary recommendation for children under the age of 18? Canadian Dietary Recommendations are targeted to adults 18 years of age and older. There is an ongoing, heated debate in the US scientific community on whether current dietary guidelines are appropriate for individuals 2 years of age and older. Secondly, education and communication issues center on defining the principles of healthy eating and healthy exercise regimens that children need to follow and how children will be motivated to follow them.

Meanwhile, the consumer press reflects the spectrum of the debate from Dr. Charles Attwood's book, *Lowfat Prescription for Kids*, an extension of Dr. Dean Ornish's work espousing a diet consisting of 10 to 15% calories from fat, to Dr. Ronald Kleinman's more commonsense approach to children's dietary habits described in *Let Them Eat Cake: The Case Against Controlling What Your Children Eat*. (New York: Villard Books, 1994.)

A number of activities in the health professional arena are going to keep this issue alive in 1996. The public health community's Partnership to Improve the American Diet may be resurfacing to take "action" on the development of kids' nutrition and health messages. White papers from the Children's Conference were published in the October 1995 *Journal of Nutrition Education*. The ADA has embraced kids' nutrition in a big way: Kellogg's and ADA have partnered to launch the Child Nutrition and Health Campaign that will encompass activities in research, policy, communications, and curriculum development. In addition, a M&M/Mars partnership with the National Association of Secondary School Principals is awarding monetary grants to school teams that address creative approaches to food served at school, physical activity, and innovative curricula on science of nutrition. School food service operations are charged with working to meet the new regulations for school meals.

Overall, the increased incidence of obesity in kids and adolescents in the United States and the level of policy and health professional activity creates a sense of urgency to resolving some of these issues in nutrition in 1996.

5. Antioxidants and Phytochemicals in the Light of "The Dawn of Nutraceuticals". This issue has moved up in the listing as consumer awareness appears to be heightened from all influencer groups. Hundreds of natural substances in plant foods are being in-

vestigated for health-promoting potential in the scientific arena. According to Dr. Charles Hennekens of Harvard,[9] the scientific literature on the role of the antioxidants betacarotene, vitamin E, and vitamin C is still promising, but theories are as yet unproven. However, going into 1996, researchers will have more information on betacarotene when data is released from Dr. Henneken's Physicians Health

> *Obesity in kids and adolescents creates a sense of urgency to resolving kids' nutrition issues in 1996.*

Study investigating the use of antioxidant supplements in 22,000 doctors in the United States. Dietary supplement and health claim issues are being debated in the regulatory arena into 1996. There is an increased interest in herbals and botanicals, as evidenced by the increased frequency of stories in consumer magazines over the past 3 years.[10]

Meanwhile, there continues to be an appealing consumer message as these activities move forward: there is support for what mother told you all along—"to eat your fruit and vegetables."

6. Food Safety Remains Important. The safety of the food supply remains an important concern for consumers. However, this issue has dropped down on this year's list as Americans' confidence in the food supply rose dramatically according to the Food Marketing Institute 1995 Trends.[7] The confidence level in the safety of the food supply is at 77%, the highest it has been since 1991; pre-Alar scare levels.[7] As the regulatory community debates changes in meat and poultry inspection for 1996, this issue will remain in front of consumers.

7. Calcium Yet to Take Center Stage. Although all the activity within influencer groups points to the need to increase calcium in the

diet, consumers have yet to embrace it. New food products entering the marketplace in early 1995 touting calcium claims are minimal in comparison with those carrying fat and calorie claims.[11] Although the 1995 Dietary Guidelines Committee considered adding a guideline to address calcium specifically, it did not make it to the final report. Interest in the health claim petition linking calcium with hypertension could help to heighten consumer awareness on the need for increasing calcium in the diet. In addition, the high visibility release of new drugs which can be used as alternatives to estrogen for treating and preventing osteoporosis may also stimulate consumers' interest in dietary calcium.

> *Although most dietary guidance points to the need for increased dietary calcium, consumers have yet to embrace this recommendation.*

8. Advances in Genetics Drive Potential for Individualized Dietary Recommendations. In the scientific and health professional communities, attention is being drawn to the potential role nutrition/nutrients may play in molecular genetics. The focus on an individual's genetic makeup and the acknowl-

> *Genetically determined variability in human nutrient needs suggests individualized dietary recommendations.*

edgement of variability in human nutrient needs is driving the potential for developing dietary recommendations for individuals. Universal dietary recommendations for control of chronic disease may not be appropriate given the advances in molecular genetics linked with predisposition to chronic diseases.[12]

9. Biotechnology Lags Behind. Bioengineered foods are making their way into the marketplace with minimal fanfare. When asked, a majority (65%) of shoppers have heard little or nothing at all about biotechnology. Of those who are aware of biotechnology, more shoppers are likely to buy produce modified by biotechnology to resist insect damages (74%) than modified to taste better or fresher (62%). Meanwhile, it appears that the scientific, industrial, regulatory, and health professional communities will continue working together to try to manage public communication efforts without evoking fear of science.

CONCLUSION

With some modifications, the nine consumer nutrition and food safety trends identified in 1995 will continue to stay in the spotlight in 1996. Major forces that will influence the 1996 consumer nutrition environment have been highlighted to put into perspective what lies ahead for consumers in 1996.

REFERENCES

1. McMahon KE. Consumer nutrition and food safety trends. *Nutr Today*, 1995;30:152–6.
2. American Dietetic Association. *The American Dietetic Association Nutrition Trends Survey*, 1995.
3. Pate RR, Pratt M, Blair SN, et al. Physical activity and public health: A recommendation from the Centers for Disease Control and Prevention and the American College of Sports Medicine. *JAMA*, 1995;273:402–7.
4. Report of the Dietary Guidelines Advisory Committee on the Dietary Guidelines for Americans, 1995.
5. Brody JE. Even moderate weight gain can be risky, a study finds. *The New York Times*, September 14, 1995.
6. Kennedy ET, Ohls J, Carlson S, Fleming K. The healthy eating index: Design and applications. *J Am Diet Assoc*, 1995;95:1103–8.
7. Food Marketing Institute. Trends in the United States: Consumer Attitudes and the Supermarket. *Food Marketing Institute*, 1995.
8. Food Marketing Institute and Prevention Magazine. Shopping for Health: New Food Labels, Same Eating Habits? *Food Marketing Institute and Prevention Magazine*, 1995.
9. Chase M. Health Journal: Food specialists seek just the right recipe for cancer-smart diet. *The Wall Street Journal*, May 8, 1995;
10. McNutt K. Medicinals in food, Part 1: Is science coming full circle? *Nutr Today*, 1995;30:218–22.
11. Friedman M. Health benefit new products war cry: "Fat freedom now." *New Product News*, May 11, 1995;
12. Simopoulos AP. Genetic variation and nutrition, Part 1: Population differences due to single gene defects and population differences in multifactorial diseases due to polygenic effects. *Nutr Today*, 1995;30:157–67.

THE 1995 DIETARY GUIDELINES: CHANGES AND IMPLICATIONS

INTRODUCTION

The Fourth edition of *Nutrition and Your Health: Dietary Guidelines for Americans* (1), published jointly by the U.S. Department of Agriculture (USDA) and the U.S. Department of Health and Human Services, has just been released to the public. These guidelines are intended to be a source of dietary information for healthy Americans 2 years of age and over (1).

The *Dietary Guidelines* was first published in 1980 (2) and revised in 1985 (3), 1990 (4), and most recently in 1995 (1). Beginning with the 1995 edition, the *Dietary Guidelines* must be reviewed and, if necessary, revised at least every five years (5).

The fourth edition of the *Dietary Guidelines* (1), which is based on recommendations of the 11 member Dietary Guidelines Advisory Committee (6), for the first time, includes USDA's Food Guide Pyramid (7) and the federal government's new Nutrition Facts Label (8,9). This *Digest* reviews the 1995 *Dietary Guidelines* (1), including changes from the previous edition (4), reasons for the changes, and efforts underway to communicate the *Dietary Guidelines* to the public.

DIETARY GUIDELINES FOR AMERICANS, 1995

The new *Dietary Guidelines* promotes a positive approach towards diet with an emphasis on the pleasures of eating. The *Guidelines* bulletin points out that there are a variety of ways to obtain healthful diets consistent with individuals' culture, taste, and calorie and nutrient needs (1). A healthful diet is important at all stages of life and interacts with genetic and other environmental factors to influence health (1).

All nutrients in foods are required for overall health. For example, adequate calcium is required for optimal bone health, but many other nutrients also are involved. In addition to a healthful diet, increased physical activity is important. In the discussion of the distinction between the *Dietary Guidelines* and the Recommended Dietary Allowances (RDAs) (10), the *Guidelines* clearly states that both apply to diets consumed over several days, and not to single meals or foods (1).

Eat A Variety Of Foods. The wording and priority of this guideline have remained the same in all four editions of the *Dietary Guidelines*. The 1995 edition emphasizes that a narrow set of food choices may result in inadequate intakes of essential nutrients (1,6). No single food can supply all nutrients in amounts needed.

The guideline to eat a variety of foods includes the phrase, "and other substances needed for good health" to communicate the idea that components (e.g., fiber) not covered in the term "nutrients" may be beneficial to health (1,6). Eating a variety of foods means choosing the recommended number of daily servings from each of the five major food groups displayed in the Food Guide Pyramid (7) and choosing different foods within each food group.

The new *Dietary Guidelines* (1) recognizes that vegetarian diets can be consistent with the *Dietary Guidelines* and can meet the RDAs. However, vegetarians need to pay special attention to their intake of iron, zinc, and B vitamins (1). Also, vegetarians who consume only foods of plant origin (i.e.,

The Dietary Guidelines *is designed to provide advice for healthy Americans age 2 years and over about food choices that promote health and prevent disease.*

vegans) have difficulty meeting their calcium needs without dairy foods in their diet (11). Vegans need to supplement their diet with vitamin B_{12}, a nutrient found only in animal products. Children who consume vegan diets need to make sure that they obtain adequate amounts of vitamin D and calcium, which most Americans obtain from milk products. This advice is consistent with that issued by The American Dietetic Association (12).

The special nutrient needs of growing children, teenage girls, and women are acknowledged (1). The *Guidelines* states that many women and adolescent girls need to consume calcium-rich foods to get the calcium needed for healthy bones throughout life (1). This advice supports the growing body of evidence that demonstrates calcium's beneficial role in reducing the risk of osteoporosis (13), as well as other diseases such as hypertension (14) and some forms of cancer. Good sources of calcium as well as iron may be in short supply in the diets of young children, teenage girls, and women of childbearing age (1,15,16). Dairy foods (e.g., milk, cheese, yogurt) are the major source of calcium in the U.S., contributing three-quarters of the calcium available in the food supply (17).

The 1995 *Dietary Guidelines* recognizes that fortified foods may be used to meet special dietary needs, but how these foods fit into the total diet depends on the amounts consumed and other foods in the diet (1). National policy dictates that some foods be enriched with specific nutrients, for example, milk with vitamin D. The *Dietary Guidelines* cautions that supplements of vitamins, minerals, or fiber do not supply all of the nutrients (as well as other substances present in foods) important to health. Further, supplements may be potentially harmful and are usually unnecessary for people who eat a variety of foods (1). Possible exceptions include vitamin D for some older adults, and folic acid and iron for women of childbearing age (1). The American Dietetic Association maintains that "the best nutritional strategy for promoting optimal health and reducing risk of chronic disease is to obtain adequate nutrients from a wide variety of foods" (18).

Balance The Food You Eat With Physical Activity—Maintain Or Improve Your Weight. For the first time, this guideline advises against weight gain in adulthood (1). The recent well-documented increase in the prevalence of obesity (19,20) demands that more attention be directed toward weight control. Weight maintenance represents the necessary first step to achieve a healthy weight. Both overweight and adult weight gain are associated with increased risk of major chronic diseases (1). Being too thin is also associated with health problems including osteoporosis in women (1).

For individuals who need to lose weight, a loss of only 5 to 10% of body weight may improve many health problems associated with overweight. A slow, steady weight loss of ½ to 1 pound a week is recommended (1).

The 1995 guideline (1) emphasizes physical activity for both weight control and health. Because physical activity expends calories, Americans of all ages are advised to spend more time being physically active. Thirty minutes or more of moderate intensity physical activity on most, and preferably all, days of the week is recommended (1). This recommendation is consistent with that of others (21–24).

Children need enough food for normal growth and development. Therefore, caution is warranted in helping overweight children achieve a healthy weight (1). To promote growth and development, children must be encouraged to consume recommended servings of foods from the five food groups and to participate in vigorous activity. Fat intake should *not* be restricted for children younger than 2 years of age. For older overweight children, modest reductions in dietary fat are not harmful as long as growth is regularly monitored (1).

For older people who begin to lose weight as they age, maintaining weight is important (1). Because some of the weight lost with advancing age is muscle, emphasis is placed on regular physical activity. Physical activity not only helps to maintain muscle and improve older adults' well-being, but it also helps to reduce the risk of falls and fractures (1). The American College of Sports Medicine (25) agrees with this advice.

For all Americans, "more physical activity is better than less, and any is more than none" (1).

Choose A Diet With Plenty of Grain Products, Vegetables, and Fruits.

A major change is the movement from fourth to third place on the list of guidelines (1,4). This guideline is more prominently displayed to emphasize the message that grain products, vegetables, and fruits are the foundation of a healthful diet, as indicated in the Food Guide Pyramid (1,7).

The contribution of these foods to total nutrient intake is stressed. Specifically, grain products, vegetables, and fruits are highlighted as sources of vitamins C and B_6, carotenoids and other antioxidant nutrients, folate, potassium, calcium, and magnesium, and as foods typically low in fat. Unfortunately, most Americans consume less than the recommended number of servings of grains, vegetables, and fruits (17,26).

Choose A Diet Low In Fat, Saturated Fat, And Cholesterol.

In 1995, this guideline appears in fourth rather than third place as in previous editions. The introductory paragraph describes both the positive and negative aspects of dietary fat to the total diet (1). Americans are consuming less total fat, saturated fat, and cholesterol today than three decades ago (17,26–28). This guideline emphasizes the continued importance of choosing a diet with less total fat, saturated fat, and cholesterol (1).

The revised guideline recommends a diet that provides "no more than 30% of total calories from fat" (1) rather than "30% or less of calories from fat" as stated in the 1990 edition (4). This change in wording is intended to minimize the implication that "the lower the fat intake the better" (6).

In the advice for children, the new guideline emphasizes that the recommendation to choose a diet low in fat, saturated fat, and cholesterol (as well as other dietary guidelines) does *not* apply to infants and toddlers below the age of 2 years, in keeping with recommendations by other authorities (29). After 2 years of age, the guideline recommends that children *gradually* adopt a diet that, by about 5 years of age, contains no more than 30% of calories from fat (1).

This departure from the traditional recommendation that lowfat diets be implemented at about age two was made to coincide with the time at which children start school, to ensure uniformity with school feeding programs, and to recognize children's need for intake of higher calorie, nutrient dense foods (30).

This guideline change regarding dietary fat represents a first step toward creating separate dietary guidelines for children in the future. Age-targeted guidelines, particularly for children, are gaining favor among health professionals (13,31–37). A Working Group convened by Health Canada and the Canadian Paediatric Society (31) recommends that from the age of two until the end of linear growth (about age 18), there should be a gradual transition from the higher fat diet of infancy to a diet which includes no more than 30% of energy as fat and no more than 10% of energy as saturated fat. During this transition, energy intake must be a priority to achieve normal growth and development (31). In the U.S., health professional organizations such as The American Dietetic Association (33,34) support the development of specific dietary recommendations for healthy children. The 1995 Dietary Guidelines Advisory Committee (6), when considering ways to improve future editions of the *Dietary Guidelines*, also recommended consideration of separate dietary guidelines for healthy children. And according to a recent National Dairy Council-sponsored survey of leading health care and nutrition professionals, nearly three out of four survey respondents favored separate dietary guidelines for children (37). In addition to fat, separate dietary guidelines for calcium (13), weight (35), and fiber (36) for children have been recommended by health professionals.

Choose A Diet Moderate In Sugars.

In all editions of the *Dietary Guidelines* (1–4) this guideline states that sugars and foods that contain primarily sugars supply calories but few nutrients. In addition, sugar and starches can promote tooth decay. In 1995, the title of this guideline is reworded to better convey the *Dietary Guidelines'* overall

The 1995 Dietary Guidelines recommends changes that, for the first time, begin to recognize the unique dietary needs of children.

goal which is to help Americans "focus on total diet in a more positive way" (6). Compared to the 1990 guideline (4), the new edition provides more information about the various forms and roles of sugars.

With respect to sugars and health, scientific evidence indicates that diets high in sugars do not cause hyperactivity or diabetes (1). Nor will avoiding sugars alone correct overweight. For very active people with high calorie needs, sugars can be an additional source of energy (1).

The 1995 guideline (1) cautions people that, while sugar substitutes do not provide significant calories, foods containing sugar substitutes are not always lower in calories than similar sugar-containing products (1). In the discussion of sugars and dental caries, frequent consumption of foods high in sugars and starches, especially as between meal snacks, is identified as harmful to teeth. To help prevent tooth decay, regular daily dental hygiene and adequate intake of fluoride, preferably from fluoridated water, is recommended (1). The information on sugars and health, as described in this guideline, is consistent with findings presented at a recent symposium on the nutrition and health aspects of sugars (38).

Choose A Diet Moderate In Salt And Sodium. The wording of this guideline has been changed to make it clear that foods (processed, prepared, and preserved) are the source of most dietary sodium, as opposed to salt from the salt shaker, and to be consistent with other guidelines to "choose a diet." The revised guideline emphasizes the positive role of sodium as well as potentially negative effects of overconsuming dietary sodium.

Although the debate continues among scientists regarding the association between salt and/or sodium intake and risk of developing high blood pressure (39–42), the 1995 guideline supports the recommendation to choose a diet moderate in salt and sodium (1).

The new edition (1) acknowledges that a number of dietary factors influence blood pressure (1). Not only consuming less salt or sodium, but also following other guidelines in the *Dietary Guidelines* may help reduce the risk of high blood pressure (1). For example, weight reduction and increased intake of fruits and vegetables, because of their low sodium and fat and high potassium content, offset the effects of sodium on blood pressure and may help to reduce blood pressure (1). Milk and yogurt are identified as other good sources of potassium (1). Increased physical activity and reduced alcohol intake also are associated with a beneficial effect on blood pressure. In addition, reducing salt intake is recommended because high salt intakes may increase the amount of calcium excreted in the urine, thereby increasing the body's need for calcium (1,43,44).

If You Drink Alcoholic Beverages, Do So In Moderation. While not endorsing alcohol intake, this guideline recognizes that moderate alcohol intake can enhance meal satisfaction and may reduce the risk of coronary heart disease in some individuals (1). However, when consumed in excess, alcohol is harmful to health and may alter judgement and lead to addiction. Compared to the 1990 edition (4), the number of alcohol-related health problems mentioned is increased. And the list of who should not drink has been reordered to place children and adolescents at the top. The prudent advice that women who are trying to conceive or who are pregnant should avoid drinking alcoholic beverages is retained in the 1995 edition (1).

COMMUNICATING THE 1995 DIETARY GUIDELINES TO AMERICANS

Although many Americans have received the message that what they eat affects their health and have made some changes towards a more healthful diet (26), the average American is still confused about nutrition (4,26,45–47). It is clear that nutrition and other health professionals face a major challenge in

Only when individuals tailor the Dietary Guidelines *to their needs can long-term health benefits be realized.*

helping Americans improve their eating and other lifestyle habits.

Tools such as the Food Guide Pyramid (7) and the Nutrition Facts Label (48) can help the public put the dietary guidelines into practice. However, a number of other factors such as taste, knowledge, food preparation skill, age, culture, and medical problems can influence food choices and health behaviors. When individualized approaches to dietary and other lifestyle changes are not realized, long-term health benefits cannot be expected. Only approaches that allow personal choices and trade-offs can be maintained.

The American public needs not just knowledge about what constitutes a healthful lifestyle, but also the motivation and assistance, for example by registered dietitians, to adapt the *Dietary Guidelines* to their individual needs. To help consumers implement the 1995 *Dietary Guidelines* (1), an alliance has been formed among the food industry and government and health organizations (49). Effective messages consistent with the 1995 *Dietary Guidelines* are being developed by the alliance to increase the public's understanding that with balance, variety, and moderation, all foods can fit into a healthful diet and that nutrition, good taste, and physical activity are inseparable for a healthy life.

REFERENCES

1. U.S. Department of Agriculture and U.S. Department of Health and Human Services. *Nutrition and Your Health: Dietary Guidelines for Americans.* 4th edition. Home and Garden Bulletin No. 232. Washington, DC: U.S. Government Printing Office, December 1995. (To order a single copy, send your name, address, and $.50 to: Consumer Information Center, Department 378-C, Pueblo, CO 81009).

2. U.S. Department of Agriculture and U.S. Department of Health, Education and Welfare. *Nutrition and Your Health: Dietary Guidelines for Americans.* Home & Garden Bulletin No. 232. Washington, DC: U.S. Government Printing Office. February 1980.

3. U.S. Department of Agriculture and U.S. Department of Health and Human Services. *Nutrition and Your Health: Dietary Guidelines for Americans.* 2nd edition. Home and Garden Bulletin No. 232. Washington, DC: U.S. Government Printing Office, August 1985.

4. U.S. Department of Agriculture and U.S. Department of Health and Human Services. *Nutrition and Your Health: Dietary Guidelines for Americans.* 3rd edition. Home and Garden Bulletin No. 232. Washington, DC: U.S. Government Printing Office, November 1990.

5. National Nutrition Monitoring and Related Research Act of 1990. Public Law 101-445. Section 301. October 22, 1990.

6. U.S. Department of Agriculture, Agricultural Research Service, Dietary Guidelines Advisory Committee. *Report of the Dietary Guidelines Advisory Committee on the Dietary Guidelines for Americans, 1995, to the Secretary of Health and Human Services and the Secretary of Agriculture.* September 1995, 58 pp.

7. U.S. Department of Agriculture, Human Nutrition Information Service. *The Food Guide Pyramid.* Home and Garden Bulletin No. 252. Washington, DC: Government Printing Office, August 1992.

8. U.S. Department of Health and Human Services, Food and Drug Administration. Fed. Register 58(3): 2066, 1993.

9. U.S. Department of Agriculture, Food Safety and Inspection Service. Fed. Register 58(3): 632, 1993.

10. National Academy of Sciences, National Research Council, Food and Nutrition Board. *Recommended Dietary Allowances,* 10th edition. Washington, DC: National Academy Press, 1989.

11. Weaver, C.M., and K.L. Plawecki. Am. J. Clin. Nutr. 59 (suppl): 1238s, 1994.

12. The American Dietetic Association. J. Am. Diet. Assoc. 93: 1317, 1993.

13. Optimal Calcium Intake. NIH Consensus Statement. June 6–8; 12(4): 1–31, 1994.

14. Hamet, P.J. Nutr. 125 (2S): 311, 1995.

15. Alaimo, K., M.A. McDowell, R.R. Briefel, et. al. Dietary intake of vitamins, minerals, and fiber of persons ages 2 months and over in the United States: Third National Health and Nutrition Examination Survey, Phase 1, 1988–91. Advance Data from Vital and Health Statistics; No. 258. Hyattsville, MD: National Center for Health Statistics, 1994.

16. Tippett, K.S., S.J. Mickle, J.D. Goldman, et. al. Food and Nutrient Intakes by Individuals in the United States, 1 Day, 1989–91. Continuing Survey of Food Intakes by Individuals, 1989–91, Nationwide Food Surveys Rep. No. 91-2. September 1995, 263 pp.

17. Zizza, C., and S. Gerrior. Food Rev. 18(1): 40, 1995.

18. The American Dietetic Association. J. Am. Diet. Assoc. 96: 73, 1996.

19. Kuczmarski, R.J., K.M. Flegal, S.M. Campbell, et. al. JAMA 272: 205, 1994.

20. McGinnis, J.M., and P.R. Lee. JAMA 273: 1123, 1995.

21. U.S. Public Health Service. *Healthy People 2000: National Health Promotion and Disease Prevention Objectives.* Publication PHS 91-502112. Washington, DC: U.S. Department of Health and Human Services, 1991.

22. Pate, R.R., M. Pratt, S.N. Blair, et. al. JAMA 273: 402, 1995.

23. National Institutes of Health Consensus Development Conference Statement. *Physical Activity and Cardiovascular Health.* December 18–20, 1995.

24. Borra, S.T., N.E. Schwartz, C.G. Spain, et. al. J. Am. Diet. Assoc. 95(7): 816, 1995.

25. American College of Sports Medicine. Med. Sci. Sports Exerc. 27(4):I, 1995.

26. Tippett, K.S., and J.D. Goldman. Food Rev. 17(1): 8, 1994.

27. Centers for Disease Control and Prevention. JAMA 443: 116, 1994.

28. McDowell, M.A., R.R. Briefel, K. Alaimo, et. al. Energy and macronutrient intakes of persons ages 2 months and over in the United States. Third National Health and Nutrition Examination Survey, Phase 1, 1988–91. Advance Data from Vital and Health Statistics No. 255. Hyattsville, MD: National Center for Health Statistics, 1994.

29. National Cholesterol Education Program (NCEP). *Report of the Expert Panel on Blood Cholesterol Levels In Children and Adolescents.* Bethesda, MD: U.S. Department of Health and Human Services, Public Health Service, National Institutes of Health, National Heart, Lung, and Blood Institute, April 1994.

30. U.S. Department of Agriculture, Food and Consumer Service. Fed. Register 60(113): 31188, 1995.

31. Report of the Joint Working Group of the Canadian Paediatric Society and Health Canada. *Nutrition Recommendations Update…Dietary Fat and Children.* Ottawa, Canada: Publications Distribution, Health Canada 1993.

32. Olson, R.E. Nutr. Today 30(6): 234, 1995.

33. Forgac, M.T. J. Am. Diet. Assoc. 95: 370, 1995.

34. ADA testifies on revised Dietary Guidelines for Americans. J. Am. Diet. Assoc. 95(4): 420, 1995.

35. Report of the American Institute of Nutrition (AIN) Steering Committee on Healthy Weight. J. Nutr. 124: 2240, 1994.

36. Williams, C.L., M. Bollella, and E. L. Wynder. Pediatrics 96(5): 985, 1995.

37. *Kids They're Not Little Adults.* Rosemont, IL: National Dairy Council, 1995.

38. Clydesdale, F.M. Am. J. Clin. Nutr. 61(1S): 161s, 1995.

39. Stamler, J. Perspectives in Appl. Nutr. 3(2): 116, 1995.

40. Dennis, B.H. Perspectives in Appl. Nutr. 3(2): 121, 1995.

41. Stern, J.S. Perspectives in Appl. Nutr. 3(2): 127, 1995.

42. Oparil, S. Perspectives in Appl. Nutr. 3(2): 131, 1995.

43. Nordin, B.E.C., A.G. Need, H.A. Morris, et. al. J. Nutr. 123: 1615, 1993.

44. Matkovic, V., J.Z. Llich, M.D. Andon, et. al. Am. J. Clin. Nutr. 62: 417, 1995.

45. The American Dietetic Association and Kraft Foods, Inc. *1995 Nutrition Trends Survey.* Chicago, IL: The American Dietetic Association, 1995.

46. Morreale, S.J., and N.E. Schwartz. J. Am. Diet. Assoc. 95: 305, 1995.

47. *How Are Americans Making Food Choices? 1994 Update.* Conducted for: The American Dietetic Association and International Food Information Council. Prepared by: The Gallup Organization. April 1994.

48. Saltos, E., C. Davis, S. Welsh, et. al. *Using Food Labels to Follow the Dietary Guidelines for Americans: A Reference.* U.S. Department of Agriculture, Agricultural Information Bulletin No. 704, 1994, 84 pp.

49. The Dietary Guidelines Alliance. For information, contact The American Dietetic Association at (312) 899-0040, ext. 4761.

The Food Pyramid: How to make it work for you

The Government's nutritional tool can lead you toward a healthy diet—but you need to know more than it tells you.

Five years ago, the U.S. Department of Agriculture introduced the Food Guide Pyramid, designed to convey a simple, graphic message: Grains, fruits, and vegetables are the cornerstone of a healthy diet. That message, reinforced by specific recommendations on how many servings per day to get from each food group, has increased many Americans' awareness of the need to eat lots of plant foods. But the pyramid offers no specific recommendations about which items to choose *within* each food group. So it's quite possible to get the appropriate number of servings for each group and still end up with an unbalanced, unhealthy diet.

Cracks in the pyramid

The pyramid falls short in two areas: fiber and fat. First, nutrition experts recommend you consume 20 to 35 grams of fiber per day. But the pyramid makes no distinction between refined-grain products such as white rice and white bread, which contain little fiber, and whole-grain foods like brown rice and whole-wheat bread, which pack a lot of fiber.

The tip of the pyramid advises people to use fats, oils, and sweets sparingly. But that advice apparently lumps together two very different groups of fat. The first includes the nontropical oils, such as olive or corn oil, which are harmless unless you're watching your waistline. The second includes items that are bad for both the waistline and the heart: butter, cream, lard, and tropical oils, rich in artery-clogging saturated fat; plus margarine and shortening, which are rich in artery-clogging trans fat.

The pyramid uses tiny circles and triangles as symbols to suggest that each of the other five food groups may also contain fats (and sweets). But it offers no explicit advice about how to limit fat consumption in those groups. For example, it doesn't distinguish between high- and low-fat dairy products. And it doesn't exclude from the grain group fatty items like fried rice, fettucini Alfredo, or garlic bread; or, from the veg-etable group, such items as cauliflower au gratin, creamed spinach, or even french fries.

The group containing meat and meat substitutes (eggs, nuts, and beans) fails to separate typically lean foods like beans, fish, and skinless poultry breast from fatty items like hot dogs and hamburgers. And the recommendation to eat two to three servings per day works for meat but not for the meat substitutes. A better standard, mentioned in the seldom-read brochure that accompanies the pyramid, is a daily maximum of 5 to 7 ounces of either meat, an equivalent quantity of meat substitutes, or both combined. (One egg, 1/2 cup of cooked dried peas or beans, 2 tablespoons of peanut butter, and 1/3 cup of nuts are each considered the equivalent of 1 ounce of meat).

Fixing the flaws

To help you meet the pyramid's requirements in a healthy way, we've prepared the detailed table on the facing page. It not only lists the recommended number of servings for each food group but also breaks each group down into three categories:

■ Foods you should choose **often**, since they're nutritious, lean, and, where applicable, high in fiber.

■ Those you should choose **sometimes**, since they're either somewhat fattier, less nutritious, lower in fiber, or, in the case of some seafood, higher in potentially hazardous chemicals than foods in the "often" category. For example, canned vegetables are listed as "sometimes" because they contain fewer nutrients than fresh or frozen vegetables. And several kinds of fish are listed there because they often contain significant amounts of such chemicals as mercury or PCBs—and, in most cases, are also fairly fatty.

■ Those you should **seldom** choose, since they're either high in fat or low in nutrients and fiber. Coconut, for example, is loaded with saturated fat. And regular biscuits, crackers, and sweetened muffins typically offer an undesirable combination of low fiber, mediocre nutrient levels, and moderately high fat.

If you eat many foods more or less often than the table recommends, you're probably eating too much fat and possibly too little fiber. Try to adjust your diet gradually, choosing more foods from the often column and fewer from the seldom column.

How to get more

Our table leaves one important aspect of the pyramid virtually unchanged: the recommended number

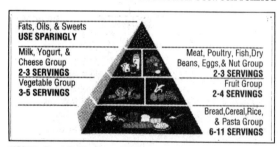

USDA's Food Guide Pyramid The pyramid shows how many servings to eat from each food group, but it offers no specific guidance on which foods to eat within each group.

For more information

■ "The M *FIT* Grocery Shopping Guide," University of Michigan, 1995. Extensive listings of brand-name and other foods, according to their overall nutritional value. $18.95. Call 313-998-7645.

Beyond the pyramid: Healthy choices for a healthy diet

Choose often	Choose sometimes	Choose seldom
Fats, oils, and sweets: Use sparingly		
While all regular fats and oils should be used sparingly, some alternatives to those items, such as nonfat spreads or salad dressings, can be used often.	Fruit-snack candies, fruit drinks (not juices), hard candies (particularly sugarless), honey, jelly, molasses, soda, sorbet, refined sugar, syrups. Nonfat or low-fat cookies, cakes, and other desserts. Mayonnaise. Light margarine; other reduced-fat spreads with less than 2 grams of saturated fat per serving. Nontropical vegetable oils, such as olive and canola. Salad dressing.	Candy bars; chocolate; regular cakes, cookies, and pies; and other rich desserts. Butter, lard, stick margarine. Coconut, palm, and other tropical oils.
Dairy: 2 to 3 servings per day		
Milk, buttermilk, and cottage cheese: skim or 1% fat. Nonfat or low-fat yogurt. Nonfat cheese. Nonfat or low-fat frozen dairy desserts.	Milk, buttermilk, and cottage cheese: 2% fat. Low-fat cheese. Reduced-fat dairy desserts.	Whole milk, whole-milk yogurt. Regular cheese; cottage cheese: 4% fat. Regular frozen dairy desserts.
Meat and meat substitutes: 5 to 7 ounces per day		
Any unground meats labeled "extra lean." **Beef:** Eye of round, top round. **Veal:** All kinds not listed in next two columns. **Pork:** Tenderloin, 95% lean ham. **Lamb:** Foreshank. **Chicken:** Skinless breast. **Turkey:** Breast, drumstick, or wing without skin. **Fish:** Lean varieties such as bass, cod, flounder, halibut, monkfish, pollack, trout. **Shellfish.** **Nonfat or low-fat lunch meats or hot dogs**, with up to 3 grams of fat per serving. **Meat substitutes:** Beans, peas, and lentils; tofu; eggs [2] or egg substitutes.	Any unground meats labeled "lean." **Beef:** Tip or bottom round, sirloin, chuck pot roast, top loin, tenderloin, flank, T-bone, ground sirloin, extra-lean ground. **Veal:** Loin, loin chop, ground. **Pork:** Sirloin chop, top or center loin chop, rib chop, ham, Canadian bacon. **Lamb:** Shank, leg, loin chop, sirloin. **Chicken:** Skinless drumstick, thigh, or wing; breast with skin. **Turkey:** Any piece with skin; thigh without skin; extra-lean ground. **Fish:** Bluefish, catfish, herring (including sardines), mackerel, pompano, salmon, shad, swordfish, tuna.[1] **Reduced-fat lunch meats or hot dogs**, with 4 to 5 grams of fat per serving. **Meat substitutes:** Nuts; nut butters.[3]	**Beef:** All cuts not listed in first two columns (such as brisket, rib roast, chuck blade roast, lean and regular ground). **Veal:** Rib roast. **Pork:** All kinds not listed in first two columns (such as spareribs, sausage, ground). **Lamb:** All kinds not listed in first two columns (such as rib chop, arm, blade, shoulder, ground). **Chicken:** Drumstick, thigh, or wing with skin; liver. **Turkey:** Lean or regular ground. **Duck, goose.** **Regular lunch meats or hot dogs**, with more than 5 grams of fat per serving.
Vegetables: 3 to 5 servings per day [4]		
Fresh or frozen vegetables not listed in third column. Vegetable juice [5] (except canned).	Canned vegetables. Canned vegetable juice.	Vegetables in cheese, cream, or other fatty sauces. French fries, onion rings, other deep-fried vegetables.
Fruit: 2 to 4 servings per day		
Fresh or frozen fruit not listed in next two columns. Fruit juice. [5]	Canned fruit; dried fruit. Avocado, olives. [3]	Coconut.
Grains: 6 to 11 servings per day		
Higher-fiber foods: Amaranth, barley, brown or wild rice, cracked or bulgur wheat, kasha, quinoa. Low-fat popcorn or unbuttered air-popped popcorn. Rice cakes, corn or whole-wheat tortillas. **Higher-fiber versions** (Any of the following items that are labeled "whole wheat" or "100% whole grain"; that make a claim about fiber, such as "high fiber" or "good source of fiber"; or that contain at least 2 grams of fiber per serving): Bread, bagels, English muffins, rolls. Pasta, couscous. Cereals with up to 3 grams of fat per serving. Bread sticks, pretzels. Nonfat or low-fat biscuits, crackers, or sweetened muffins.	Any item in the first column, under "higher-fiber versions," that does not bear those labels, make those claims, or contain that much fiber. White rice. Regular popcorn flavored with or popped in nontropical oils. Wheat tortillas. Whole-wheat biscuits, crackers, or sweetened muffins that are not low-fat or nonfat. Whole-wheat pancakes, waffles, or French toast. Higher-fiber cereals with more than 3 grams of fat per serving, such as granola or muesli.	Fried rice; any grain dish with fatty sauce. Regular popcorn flavored with butter or popped in tropical oils. Biscuits, crackers, or sweetened muffins that are not high-fiber, low-fat, or nonfat. Croissants, Danish, donuts. Regular pancakes, waffles, or French toast.

[1] Young children and women who are or may become pregnant should avoid bluefish, salmon, swordfish, tuna, and probably other large predatory fish, which may contain high levels of hazardous chemicals and heavy metals. Other people should eat those fish no more than once a week.

[2] These are high in cholesterol, which can raise blood-cholesterol levels in some people. Eat eggs only sometimes—no more than four yolks per week—if you have borderline or high cholesterol.

[3] Although these foods contain little saturated fat, the artery-clogging kind, they do contain a significant amount of other fats and, in turn, calories. People who are watching their weight may want to eat these foods seldom rather than sometimes.

[4] Includes beans and potatoes. Note that beans are included in both the meat and vegetable groups. (But count each serving only once.)

[5] Count as only one serving per day. You still need to eat lots of whole fruits and vegetables, since whole produce, unlike juice, supplies lots of fiber.

of servings. Americans typically have the most trouble meeting those recommendations for fruits and vegetables, which call for a combined total of 5 to 9 daily servings. Many people also find it hard to get the recommended 6 to 11 servings of grains. (Where you fit within those ranges depends on your caloric needs; the low ends, for example, are appropriate for most inactive women and older people, the high ends mainly for active younger men.)

But getting enough servings may be easier than you think, since standard serving sizes are typically small. For example, one slice of bread, half a muffin, a half-cup of cooked or chopped vegetables or fruit, and a small glass of fruit or vegetable juice each equal one serving. (For more details on serving size, see the series in "A Picture of Health" in our April through July issues.)

Here are some strategies that can help you meet your daily quotas:

Produce

■ Get two servings of fruit at breakfast by drinking a small glass of orange juice and finishing the meal with, say, a nectarine. (But count only one serving of juice per day.)

■ Add fruits and vegetables to other foods—berries in pancakes, peaches in yogurt, peppers and onions in omelets, shredded carrots in sandwiches.

■ Take double servings of vegetables.

■ Snack on raw vegetables or fruit.

■ Thicken soups with pureed vegetables.

Grains (preferably whole wheat or whole grain)

■ Eat cereal for breakfast and add bread or rolls to any meal.

■ Cook whole grains in soup stock and season with herbs. Toss with cooked vegetables and beans.

■ Make cold salads from cooked grains plus chopped raw vegetables.

■ Add cereals to yogurt.

■ Add cooked grains or wheat germ to soup.

Summing up

To get the most benefit from the food pyramid, you need to know more than just the number of servings in each food group.

What to do:

■ Consult our table, which shows the ideal balance among various foods in each category, based on their fat, fiber, and nutritional content.

■ If your diet doesn't conform to that ideal, try to eat more of the "often" foods and fewer of the "seldom" items. More generally, aim to boost your intake of lean, high-fiber foods, and to eat fewer fatty, highly refined, or processed foods.

■ If your diet doesn't include enough servings of produce or grains, look for creative ways to get more, such as adding chopped fruits or vegetables to other dishes.

THE NOT-SO-GREAT MEDITERRANEAN DIET PYRAMID

Kathleen Meister

KATHLEEN MEISTER, M.S., IS A FREELANCE MEDICAL WRITER AND FORMER ACSH RESEARCH ASSOCIATE.

Proponents of the Mediterranean Diet Pyramid claim that it is a better guide to healthful eating than the U.S. government's food pyramid. Many nutrition scientists disagree.

■ It doesn't seem fair, does it? Just when you were getting used to the U.S. government's food pyramid, people have started talking about another food pyramid—a distinctly different one based on the traditional cuisines of the Mediterranean. The key characteristics of this pyramid (see illustration) include:

· a heavy reliance on foods from plant sources (grains, legumes, vegetables and fruits);
· the use of olive oil as the principal fat;
· moderate daily intake of wine;
· daily consumption of small amounts of cheese or yogurt; and
· relatively infrequent intake of other foods of animal origin, especially red meat.

Would it be better for Americans to eat in this way, instead of according to the food pyramid promoted by the U.S. government? The proponents of the Mediterranean pyramid believe it would be. They point to evidence showing that population groups who eat in the traditional Mediterranean fashion have lower heart disease rates and higher life expectancies than Northern and Western European population groups. Other scientists argue, however, that the Mediterranean pattern may not be the only desirable eating plan in the world or necessarily the best one for Americans.

Does It Travel?

In the words of Joan Gussow, Ed.D., of Columbia University, a speaker at a recent symposium on Mediterranean diets, "The most basic question to ask about the Mediterranean diet is, does it travel?" Are Mediterranean food habits as healthful for people with typical Western lifestyles as they are for the rural Mediterranean population groups who have followed them for generations? Are they culturally and agriculturally feasible in regions other than the ones where they originated? Some experts say no.

"No one is saying that the Mediterranean diet as practiced in Mediterranean countries is unhealthful," says Joyce Nettleton, D.Sc., R.D., of the Chicago-based Institute of Food Technologists (IFT). "But it's overly simplistic to transfer observations from Mediterranean countries and say that they will work here."

THE MEDITERRANEAN PATTERN MAY NOT BE THE ONLY DESIRABLE EATING PLAN IN THE WORLD OR NECESSARILY THE BEST ONE FOR AMERICANS.

Many nutrition scientists object to the Mediterranean pyramid because it does not emphasize reduction of total fat. The pyramid, in fact, specifically encourages the consumption of one type of fat—olive oil.

This advice "runs counter to U.S.

dietary recommendations endorsed by virtually all health agencies," says Christine Bruhn, Ph.D., of the University of California, Davis. "I'm concerned about the idea of recommending that people deliberately seek out and consume a particular type of fat. It is more appropriate to try to reduce fat intake to less than 30 percent of total calories."

Mediterranean population groups seem to have low rates of heart disease despite their relatively high fat intake because most of the fat in their diets is monounsaturated. In terms of blood cholesterol levels and heart disease risk, a diet high in monounsaturated fat may be at least as desirable as a diet low in total fat. Indeed, the American Diabetes Association recently recommended a high-monounsaturate diet for those diabetics who have high levels of certain blood fats (triglycerides and very-low-density lipoprotein [VLDL] cholesterol) because the diet improves these cardiovascular risk factors. A high-monounsaturate diet may not suit everyone, however.

Fat, Calories and Obesity

People who need to watch their weight—a category that includes most American adults—should probably avoid diets high in any kind of fat. Ounce for ounce, fat has more than twice as many calories as protein and carbohydrate. A serving of high-fat food takes up much less room on the plate than a serving of low-fat food supplying the same number of calories. For very active people with high calorie needs, such as traditional Mediterranean farmers, this may not matter. But for inactive, overweight Americans who need to keep calorie intake down, it is an important issue. If portions seem too small, people may feel unsatisfied even though they have consumed sufficient calories, and they may be tempted to overeat.

The recommendation to con-

sume olive oil in preference to all other fat sources has also been criticized. Other foods, such as canola oil, nuts and avocados, also provide monounsaturated fatty acids, and many other vegetable oils provide essential fatty acids and vitamin E.

MANY NUTRITION SCIENTISTS OBJECT TO THE MEDITERRANEAN PYRAMID BECAUSE IT DOES NOT EMPHASIZE REDUCTION OF TOTAL FAT.

Also, substantially increasing the use of olive oil in the U.S. may be impractical for agricultural and economic reasons, as Dr. Gussow explains. "Olive trees are not hardy in much of the United States," she says. "If we are going to eat Mediterranean, a good deal of the U.S. will have to depend heavily on imported foods." Translation: expensive foods. In U.S. supermarkets, olive oil usually costs at least twice as much as soybean or canola oils.

The Wine Question

The Mediterranean pyramid's recommendation for daily wine consumption has created intense controversy. Oldways Preservation and Exchange Trust, a nonprofit organization involved in the pyramid's development and promotion, says it would be "intellectually dishonest" to omit wine from any depiction of traditional Mediterranean diets. According to Walter Willett, M.D., Dr.P.H., of the Harvard School of Public Health, one of the pyramid's originators, "We can't take it out of the picture because it really is a traditional part of meals in the Mediterranean and almost certainly is an important contributor to the low rate of coronary heart disease in that population."

The inclusion of wine may be

accurate, but it thrusts the Mediterranean pyramid into the middle of one of the thorniest controversies

THE MEDITERRANEAN PYRAMID'S RECOMMENDATION FOR DAILY WINE CONSUMPTION HAS CREATED INTENSE CONTROVERSY.

in public health. Even though the death rates of moderate drinkers are lower than those of abstainers, health authorities have been extremely reluctant to promote alcohol consumption because some people cannot drink in moderation, and immoderate drinking poses extreme risks to health and safety.

Balancing the benefits of alcohol against its risks is extraordinarily difficult. Indeed, some experts believe that it is impossible to issue one all-purpose guideline on alcohol intake for everyone. In the views of many policy makers and health professionals, the best decisions about the use of alcohol are those made on an individual basis, considering the health risk factors and alcohol consumption history of each person.

To their credit, the Mediterranean pyramid proponents acknowledge these complexities. In the written explanations accompanying the pyramid, they carefully specify the meaning of moderation (one or two drinks per day for men, one for women) and state that "from a contemporary public health perspective, wine should be considered optional in a Mediterranean-style diet and avoided whenever consumption would put the individual or others at risk, including during pregnancy and before driving."

Such subtleties tend to disappear, however, when people translate lengthy explanations into simple graphics. Take a look at the picture **of the pyramid printed in this article. This is very similar to the version of the pyramid currently distributed by**

Q: WHEN IS AN ENDORSEMENT NOT AN ENDORSEMENT?

A: WHEN IT NEVER HAPPENED

The May/June 1994 issue of *Health* magazine says that the Mediterranean Diet Pyramid was "developed and endorsed" by the Harvard School of Public Health, Oldways Preservation & Exchange Trust (a Boston-based non-profit organization) and the World Health Organization's European Regional Office.

The June 8, 1994, issue of *The Washington Post* calls the pyramid "a joint effort" of these three organizations. Similarly, the July 4, 1994, issue of *U.S. News & World Report* refers to it as "the brainchild" of this "unlikely trio."

An Oldways news release dated March 1, 1994, describes the pyramid project as "an ongoing public education initiative" of the Harvard School of Public Health and Oldways. A preliminary version of the pyramid distributed with the news release carries three logos—those of Harvard, Oldways and WHO—and states that the three organizations "developed and endorsed" the pyramid.

DID HARVARD REALLY ENDORSE THE PYRAMID?

These references to a Harvard "endorsement" came as a considerable surprise to Fredrick Stare, M.D., Ph.D., an ACSH director. Dr. Stare founded the Department of Nutrition at the Harvard School of Public Health and served as its chairman for many years. He knew very well that Harvard had a policy of not endorsing any particular diet plan.

Has that policy changed recently? *Priorities* checked with the News Office of the Harvard School of Public Health and found that the answer is no. The school maintains its tradition of never endorsing any specific diet. It does not endorse the Mediterranean Diet Pyramid.

Beverly Freeman, a spokesperson for the Harvard School of Public Health, told *Priorities* that Dr. Walter Willett, current chairman of the school's Department of Nutrition, collaborated with Oldways in the development of the pyramid. Ms. Freeman also said that Oldways and Harvard have cosponsored meetings at which scientists presented and discussed the pyramid. Neither of these actions, however, constitutes a Harvard "endorsement."

Oldways has responded to the complaints from Dr. Stare and others about its inaccurate use of the Harvard name. The current version of the Mediterranean Diet Pyramid, released at a San Francisco food symposium in June 1994, no longer carries the Harvard logo, and current Oldways literature no longer refers to the nonexistent Harvard "endorsement." It is too late, however, to change the misstatements that appeared in nationally prominent publications or to correct the impression that Oldways is—at the very least—unprofessional, careless and excessively eager to cite the Harvard name in every possi-ble context. (One of Oldways' news releases—a one-page document—mentions the word "Harvard" six times.)

WHAT ABOUT WHO?

Since Oldways has misused the name of one prestigious institution, *Priorities* can't help but wonder about the validity of the supposed "endorsement" of the pyramid by another distinguished organization—the European Regional Office of WHO. *The Wall Street Journal*, the *San Francisco Examiner* and other publications have reported this endorsement as a fact. But we are skeptical.

Does WHO officially back the pyramid, or is it just that Elisabet Helsing, Dr. Med. Sci., of the WHO European Regional Office promotes it, just as Harvard's Dr. Willett does? Would WHO—an organization with a long history of crusading against alcohol abuse and a formal goal of reducing alcohol intake—really accept the idea of endorsing a document that calls for daily wine drinking?

Despite extensive inquiries, Dr. Stare has been unable to confirm whether WHO has endorsed the Mediterranean Diet Pyramid. So we're asking K Dun Gifford, President of Oldways, to clarify the situation for us. Mr. Gifford, could you please provide written confirmation of WHO's endorsement of the Mediterranean Diet Pyramid? (On WHO stationery, please, and over the signature of an appropriate top-level official from WHO headquarters in Geneva.) If you can do this, we will publish it in the next issue of *Priorities.* *

Oldways. It does not mention that wine is "optional" or define the quantitative meaning of "moderate." What kind of message about wine drinking will people receive if this graphic is all they see?

And why recommend wine, but not beer or hard liquor? Wine may be the traditional beverage of the Mediterranean region, but most epidemiological studies have associated all types of alcoholic beverages with reduced cardiovascular risk. Some scientists have suggested that antioxidants in wine may contribute to its protective effect, but no one has proven that this is true. There's no compelling reason to urge beer or spirits drinkers to switch to wine, yet this is what the Mediterranean pyramid seems to

suggest. Worse yet, if these drinkers interpret the Mediterranean pyramid as suggesting that they drink wine in addition to their preferred beverages, they could find themselves in serious trouble.

Where's the Milk?

Wine has a place in the Mediterranean pyramid, but another beverage—milk—is conspicuously absent. This omission reflects traditional Mediterranean food patterns. "Milk was not included in the Mediterranean diet pyramid for the simple reason that, historically, it was only a minor component of the diet," according to Oldways. "Milk goes sour quickly in hot, Mediterranean climates, so early on traditions of

preserving milk—in the form of cheese and yogurt—were developed."

While the omission of milk is historically accurate, it is bad advice for the American public. In the U.S. diet, milk is the principal source of calcium, a mineral crucial to bone health. Calcium is one of the most underconsumed nutrients, placing some American women at risk for osteoporosis. In June 1994, the National Institutes of Health recommended that both pre-menopausal and postmenopausal women should substantially increase their calcium intakes. Women can't do this if they avoid drinking milk because it doesn't fit into a Mediterranean meal pattern.

"Consumers should be encour-

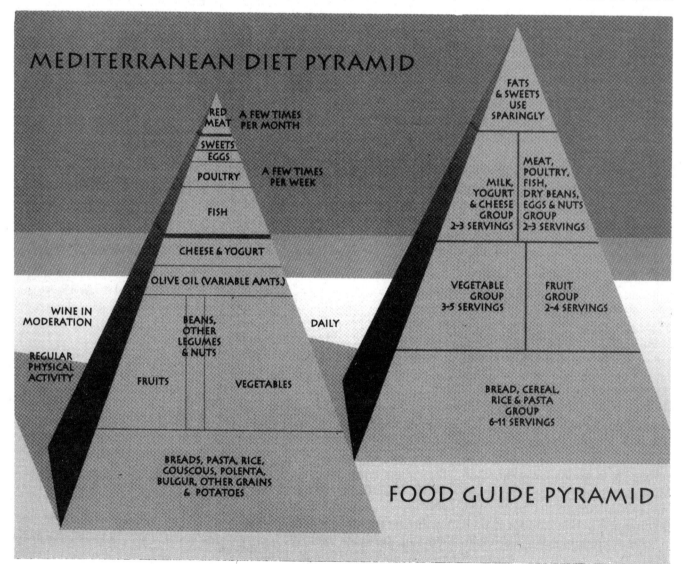

aged to obtain calcium from a wide range of sources, not just cheese and yogurt," Dr. Bruhn says. In her view, the lack of low-fat milk in the Mediterranean pyramid is a glaring omission. There is no scientific rationale for urging the avoidance of low-fat milk. Indeed, many nutrition authorities consider low-fat milk to be a more desirable food than cheese because most cheeses are high in total and saturated fat.

Another aspect of the Mediterranean pyramid that has prompted criticism is the extreme limitation on red meat. Meat is a key source of iron, a nutrient often in short supply in the diets of children, adolescents, women of childbearing age and the elderly. Meat also provides substantial amounts of zinc and copper. The U.S.D.A. Food Guide Pyramid and the federal government's Dietary Guidelines for Americans deal with the problem of saturated fat in meat by limiting serving sizes and recommending the consumption of lean, well-trimmed meat. This approach is more likely to be acceptable to American consumers than the Mediterranean pyramid's more drastic advice to limit red meat intake to no more than 12 to 16 ounces per month.

Choosing a Nutritionally— and Culturally—Acceptable Diet

In a culturally and ethnically diverse population, such as that of the United States, no single, narrowly defined dietary pattern should be recommended for everyone. "When formulating dietary advice for the public, it is important to make an attempt to accommodate popular food habits and preferences, so that your advice is acceptable within the cultural framework," says IFT's Dr. Nettleton. The U.S.D.A.'s Food Guide Pyramid and its companion Dietary Guidelines do this very effectively. The Mediterranean pyramid does not.

The Mediterranean way of eating can be a healthy one—if you're careful to limit your portions of high-fat foods so that you don't get too many calories, if you make an effort to include plenty of calcium and iron sources in your Mediterranean-style meals and if you make your personal decision about wine drinking with care. However, the Mediterranean way should not be regarded as the only way.

People can eat healthfully with a wide range of food choices from a variety of cuisines. No one food pattern is the "best." Americans would be better advised to choose a nutritionally balanced diet compatible with their personal, cultural and ethnic traditions, rather than trying to follow an unfamiliar, very foreign eating pattern that overemphasizes some types of foods and unnecessarily limits the consumption of others.

"In *Priorities*, Vol. 7, No. 2, 1995 (pp. 3 and 46), the author, Kathleen Meister responds to correspondence from K. Dun Gifford, President of Oldways Preservation & Exchange Trust and Joan Gussow, Professor Emeritus at Teachers College, Columbia University. Also, in an Editor's Note, the following is presented: "In further correspondence, K. Dun Gifford provided evidence of the endorsement of the Mediterranean Diet Pyramid by WHO and clarified the relationship between Harvard and Oldways.

Geneviéve Pinet, Senior Legal Adviser in the Office of the WHO Legal Counsel in Geneva, in a letter dated October 15, 1993 state[s]: 'We are fully satisfied with the information . . . and hereby authorize the use of the WHO logo on the Mediterranean Diet Pyramid.'

The Harvard School of Public Health Office of Public Affairs approved a press release dated May 1, 1994 stating: 'The World Health Organization (WHO) European Regional Office has joined with the WHO/FAO Collaborating Center in Nutrition at Harvard School of Public Health and Oldways Preservation & Exchange Trust in releasing today The Traditional Healthy Mediterranean Diet Pyramid.' " **Ed.**

PHYTOCHEMICALS: DRUGSTORE IN A SALAD?

Researchers have long puzzled over why people who eat lots of fruits, vegetables, beans, and grains have a strikingly lower risk of coronary heart disease and cancer than people who center their diet on meat and dairy products. Part of the benefit undoubtedly stems from the fact that plant foods are low in fat and high in vitamins, minerals, and fiber. But the overall benefit seems greater than the sum of those parts.

Now an emerging body of scientific evidence is pointing to the value of plant chemicals, or phytochemicals, that are neither vitamins nor minerals. Manufacturers eager to capitalize on that research have been flooding the market with phytochemical supplements, accompanied by a host of extravagant claims (see box, "Produce in a Pill?"). Here's a more objective look at the most promising findings so far.

Hormones in grains and beans

Most beans and whole grains are good sources of phytochemicals called **saponins.** Saponins neutralize certain potentially cancer-causing enzymes in the gut; in addition, inactivating those enzymes may indirectly reduce blood-cholesterol levels.

There's stronger evidence on another group of chemicals in beans and grains: **isoflavones** and other **"phytoestrogens,"** which resemble the female hormone estrogen in several ways. For example, human estrogen lowers cholesterol levels; so can a diet rich in soy foods, which are loaded with isoflavones. When researchers remove the phytoestrogens, soy loses most of its cholesterol-cutting power. Some preliminary evidence suggests that isoflavones, like human estrogen, may even help ease hot flashes and slow the bone loss that follows menopause.

In some ways, paradoxically, phytoestrogens may have the opposite effect of human estrogen—and that may also be beneficial. For example, researchers have found that animals fed a high-soy diet and humans who eat a lot of tofu, or soybean curd, have a

reduced risk of cancer. Two possible reasons: Isoflavones entering the cells in the breasts or ovaries may crowd out the animal or human estrogen, which is thought to fuel the growth of certain cancers; and one particular isoflavone, called **genistein,** may inhibit the cellular enzymes and suppress the new blood vessels that help cancers multiply.

Garlic and onions: Sulfur power

Allium vegetables—garlic, onions, chives, leeks, and scallions—seem like nutritional weaklings, according to the standard vitamin and mineral tables. But they're rich in beneficial sulfur compounds. For example, **allicin** seems to reduce production of cholesterol in the liver. Consuming just half a clove of garlic per day may indeed cut cholesterol levels, by an average of about 10 percent.

Other sulfur compounds in allium vegetables, particularly **sulfur-allyl cysteine,** help the liver to detoxify chemicals that may cause cancer. A diet that's rich in either garlic or sulfur-allyl cysteine reduces the risk of various cancers in animals. More significant, a five-year retrospective study of some 42,000 women from Iowa found that those who ate garlic at least once a week had one-third less risk of developing colon cancer than those who never ate it. Smaller studies have linked both onions and chives with a comparably reduced risk of colon cancer.

Broccoli, cabbage, and more

There is strong evidence that cruciferous vegetables—including broccoli, Brussels sprouts, cabbage, cauliflower, kale, and turnips—help ward off cancer. In addition to the possibly cancer-fighting antioxidant vitamins, cruciferous vegetables contain at least two potent phytochemical groups.

One is the **indoles,** which help the body convert one type of estrogen into a harmless form of the hormone, rather than into the potentially cancer-fueling

Scientists are unearthing a wealth of obscure, potentially protective chemicals in plant foods.

Summing up

Plant foods offer far more than just vitamins and minerals. Researchers have now identified dozens of apparently disease-fighting chemicals in those foods—and they've barely scratched the surface.

What to do

- Eat a wide variety of plant foods. Try to include cruciferous vegetables, citrus fruits, and grains and beans, which all contain beneficial phytochemicals. Flavoring your meals with allium vegetables such as garlic or onions should boost their health value, too.
- Aim for 5 to 9 servings per day of fruits and vegetables, 6 to 11 servings of grains and beans.
- Forget "whole food" supplements, which can't possibly offer all the benefits that whole produce does (see box at right).

kind. Indoles sharply retard the growth of malignant breast tumors in animals.

Cruciferous vegetables also contain **isothiocyanates,** yet another group of sulfur compounds. Modest doses of one such chemical, **sulforaphane,** cut the risk of breast cancer in rats by more than half, in theory by boosting the liver's detoxifying power.

Pulp fact

People who eat a lot of oranges and other citrus fruits—or who drink the juice of those fruits—have a clearly reduced risk of cancer. While the vitamin-C content of those fruits may be at least partly responsible, their skin is loaded with apparently potent anti-cancer chemicals known as **terpenes,** which do end up in the juice. Large doses of one terpene, **limonene,** actually shrink breast cancers in animals; in fact, concentrated limonene may work much like another terpene, the breast-cancer drug tamoxifen (*Nolvadex*).

Antioxidants in a glass

One potent group of phytochemicals—the **flavonoids,** which combat oxidation and blood clots—crops up in lowly or unlikely places. Flavonoids are found in apples, celery, cranberries, grapes, and onions, which are low in most vitamins and minerals. They're particularly abundant in two beverages that contain even fewer nutrients: tea and red wine.

Tea. The "bad" LDL cholesterol seems to clog the arteries only when it has been chemically damaged by oxidation. A two-cup dose of green or black tea temporarily reduces such oxidation. And a retrospective Dutch study of some 800 men found that those who consumed the most flavonoids, mainly from black tea, had two-thirds less risk of coronary disease than those who consumed the least.

Tea flavonoids clearly help ward off cancer in animals, in theory by blocking cancer-causing oxidation of the DNA that controls cell growth. The evidence in humans is mixed, but some studies suggest that regular tea drinkers may have up to 50 percent less risk of certain cancers than other people have.

Red wine. Researchers have shown that moderate consumption of any alcoholic beverage reduces the risk of coronary disease, apparently by boosting levels of the "good" HDL cholesterol and reducing the chance of blood clots. Now some studies are bolstering the suspicion that red wine may protect the heart better than other alcoholic beverages. Several reports have found that red wine but not white wine minimizes both LDL oxidation and blood clotting. One likely reason: Flavonoids are concentrated in grape skins, which are not used in white wine.

Fruit salad, mixed vegetables

Some apparently protective chemicals occur in a wide variety of plant foods. Among the most common are **carotenoids,** which fight disease-causing oxidation. Until recently, researchers have focused almost exclusively on one carotenoid, **beta-carotene.** Last year, Harvard researchers presented the best evidence so far linking carotenoids other than beta-carotene with a reduced risk of disease. Their retrospective study found that people who consume the most **lutein** and **zeaxanthin,** found in green leafy vegetables, had roughly 50 percent less risk of macular degeneration, the leading cause of blindness after age 65, than those who consume the least.

PRODUCE IN A PILL?

"Over 200 pounds of vegetables in a bottle," claims an ad for *Vegetable Essence,* a nutritional supplement from Great Life. For people who know they should eat more produce but can't bring themselves to do it, *Vegetable Essence* and scores of similar new supplements sound too good to be true.

They are. It turns out that the new "whole food" supplements are far from whole; instead, most of them offer just one or two of the most promising phytochemicals. Schiff's *Broccoli Concentrate,* for example, contains only sulforaphane, a potentially cancer-fighting chemical in cruciferous vegetables such as broccoli. But you'd have to swallow roughly 100 pills, at a cost of about $20, to get as much sulforaphane as a single serving of broccoli provides. And you'd miss the dozens of other potentially beneficial phytochemicals in broccoli—as well as the vitamins, minerals, and fiber.

At least one of the new supplements, Great Life's *Vegetable Essence,* takes a different approach, offering a blend of powdered vegetables. The manufacturer doesn't know the phytochemical content of its pills. So we asked researchers at Rutgers University and the University of Illinois who specialize in phytochemicals and food processing. They told us it's currently impossible to condense large amounts of produce into a pill without losing large amounts of nutrients, including the phytochemicals.

Taking Soy to Heart

Oat bran was the first headline-grabbing dietary weapon against heart disease, quickly followed by garlic, red wine, olive oil, and an ever-lengthening list of vitamins. Now the spotlight is on soy protein, a part of the humble bean that in the United States has been valued more as animal fodder than as human fare.

Its low profile is bound to change now that some experts say soy's ability to clear cholesterol from the circulation is unsurpassed by any other foodstuff. Learning to love this little leguminous bean may be especially important for the 37.2 million Americans with cholesterol levels above 240 mg/dl, because soy protein appears to magnify the benefits of a low-fat diet.

Good dietary sources of this protein are tofu (soy bean curd), soy flour, and other dry and moist preparations. Soy sauce contains only a trace and has the drawback of being loaded with sodium.

The soy story

When researchers from the University of Kentucky at Lexington analyzed data from 38 clinical trials examining the impact of a high-soy diet on cholesterol level, they found that people who ate an average of 47 grams daily had a 12.9% fall in harmful low-density lipoprotein (LDL) and a 9.3% drop in total cholesterol. Their levels of beneficial HDL-cholesterol stayed about the same. Moreover, soy had the greatest effect in people whose cholesterol readings were highest to begin with, the researchers reported in the *New England Journal of Medicine*.

These results should probably be taken with a grain of salt — or a teaspoon of soy sauce — because they depend on *meta-analysis*. This method groups together data from many small trials and then uses statistical manipulation to look for meaningful differences. Such groups are almost always made up of studies that vary considerably in their design and results.

Still, the idea that soy somehow cleans cholesterol out of the bloodstream has a long history. Some 30 years ago, an American researcher gave soy protein to prison inmates and wrote about the falls in serum cholesterol that he observed. His groundbreaking research went largely unnoticed in this country.

Italy is the epicenter of soy protein science and studies there have yielded the most compelling evidence that soy selectively lowers LDL cholesterol, which is a major contributor to atherosclerosis and heart attack. Italian researchers have repeatedly seen LDL plummet by 22–25%, and total cholesterol fall by as much as 23%. As in the recent meta-analysis done in the United States, a high-soy diet worked best for people with the highest initial cholesterol levels.

Italian studies yielded such dramatic results because they enrolled only patients with elevated cholesterol levels, while some U.S. investigations also included participants in the normal range (200 mg/dl or less). Soy protein probably only works for people with cholesterol levels above 240 mg/dl, said Cesare R. Sirtori, a professor of clinical pharmacology at the University of Milan and an international leader in the field for more than two decades.

Cardiologists in Italy find the benefits of a high-soy diet so convincing that they have long prescribed soy protein to both children and adults with some inherited forms of *hypercholesterolemia* (elevated cholesterol). The Italian National Health Service even provides it free to some families.

How does it work?

So far, the evidence suggest that soy boosts the activity of LDL receptors, special snares that snatch bad cholesterol from the bloodstream and deliver it to the liver where it is broken down for excretion. Scientists don't know exactly how soy does this, but they do know it's loaded with *genistein* and *daidzein*, two *phytoestrogens* (plant hormones) that don't occur in other vegetation. When monkeys were fed two types of soy protein — with and without these phytoestrogens — the feed that was rich in them caused cholesterol levels to fall significantly. Based on these studies, experts estimate that 60–70% of soy's cholesterol-lowering ability comes from phytoestrogens.

These plant hormones may also help prevent heart disease in other ways, even in people with normal cholesterol. They appear to protect particles of LDL against oxidation, making them less likely to adhere to the lining of the coronary arteries. Genistein may also prevent the proliferation of smooth muscle cells in the artery walls and keep platelets from clumping together, two processes that contribute to coronary blockages. If these early findings hold up, high-soy diets may turn out to lower the risk for heart disease not only for people with elevated cholesterol but for everyone.

It's unclear how much soy protein is needed. Although the meta-analysis showed positive results for people who ate 47 grams of soy protein daily, experts believe that 20 to 25 grams (or 5 to 6 ounces of firm tofu) may be enough to lower cholesterol levels.

For those who find tofu rubbery or tasteless, there are lots of culinary alternatives. Soy milk can be used as a beverage, soy flour can be added to baked goods, and isolated soy protein or textured vegetable protein can be stuffed into ravioli, lasagna, and other dishes (the Italians' approach to high-soy eating).

An alternative to drugs?

Experts don't yet know if soy protein can eliminate the need for cholesterol-lowering

---

> ### Singing the Praises of Soy
>
> In addition to possibly reducing the risk of heart disease, soy has many other virtues. There is increasing evidence that people who eat a diet rich in soy products are less likely to develop cancer (especially of the breast or prostate), osteoporosis, or kidney disease or to suffer troubling symptoms at menopause. It appears that people who eat about 3 ounces of tofu (or the equivalent) daily may realize these benefits. In addition, soy is high in folate, protein, omega-3 fatty acids, and minerals.

---

medications in people with dangerously high levels. Researcher Ronald Krauss, who studies cholesterol and chairs the American Heart Association's Nutrition Committee, says that physicians generally ask people to lower their cholesterol by dietary means before prescribing drugs. "Soy in combination with a low-fat, low-cholesterol diet may indeed obviate the need for cholesterol-lowering drugs in some people. However, they must have close follow-up to see if this strategy works," said Dr. Krauss, head of molecular medicine at Lawrence Berkeley National Laboratory, University of California.

One thing's for certain: soy is no panacea. While it may lower cholesterol levels more effectively than a heart-healthy diet alone, no amount of soy can counteract the effects of eating lots of fat, being overweight, or being sedentary. Those who've been told that their cholesterol is too high should first focus on carving out a low-fat regimen they can stick to and then figure out how to replace some of the animal protein they're eating with soy.

The soybean has been cultivated in China for nearly 5,000 years, and it is so important there that the Chinese name for it is *ta-tou*, which means "greater bean." Perhaps we're beginning to understand why.

— *KRISTINE NAPIER, M.P.H., R.D.*

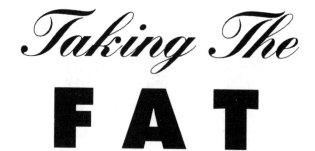

Taking The FAT Out Of Food

*Whipping up fat-free cakes and lower fat cookies is possible
with today's fat replacers.*

Paula Kurtzweil

*Paula Kurtzweil is a member of FDA's
public affairs staff.*

Food manufacturers are making it easier for fat-conscious consumers to have their cake and eat it, too—and their cheeses, chips, chocolate, cookies, ice cream, salad dressings, and various other foods that are now available in lower fat versions.

These products can help adult consumers reduce their fat intakes to recommended levels while allowing them to enjoy foods traditionally high in fat. A diet high in fat can contribute to heart disease and some forms of cancer and, because fats are calorie-dense, to excessive body weight.

A host of fat substitutes that replaces most, if not all, of the fat in a food, makes these lower fat foods possible. Most of these fat replacers are ingredients already approved by the Food and Drug Administration for other uses in food. For instance, starches and gums are approved as thickeners and stabilizers. New compounds, such as olestra,

have undergone or will undergo close scrutiny by FDA to assess their safety.

In theory, the perfect fat replacer is one that contributes everything fat does in a food but without the calories, saturated fat, and cholesterol. The question remains: Can fat-reduced products actually reduce people's overall calorie intake and have a significant impact on their total fat intake?

Fat in the Diet

Fat is a difficult substance to replace because it has many important functions. A major nutrient, it is important for proper growth and development and maintenance of good health. Fats carry the fat-soluble vitamins A, D, E, and K and aid their absorption in the intestine. They are the only source of the essential fatty acids linoleic and linolenic acids. They are an important source of calories for many adults and for infants and toddlers, who have the highest energy

needs per kilogram of body weight of any age group. Fat provides 9 calories per gram, compared with 4 calories per gram for protein and carbohydrates.

As a food ingredient, fat is important in food preparation and consumption because it gives taste, consistency, stability, and palatability to foods and helps us feel full so we stop eating.

But there are limits on the amount we should eat because of fats' link to heart disease, cancer and overweight. The Dietary Guidelines for Americans recommend limiting total fat intake to no more than 30 percent of calories and saturated fat to no more than 10 percent. Cholesterol intake should be limited to no more than 300 milligrams a day. Saturated fat and cholesterol are the substances in fat that contribute to the formation of plaque, which clogs arteries, leading to heart disease.

Americans appear to be heeding the experts' advice because, according to a

1995 annual survey by the Food Marketing Institute—an organization of grocery retailers and wholesalers—65 percent of the consumers surveyed—the highest level to date—rated fat as their No. 1 nutrition concern. More than three-fourths of the consumers said they stopped buying a specific food because of the amount of fat listed on the nutrition label.

A 1995 survey by the Calorie Control Council—an international association of manufacturers of low-calorie, low-fat, and diet foods and beverages—found that 72 percent of respondents who said they look for "light" foods said they are most attracted to food products claiming to be "reduced in fat."

Manufacturers are responding by adding more and more reduced-fat foods to their product lines. That corresponds to the Department of Health and Human Services' Healthy People 2000 goal of increasing to 5,000 from 2,500 in 1986 the number of brand items reduced in fat and saturated fat.

Regulation

Fat replacers can help reduce a food's fat and calorie levels while maintaining some of the desirable qualities fat brings to food, such as "mouth feel," texture and flavor.

Under FDA regulations, fat replacers usually fall into one of two categories: food additives or "generally recognized as safe" (GRAS) substances. Each has its own set of regulatory requirements.

Food additives must be evaluated for safety and approved by FDA before they can be marketed. They include substances with no proven track record of safety; scientists just don't know that much about their use in food. Examples of food additives are polydextrose, carrageenan and olestra, which are used as fat replacers. Manufacturers of food additives must test their products, submit the results to FDA for review, and await agency approval before using them in food.

GRAS substances, on the other hand, do not have to undergo rigorous testing before they are used in foods because they are generally recognized as safe by knowledgeable scientists, usually because of the substances' long history of

Most of these fat replacers are ingredients already approved by the Food and Drug Administration for other uses in food.

safe use in foods. Many GRAS substances are similar to substances already in food. Examples of GRAS substances used as fat replacers are cellulose gel, dextrins, guar gum, and gum arabic.

Sources

Fat replacers may be carbohydrate-, protein- or fat-based substances.

The first to hit the market used carbohydrate as the main ingredient. Avicel, for example, is a cellulose gel introduced in the mid-1960s as a food stabilizer. Carrageenan, a seaweed derivative, was approved for use as an emulsifier, stabilizer and thickener in food in 1961. Its use as a fat replacer became popular in the early 1990s. Litesse (polydextrose) came on the market in 1981 as a humectant, which helps retain moisture. Others in this category include dextrins, maltodextrins, fiber, gums, starch, and modified food starch. FDA has affirmed many carbohydrate-based fat replacers as GRAS.

Although their original intent was to perform certain technical functions in food that would improve overall quality, some carbohydrate-based fat replacers are now used specifically to reduce a food's calorie content. They provide from zero to 4 calories per gram. They are used in a variety of foods, including dairy-type products, sauces, frozen desserts, salad dressings, processed meats, baked goods, spreads, chewing gum, and sweets.

Protein-based fat substitutes came along in the early 1990s. These and fat-

based replacers were designed specifically to replace fat in foods.

One form, Microparticulated Protein Product (MPP), such as Simplesse and Trailblazer, is made from whey protein or milk and egg protein. These fat replacers provide 1 to 4 calories per gram, depending on their water content, and are approved for use in frozen dessert-type foods. FDA has agreed that whey-based MPP conforms to FDA's definition of whey protein concentrate, such as the fat replacer Dairy-Lo, a GRAS substance. Therefore, whey-based MPP can be used in other foods, including reduced-fat versions of butter, sour cream, cheese, yogurt, salad dressing, margarine, mayonnaise, baked goods, coffee creamer, soups, and sauces.

Another type of protein-based fat replacers, called protein blends, combine animal or vegetable protein, gums, food starch, and water. They are made with FDA-approved ingredients and are used in frozen desserts and baked goods.

Olestra

Olestra is an example of a fat-based fat replacer. FDA approved olestra (brand name Olean), made by Procter & Gamble Co. of Cincinnati, in January 1996, for use in preparing potato chips, crackers, tortilla chips, and other savory snacks. Procter & Gamble said it expected to begin test-marketing olestra-containing products in 1996.

Olestra has properties similar to those of naturally occurring fat, but it provides zero calories and no fat. That's because olestra is undigestible. It passes through the digestive tract but is not absorbed into the body. This is due to its unique configuration: a center unit of sucrose (sugar) with six, seven or eight fatty acids attached.

Olestra's configuration also makes it possible for the substance to be exposed to high temperatures, such as frying—a quality most other fat replacers lack.

As promising as olestra sounds, it does have some drawbacks. Studies show that it may cause intestinal cramps and loose stools in some individuals.

Also, according to clinical tests, olestra reduces the absorption of fat-soluble nutrients, such as vitamins A, D, E, and K and carotenoids, from foods

Favorite Foods Containing Fat Replacers Among People Who Use 'Light' Foods

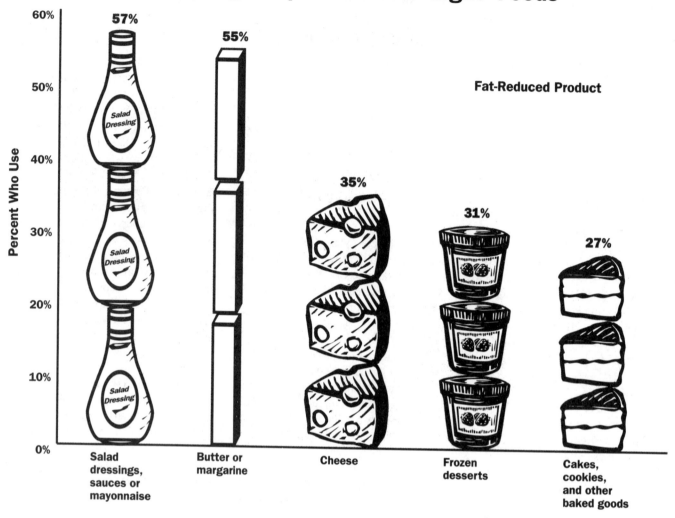

Percent Who Use

- 57% — Salad dressings, sauces or mayonnaise
- 55% — Butter or margarine
- 35% — Cheese
- 31% — Frozen desserts
- 27% — Cakes, cookies, and other baked goods

Fat-Reduced Product

(Source: 1995 Calorie Control Council national survey)

eaten at the same time as olestra-containing products. Tests by Procter & Gamble show that no reduction in absorption of fat-soluble vitamins will occur when proper levels of vitamins are added for compensation to olestra-containing foods.

To address these concerns, FDA approved olestra on conditions that vitamins A, D, E, and K be added to olestra-containing foods and that Procter & Gamble continue studies on consumption and long-term effects of olestra. These studies will be reviewed at an FDA Food Advisory Committee meeting in mid-1998.

To provide consumers with information about olestra's possible effects, FDA also required that the following interim labeling statement appear on products made with olestra:

"This Product contains Olestra. Olestra may cause abdominal cramping and loose stools. Olestra inhibits the absorption of some vitamins and other nutrients. Vitamins A, D, E and K have been added."

FDA has invited public comment on the need for such a label statement and on the statement's adequacy and clarity. The agency will evaluate those comments before issuing a final label statement.

Concern with olestra's drawbacks led one of olestra's critics, the Center for Science in the Public Interest—a nonprofit consumer advocacy organization—to file an objection to FDA's approval. FDA's response to the objection is pending.

Other Replacers

Some other fat-based replacers are being considered or developed:

• Salatrim (which stands for short and long-chain acid triglyceride molecules) is the generic name for a family of reduced-calorie fats that are only partially absorbed in the body. Salatrim provides 5 calories per gram. A petition seeking FDA's affirmation that Salatrim is GRAS was filed in June 1994. An example of its use is in Hershey Co.'s reduced-fat baking chips, semi-sweet chocolate flavor.

• Caprenin, another Procter & Gamble product, is a 5-calorie-per-gram fat sub-

How Fat Replacers Can Affect Fat Intake

Sample Menu

	Calories	Fat (grams)		Calories	Fat (grams)
Regular Diet			**Fat-Replaced Diet**		
Breakfast			**Breakfast**		
2 slices toast	128	2	2 slices toast	128	2
1 tbsp margarine	100	11	1 tbsp reduced-fat margarine	50	6
1 cup orange juice	111	0.5	1 cup orange juice	111	0.5
coffee with creamer	16	1	coffee with nonfat creamer	8	0.3
Lunch			**Lunch**		
2 slices bread	128	2	2 slices bread	128	2
1 oz American cheese	106	9	1 oz reduced-fat cheese product	73	4
2 oz bologna	180	17	2 oz fat-free bologna	40	0
1 tbsp mayonnaise	100	11	1 tbsp reduced-fat imitation mayonnaise	50	5
Banana	105	0.6	Banana	105	0.6
30 grams (about 2) chocolate cookies	140	6	30 grams (about 2) reduced-fat chocolate cookies	120	3
Snack			**Snack**		
Candy bar	251	9	Reduced-fat candy bar	170	5
Supper			**Supper**		
3½ oz baked chicken	239	14	3½ oz baked chicken	239	14
½ cup green beans	22	0.2	½ cup green beans	22	0.2
1 tsp margarine	33	4	1 tsp reduced-fat margarine	17	2
Lettuce salad	5	-	Lettuce salad	5	-
1 tbsp salad dressing	67	6	1 tbsp reduced-fat salad dressing	33	2
Baked potato	220	-	Baked potato	220	-
1 tbsp sour cream	26	2.5	1 tbsp reduced-fat sour cream	20	1
½ cup vanilla ice cream	132	7	½ cup reduced-fat vanilla frozen dessert	116	0.7
Snack			**Snack**		
Chocolate cookies	140	6	Reduced-fat chocolate cookies	120	3
Total	2,249	108.8		1,775	51.3

(Sources: food labels and *Food Values of Portions Commonly Used*, 16th edition)

stitute for cocoa butter in candy bars. A petition seeking FDA's affirmation that Caprenin is GRAS was filed in 1991.

• Emulsifiers are fat-based substances that are used with water to replace all or part of the shortening content in cake mixes, cookies, icings, and vegetable dairy products. They give the same calories as fat but less is used, resulting in fat and calorie reductions.

Other fat replacers are being developed, according to the Calorie Control Council and other organizations. These include DDM (dialkyl dihexadecylmalonate), a fat-based substance that is not absorbed into the body and can be used in frying and baking. Frito-Lay Inc. has been studying this fat substitute since 1986, although it has not yet petitioned FDA for approval. Also on the

Olestra has properties similar to those of naturally occurring fat, but it provides zero calories and no fat.

horizon is a fat substitute made by combining starches or gums with small amounts of oil. Opta Food Ingredients Inc. received an exclusive license from the U.S. Department of Agriculture last February for the process, called Fantesk. This fat replacer would give foods the taste and texture of regular fat but provide less than 0.5 grams of fat per serving.

Reducing Dietary Fat

Can these fat replacers help consumers make positive dietary changes? Can they help those who are overweight lose weight?

It may be too early to say, and studies to date give varying answers. For ex-

ample, in a study of lean non-dieting men, one group ate breakfasts of conventional fat foods, while the other ate olestra-containing foods. Those who ate the olestra-containing foods made up their usual daily calorie intake by eating more carbohydrate-containing foods. The study, sponsored partly by Procter & Gamble and published in a 1992 issue of the *American Journal of Clinical Nutrition* (Volume 56), suggested that a diet of reduced-fat foods can help reduce fat intake without affecting total calories.

Fat intake also was decreased in a study of 96 men and women "habitual snackers." One group was fed potato chips prepared with olestra, while the rest ate potato chips prepared with conventional frying oil. The group fed olestra chips ate on average 29 grams less fat and 270 fewer calories a day than those fed regular chips—even though those who knew they were eating fat-free chips ate 10 grams of chips more than those who ate regular chips. This study, done at Pennsylvania State University, also was partly sponsored by Procter & Gamble.

A possible concern about fat replacers is: Can foods claiming to be reduced in fat inadvertently influence people to eat more? Another study at Pennsylvania State University suggests they might. In this study, women were fed the same yogurt labeled either "high-fat" or "low-fat." The group fed the low-fat-labeled version ate more in a lunch that followed the yogurt than the group eating the high-fat-labeled yogurt. As a result, the group eating what they thought was low-fat yogurt took in more calories than the other group.

"It appeared that these women regarded the low-fat label as a license to overeat," wrote Debra Miller, a doctoral student in biobehavioral health and nutrition at Pennsylvania State, in an article she prepared for *Weight Control Digest*.

Still, reduced fat foods appear to be an important part of a fat-reduction diet, according to a study involving the Women's Health Trial. The study, designed to determine the role of low-fat diets in the prevention of breast cancer, found that eating "specially manufactured" low-fat foods was one of the most

Can these fat replacers help consumers make positive dietary changes? Can they help those who are overweight lose weight?

easily adopted dietary practices for those who received prior dietary instruction. Avoiding meats and giving up fats as flavorings (for example, eating bread without butter or margarine) were among the most difficult practices to adopt.

In using reduced-fat foods, the American Dietetic Association cautions consumers to realize that fat-free doesn't mean calorie-free. The calories lost in removing regular fat from a food can be regained through sugars added for palatability, as well as fat replacers, many of which provide calories, too. Consumers should refer to the Nutrition Facts panel on the food label to compare calories and other nutrition information between fat-reduced and regular-fat foods.

Many nutrition experts agree that, used properly, fat replacers can play an important role in improving adult Americans' diets. But, as with any diet or food, they emphasize variety and moderation to ensure a healthy intake.

"These [fat replacers] are truly innovative ideas," said Dennis Gordon, Ph.D., a food scientist at North Dakota State University, Columbia. "But they shouldn't be looked at as a total panacea. [The advice] is the same as with anything: Be prudent."

Fast food: Fatter than ever

The chains are beefing up their menus, leaving health-conscious patrons in a pickle.

A few years ago, the fast-food industry attempted to trim its image, in the hope that salads, seaweed-laced burgers, and other low-fat fare would attract nutrition-conscious customers. But the public didn't bite. Now the fast-food chains are heading fast in the opposite direction, unabashedly pushing fattier fare than ever.

In May, McDonald's ditched its side salads and replaced its low-fat *McLean Deluxe* burger with the high-fat *Arch Deluxe*, a quarter pound of beef topped with cheese and optional bacon. The chain is also expected to boost the size of its basic patty by 25 percent. Meanwhile, Burger King has already increased the size of its regular burger by nearly 60 percent. And Taco Bell has pruned its *Border Light* line of reduced-fat foods and introduced a new line of fattier items, such as the *Big Border Taco*, which packs twice the meat and cheese of a regular taco.

Is it time for people who care about their health to bid fast food a hasty farewell?

Fast food's fatty toll

A recent study, funded by McDonald's, showed that it's possible to eat a diet that gets just 30 percent of its calories from fat—the maximum recommended amount—while dining at McDonald's five times a week. But it sure wasn't easy. The volunteers had to eat small meals at McDonald's, featuring the few relatively lean options. Outside McDonald's, they had to curtail their fat intake to substantially less than 30 percent of calories to make up the difference.

Even a single fast-food meal can supply so many calories and so much fat that you'd have to fast for an entire day and avoid all fat for a second day to compensate. Worse, some evidence suggests that an extremely fatty meal might trigger a heart attack in people with coronary heart disease, in theory because fat pouring into the bloodstream stimulates clotting.

Those findings don't mean you should never set foot in a fast-food restaurant again. But they do mean that it's best to exercise some restraint on even an occasional fast-food foray—and a lot of restraint if you eat fast food regularly.

Fast and lean

Here are four guidelines on how to choose lean meals from fast-food menus that are glutted with fat.

■ **Think small.** Something about fast-food restaurants seems to trigger a primal urge to pig out. The chains feed that frenzy with signs like Burger King's "Go large" or McDonald's "Super size it," for just a

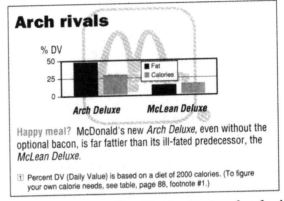

Arch rivals

Happy meal? McDonald's new *Arch Deluxe*, even without the optional bacon, is far fattier than its ill-fated predecessor, the *McLean Deluxe*.

[1] Percent DV (Daily Value) is based on a diet of 2000 calories. (To figure your own calorie needs, see table, page 88, footnote #1.)

little more money. But thinking big in a fast-food restaurant is a bad deal for both your waistline and your heart (see chart below). The smallest burgers are often especially lean—just 33 percent of calories from fat in a Wendy's *Junior*, for example—because they're not only small but plain.

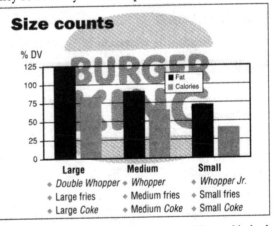

Size counts

■ **Hold the toppings.** Salad vegetables and baked potatoes have no fat, and roast beef can be quite lean. So why is the first meal in the next chart—salad, potato, and beef sandwich—loaded with well over a day's worth of fat? Because it's loaded with toppings. The sour cream, cheese, butter, and bacon bits on the potato alone add 16 grams of artery-clogging saturated fat, four-fifths of the recommended daily maximum for the average person. The blue-cheese dressing on that salad supplies nearly half a day's worth of total fat—and many people add a second packet. Salads that contain cheese can be fattier still. But if you hold the toppings or switch to low-fat alternatives (see chart), those same dishes can provide a much leaner meal.

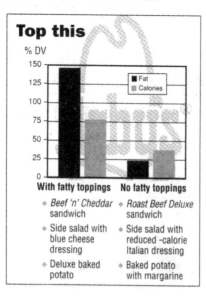

Top this

% DV

- ◆ Beef 'n' Cheddar sandwich
- ◆ Side salad with blue cheese dressing
- ◆ Deluxe baked potato

- ◆ Roast Beef Deluxe sandwich
- ◆ Side salad with reduced-calorie Italian dressing
- ◆ Baked potato with margarine

Toppings have loads of salt, too, so they're particularly bad for people who are on a low-sodium diet. The biggest offenders are often the reduced-calorie dressings, since the chains often add salt to compensate for the loss of palate-pleasing fat. Two packets of Arby's reduced-calorie Italian, for example, provide 2000 mg of sodium—nearly a full day's ration.

■ **Don't get fried.** Frying can bloat the leanest foods. The cod or pollack in Burger King's *Big Fish Sandwich*, for example, gets just 7 to 10 percent of its calories from fat. But those figures jump to an average of 37 percent after the fish has been breaded and deep fried. Add tartar sauce, and the sandwich gets more than half its calories from fat and supplies more than two-thirds the daily dose of fat.

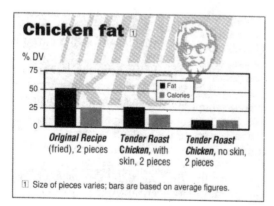

Chicken fat [1]

% DV

- *Original Recipe* (fried), 2 pieces
- *Tender Roast Chicken*, with skin, 2 pieces
- *Tender Roast Chicken*, no skin, 2 pieces

[1] Size of pieces varies; bars are based on average figures.

While there's no lean version of fast-food fish, there are good alternatives to other fried foods. In some restaurants, you can get a baked potato, topped with just a pat of margarine or butter, instead of french fries. Or you can order roasted or grilled chicken, rather than fried chicken pieces or sandwiches, which typically supply as much or more total fat—though less saturated fat—than a regular burger. For still leaner chicken, order it roasted without the skin if possible (see the bar chart above).

■ **Watch the drinks and desserts.** Regular soda adds lots of calories but no other nutrients. Shakes are more nutritious, and they're usually low in fat, since they're usually made with at least some skim milk. But they're still full of calories—up to a quarter of a day's worth for the average adult—since they're full of sugar. Better choices include diet soda, juice, or low-fat milk.

Don't expect anything healthful from fast-food fruit pies, which get nearly half their calories from fat. Sundaes, like shakes, are usually leaner than the pies, but they're still high in calories. McDonald's offers low-fat frozen yogurt; elsewhere, you might decide to skip dessert.

Best and worst

So despite the trend toward fattier fare, it's still possible to order a low-fat, reasonably low-calorie fast-food meal, such as the "lean meal" platter shown in the bar chart below. But it's usually not possible to construct a thoroughly healthful meal—one high in whole grains, fruit, and significant amounts of any vegetable other than iceburg lettuce, which contains insignificant amounts of vitamins, minerals, and fiber. (Only Wendy's offers a salad bar containing nutritious produce.) And if you break all the rules, you could end up with a belly-bloating, artery-clogging meal like the "fatty meal" shown in the chart below.

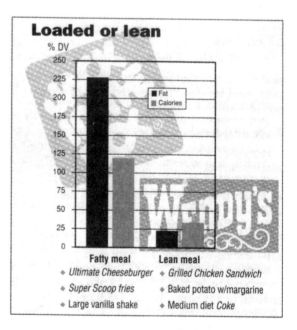

Loaded or lean

% DV

Fatty meal
- ◆ *Ultimate Cheeseburger*
- ◆ *Super Scoop* fries
- ◆ Large vanilla shake

Lean meal
- ◆ *Grilled Chicken Sandwich*
- ◆ Baked potato w/margarine
- ◆ Medium diet *Coke*

Summing up

If you want to help squeeze an occasional fast-food meal into an otherwise healthful diet, follow these guidelines:

■ Choose modest portions; go easy on the toppings; avoid fried foods; choose diet soda, juice or low-fat milk; and skip the fruit pies and other fatty desserts.

■ To identify the leaner options, see the table below, or check the brochures or wall posters found at many major fast-food chains.

Fast-food nutritional profile

	Calories	% Calories from fat	Total fat (% DV) [1]	Saturated fat (% DV) [1]	Sodium (% DV) [1]
BURGERS					
McDonald's Hamburger	270	33%	5%	18%	22%
Wendy's Jr. Hamburger	270	33	15	15	23
McDonald's Cheeseburger	320	41	22	30	31
Wendy's Plain Single w/ Everything	420	43	31	35	34
McDonald's Quarter Pounder	420	45	32	40	29
McDonald's Big Mac	530	47	43	50	40
Hardee's Quarter Pound Cheeseburger	420	48	34	55	36
McDonald's Arch Deluxe	570	49	48	55	46
Burger King Whopper Jr.	420	52	37	40	22
Jack in the Box Jumbo Jack	560	52	49	50	31
Burger King Whopper	640	55	60	55	36
Burger King Double Whopper	870	57	86	95	39
Jack in the Box Ultimate Cheeseburger	1030	69	122	130	50
CHICKEN / TURKEY					
McDonald's McGrilled Chicken Classic	260	13%	6%	5%	21%
Wendy's Grilled Chicken Sandwich	310	23	12	8	33
Arby's Roast Turkey Deluxe	260	24	11	10	53
Hardee's Chicken Fillet Sandwich	420	31	23	15	50
KFC Tender Roast Chicken, no skin [2]	114	32	6	6	19
Arby's Turkey Sub	550	44	42	35	87
Jack in the Box Chicken Caesar Sandwich	520	44	40	30	44
KFC Tender Roast Chicken, with skin [2]	185	47	14	15	22
Burger King BK Broiler Chicken Sandwich	550	47	45	30	20
McDonald's McChicken Sandwich	510	53	46	25	34
Burger King Chicken Sandwich	710	55	66	45	58
KFC Original Recipe [2]	263	61	26	21	32
ROAST BEEF					
Arby's Roast Beef Deluxe (Light menu)	296	30%	15%	15%	34%
Hardee's Regular Roast Beef	270	37	17	25	32
Hardee's Big Roast Beef	410	51	35	45	48
Arby's Beef 'n Cheddar	487	52	43	45	51
FISH					
Hardee's Fisherman's Fillet	450	40%	31%	30%	46%
McDonald's Filet-O-Fish	360	42	25	20	29
Arby's Fish Fillet	529	46	42	35	36
Burger King BK Big Fish Sandwich	700	53	63	30	41

[1] Data for percent of Daily Value (% DV) based on a diet of 2000 calories per day. To determine your own caloric needs (for maintaining current weight), multiply your weight in pounds by one of the following factors, depending on your activity level: 11, if you're nearly sedentary; 13, if moderately active; 15, if a moderate exerciser or physical laborer; 18, if an extremely active exerciser or physical laborer.

[2] Data for this item represent an average of one chicken breast, one leg, and one thigh.

GENETIC ENGINEERING

Fast Forwarding To Future Foods

John Henkel
John Henkel is a staff writer for FDA Consumer.

Take a peek into the supermarket of the near future.

At first glance, products on display won't seem much different from those you are used to. Cucumbers. Peppers. Corn. They'll still be there. But amid all the produce and other kitchen staples, you're apt to find new versions of familiar foods—ones that are custom "built" to improve quality or remove unwanted traits. Insect-resistant apples, long-lasting raspberries, and potatoes that absorb less fat are among the more than 50 plant products under study now that are likely to reside soon on grocers' shelves.

These commodities will arrive courtesy of genetic engineering, a process that allows plant breeders to modify the genetic makeup of a plant species precisely and predictably, creating improved varieties faster and easier than can be done using more traditional plant-breeding techniques. Genetic engineering already is improving lives in areas such as disease diagnostics and treatments, but at the moment it is a fledgling economic force in the commercial food business.

Though genetic engineering promises better and more plentiful products, genetically engineered foods may encounter a few obstacles to widespread public acceptance. Some consumers, along with a few advocacy groups, have voiced concern about the safety and environmental impact of these new food products. Some urge an outright ban on any genetically engineered foods. Others support mandatory labeling that discloses the use of genetic engineering. Still others advocate more stringent testing of these products before marketing.

New Foods Safe

From the standpoint of the Food and Drug Administration, the important thing for consumers to know about these new foods is that they will be every bit as safe as the foods now on store shelves, and in some instances safer. All foods, whether traditionally bred or genetically engineered, must meet the provisions of the Federal Food, Drug, and Cosmetic Act.

To let both the public and companies know how these new foods would be regulated, FDA published a detailed statement in the May 29, 1992, *Federal Register* explaining how foods derived from new plant varieties—fruits, vegetables, grains, and their byproducts, such as vegetable oil—will be regulated under the act. The statement contains a thorough scientific discussion, complete with carefully designed flow charts, to help plant developers ensure food safety in genetically engineered products.

Present Situation

To understand how FDA will oversee the safety of these new foods, it helps to know how new foods reach supermarkets today. Each year, 10,000 to 20,000 new food products are introduced. In contrast, FDA expects only 100 to 150 genetically engineered foods to be introduced over the next five years.

Except for a handful of new "food additives" such as artificial sweeteners, which must receive premarket approval from FDA before entering the marketplace, most new foods are introduced under the "postmarket" authority of the Food, Drug, and Cosmetic Act. Under this authority, foods made up of proteins, fats and carbohydrates with a history of safe use in food can be sold once companies are satisfied the new product is safe without first getting FDA permission.

This system, which has been in place for more than 50 years, has resulted in the world's safest, most abundant, and cheapest food supply. Should a problem arise with any of these products, FDA has powerful enforcement tools that enable the agency to seize a product as soon as a safety concern is identified.

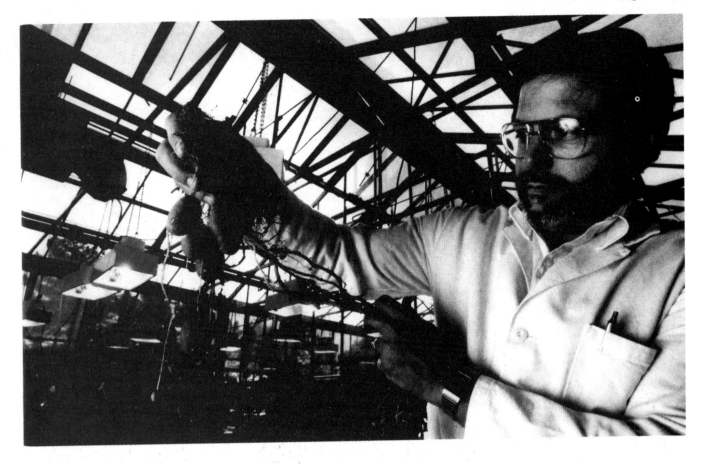

USDA microbiologist David Rockhold

harvests genetically engineered potato

tubers that will be transplanted to

Idaho fields for growing tests.

(Photos on this page and page 40

courtesy of the U.S. Department of

Agriculture)

To help assure the public that this system will work as well for genetically engineered foods as it has for the 30,000 products that can be found in the typical supermarket, FDA plans to require for the first five years that the sponsors of these products notify the agency before marketing these products. "This will ensure that FDA remains abreast of developments achieved through this rapidly evolving technology," says Jim Maryanski, Ph.D., FDA's food biotechnology coordinator.

Labeling Issues

FDA has received many inquiries asking about the labeling of genetically engineered foods. Congress has provided FDA a limited basis on which to require labeling. For FDA to require labeling there must be something tangibly different about the food that "is material with respect to consequences which may result from the use of the food."

In general, this means most genetically engineered foods will not need special labeling because they will be virtually identical to traditionally bred varieties. But there are exceptions, such as when a gene from a food that could cause an allergic reaction—peanuts, for example—is transferred into another food. In that case, FDA policy places the burden on the developer. "The food will have to be labeled so everyone will know it contains an allergen, unless the developer can show scientifically that the allergenicity has not been transferred," says Laura Tarantino, Ph.D., chief of FDA's biotechnology policy branch. "But under current methods, that would be hard to do. So this is one case where we would clearly insist on label-

ing. Fortunately, the products in front of us right now don't raise those issues."

FDA also will require labeling if a company uses genetic engineering techniques to change a food's composition significantly. For example, if a vegetable normally containing high levels of vitamin C is engineered to remove the vitamin, FDA would require labels to disclose this change.

A New Twist on an Old Idea

For the last 10 years, genetic engineering has inhabited agricultural research laboratories and only now is making its initial appearance in food stores.

Last May, the agency gave the OK to a whole food product, a slow-ripening tomato (see box). The tomato's developer, Calgene, Inc., seeking to build public understanding and confidence in the new product, decided to get FDA premarket approval for the tomato, called the Flavr Savr. Last November, FDA reviewed seven more genetically engineered foods from different companies. These products—which include three kinds of tomatoes, a squash, and a potato—did not undergo premarket

1. TRENDS TODAY AND TOMORROW

approval as did the Flavr Savr. Instead, developers used the premarket notification/postmarket authority approach that will govern the introduction of these new foods during the next five years.

FDA has also approved two genetically engineered products for use in food production—chymosin, a milk-clotting agent used to make cheese, and recombinant bovine somatotropin (rbST), a growth hormone that boosts a cow's milk yield (see "No Human Risks ..." in the May 1994 *FDA Consumer*). Several other products, especially new forms of vegetable oils, are poised for introduction. But "it'll probably be a good five years before we see genetically engineered foods really take off commercially," says Tarantino.

Though the notion of tinkering with a plant's traits is thought of as something radically new by some people, scientists have been doing it for many years in cruder, less predictable ways. For example, farmers have a long tradition of breeding desired qualities into crops. But this process took many plant generations. Researchers now can isolate a known trait from any living species—plant, animal or microbe—and incorporate it into another species. These traits are contained in genes—segments of the DNA molecules found in all living cells. The process of recombining genes bearing a chosen trait into the DNA molecules of a new host is called "recombinant DNA."

In ancient times, farmers practiced a less refined version of genetic manipulation by saving seeds from crops that proved the hardiest and most resistant to disease. By selecting which plants they would breed, these farmers "engineered" new combinations of genes, ones that would produce superior plant stock. By the 1500s, farmers were improving plants by crossing, for example, a productive crop with a wild relative resistant to disease or pests. The result was a hybrid, a new species that embodied desirable traits from both "parents."

In the mid-1800s, Austrian monk Gregor Mendel revolutionized genetic science by employing precise pollination methods and statistical analysis. Mendel's pioneering methods allowed scientists later to determine how specific

A New Tomato

The first genetically engineered whole product went on the market last May when FDA approved a tomato that can be shipped vine-ripened without rotting rapidly. The Flavr Savr is the first ready-to-eat food product available to the public that uses recombinant DNA processes. Its maker, Calgene, Inc., created the Flavr Savr on the premise that many consumers are not satisfied with most store-bought tomatoes, especially in the off-season. Surveys show that though 85 percent of U.S. households buy fresh tomatoes, some 80 percent are displeased with the quality of grocery store tomatoes.

The problem is that tomatoes need warm climates to grow, so most off-season store tomatoes must travel a long way after they are picked. To survive their journey intact, tomatoes are picked while they are still green, which is a good way to avoid bruising, but which results in a tomato that is often described as having the consistency and mouth-feel of a tennis ball.

If picked when ripe, tomatoes rot quickly. Though Calgene vine-ripens its tomatoes, the company solved the rotting problem by inserting a reversed copy—an "antisense" gene—of the DNA molecules that prompt tomato spoilage. This suppresses the enzyme that results in rotting, allowing the tomato to stay ripe, but not rot, up to 10 days—plenty of time for shipping and sale. Refrigeration is not necessary.

Though FDA policy didn't require premarket approval of the Flavr Savr tomato, Calgene sought it anyway. The company also asked FDA to approve as a new food additive the protein that produces kanamycin resistance. This marker protein allows breeders to identify early in the gene-transfer process which plant cells have successfully incorporated the new trait. Inserting the marker confers resistance to the antibi-

otic kanamycin. This is a valuable tool when trying to figure out which seeds have the new gene and which do not. But it also adds very small amounts of a new protein to diets of millions of Americans and raises concerns about issues such as antibiotic resistance.

"That was one of the scientific issues we evaluated," says Jim Maryanski, Ph.D., FDA's food biotechnology coordinator. "And we showed there really wasn't any chance the kan^r gene [marker protein] could affect the clinical effectiveness of kanamycin in people taking the drug orally."

FDA published regulations in 1994 allowing use of the kan^r gene in new plant varieties. Though not required, Calgene plans to provide point-of-sale information that describes the tomato as a genetically engineered product.

Reactions to the Flavr Savr have been largely positive, though some consumer groups have decried the product, giving it names like "Frankentomato." Others, including some restaurant chefs, have issued public criticism of all recombinant DNA-derived foods.

But industry groups are enthusiastic. Carl Feldbaum, president of the Biotechnology Industry Organization, calls the new tomato "a significant step forward for consumers in terms of the quality of the food they eat."

And Tom Stenzel, president of the United Fresh Fruit & Vegetable Association, says the genetically engineered food products now in development "will offer consumers more choices for improved quality, nutrition, and environmental benefits."

Ultimately, consumers will decide for themselves whether these new products and processes make sense. As for safety, FDA officials emphasize that these foods will be just as safe or safer than products consumers are used to finding on their store shelves.

—*J.H.*

Calgene's recipe for genetically engineered tomatoes

Ripe tomatoes contain an enzyme called PG (polygalacturonase), which causes the fruit to soften and rot. Here's what Calgene scientists did to modify this process and produce Flavr Savr:

1. Isolated and cloned the PG gene, which causes ripe tomatoes to soften and rot.

2. Reversed the PG gene sequence so that the gene is backwards (in what scientists call the "antisense orientation").

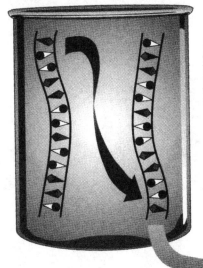

3. Put the reversed PG gene into Agrobacterium, which infects plants and is commonly used by genetic engineers to get modified or foreign genes into target cells.

Agrobacterium cell

Altered "antisense" PG gene is placed in Agrobacterium.

4. Put Agrobacteria in a petri dish with leaf pieces cut from a tomato plant. The leaves' edges absorb the Agrobacteria and antisense PG gene.

5. Antisense gene becomes part of the genetic material of the tomato plant cells.

Plant cell

9. In the genetically engineered tomato, the natural PG gene's production of the fruit-rotting PG enzyme has been repressed by the reversed gene. That gives the commercial tomato extended shelf life, allowing it to ripen more fully on the vine and still have time to get to market before it spoils.

8. Seeds are collected from the genetically engineered greenhouse tomatoes and are planted outdoors for field trials and more seed production.

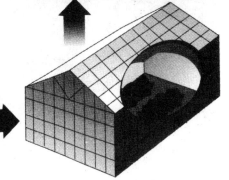

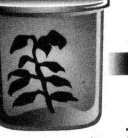

7. Plants sprout roots, are transplanted to soil, and grow to mature tomato plants.

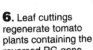

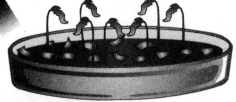

6. Leaf cuttings regenerate tomato plants containing the reversed PG gene.

Sources: Calgene Inc., Genetic Engineering of Plants, World Book Encyclopedia, © The Sacramento Bee, 1994.

FDA will require labeling if a company uses genetic engineering techniques to change a food's composition significantly.

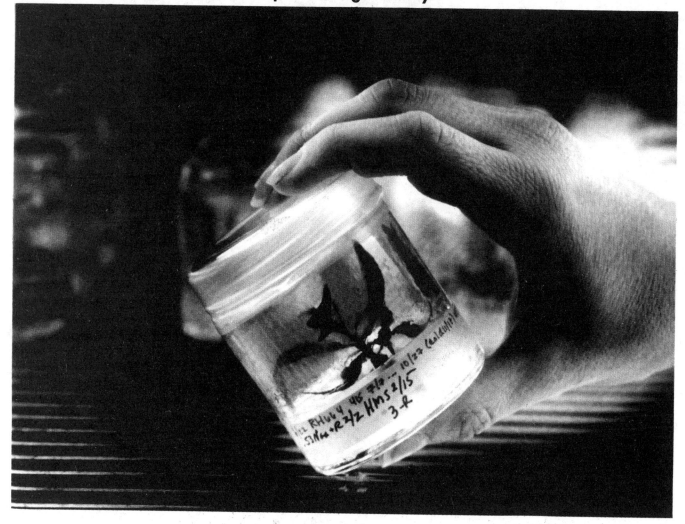

traits could be inherited into subsequent generations and to "coax" plants to swap traits they wouldn't readily exchange in nature.

Advantages and Challenges

Genetic engineering gives today's researchers considerable advantages in plant breeding programs, but it also poses new challenges. One important benefit is predictability, says Maryanski. Scientists, he says, now can identify the specific gene for a given trait, make a copy (clone) of that gene for insertion into a plant, and be certain that only the new gene is added to the plant. This eliminates the "backcrossing" traditional plant breeders must do to eliminate extraneous undesired genes that are frequently introduced when using cross-hybridization.

"The limitation," says Maryanski, "is that the scientist must be able to identify the gene for a desired trait. For example, if you wanted to improve the yield of a food crop, that trait may be encoded by several genes. Such an improvement would be very difficult to achieve at this stage of the technology." Thus, he adds, crop improvement through recombinant DNA techniques is restricted to traits for which scientists can identify the appropriate genes.

Another advantage of new methods is a significant acceleration of the development timetable. "Conventional breeders may find a plant with the traits they want," says Maryanski, "but it will likely have many other unwanted genes that come along with the desired genes. So they spend literally years trying to remove the undesirable traits and still

A jar holds the beginnings of a disease-resistant peach tree genetically engineered by U.S. Department of Agriculture researchers.

maintain those they wanted in the first place." Traditional techniques typically take 12 or more years to create a new strain, compared to about five years using recombinant DNA procedures. Despite the speed advantage, the newer methods are "not just a quick afternoon in the laboratory," Maryanski says. "There are a lot of tricks used that actually get the new plant cells to grow."

Plant breeders do not use recombinant DNA techniques exclusively. Instead, they use a combination of new and traditional methods to provide a plant with quality, yield, weather and pest resistance, and other desirable traits. For example, "the gene insertion doesn't always 'take'—that is, the gene might not stay there," Maryanski says. So recombinant DNA researchers still have to pass plants through several generations using conventional methods to ensure the desired trait truly has been incorporated, a process called stabilization.

Power Concerns Some

Another difference with recombinant DNA, which can be a benefit but which concerns some, is the "power" of genetic engineering—the ability to transfer genes from a wide variety of species. Because the chemical makeup of DNA is similar in all living things, desirable genes from any organism can be inserted into a plant species. This provides the developer with a much larger selection of valuable traits. For example, one developer has experimented with using a gene isolated from a fish, the winter flounder, to impart freeze resistance into a variety of tomato. Such research is prompting concerns among some consumers, especially vegetarians and members of certain religious groups. They wonder if the process of inserting an animal gene into a plant somehow creates a vegetable that is part animal and should be labeled.

Maryanski says most scientists don't believe this is possible because only a copy but no original material from the animal is used. "Also," he says, "you can't really confer animal life characteristics on a plant because you're only transferring one gene for a very specific trait." He acknowledges, however, that though no plant products using animal-derived genes are planned for marketing in the near future, the animal gene issue is a weighty one that deserves "considerable discussion" within the scientific community and the general public.

Public Acceptance

Whether genetically engineered foods succeed or fail ultimately depends on public acceptance. Early reports on the Flavr Savr tomato, the first recombinant DNA-derived whole food product to reach grocery shelves, are favorable. Calgene says sales in the product's first two markets—California and Illinois—are "a total success." Calgene chairman Roger Salquist says consumers "are responding with purchases and praise."

In contrast, some consumer groups have criticized the Calgene product, demanding greater FDA scrutiny of genetically engineered foods or an outright ban on all of them. Their reasons range from safety fears to ethics. One group, the Environmental Defense Fund, says, "Consumption of some of these novel foods might present new hazards. [Some genetically engineered] compounds are new food ingredients and clearly should be evaluated for their safety."

FDA scientists and others in the field blame some negative consumer reaction on the recombinant DNA technique's complexity. The technology is difficult to understand, so there is a fear of the unknown. Genetic engineering "simply sounds scary," says Maryanski. "People call FDA and say, 'We don't want anyone tinkering with our food.' Then we remind them that there's hardly a food in the grocery store that hasn't been extensively tinkered with."

He illustrates this by comparing today's foods with those in the last century. "Take corn. Those nice, juicy ears of corn we have—they didn't exist. Some kinds of corn had a hard outer shell on the kernel that you couldn't eat until it was made into flour. And the kiwi was developed from a hard little berry. We only have our present-day kiwi—and our corn and wheat and hundreds of other foods—because of extensive plant breeding."

Genetically altered states

In 1994, when the Food and Drug Administration approved the sale of the Flavr Savr tomato—the first genetically engineered food—it opened a virtual Pandora's box of controversy and fear. Consumer resistance to the concept of genetic engineering, dubbed "biotechnophobia," quickly led to boycotts and other forms of public outcry.

Now the issue is back in the spotlight with the release of a pivotal study that documents for the first time what many scientists and consumer groups have suspected all along: it's possible to pass an allergy-provoking gene from one food to another. An Iowa-based company, Pioneer Hi-Bred International, took a gene from Brazil nuts and added it to soybeans to boost the beans' nutritional profile. Soybeans, often used as animal feed, lack a certain protein component required for animal growth. But adding the Brazil-nut gene would enable farmers to grow soybeans that contained it.

The hitch is that Brazil nuts commonly cause allergic reactions in people. To determine whether transferring the nut gene to the soybeans gave the new beans the same allergy-provoking potential, the Iowa company asked scientists at the University of Nebraska to test the soybeans.

In a series of experiments, the researchers mixed blood samples from people allergic to Brazil nuts with protein extracts from the genetically engineered soybeans. Overall, the blood samples "reacted" the same way to Brazil nuts and the new soybeans. Extracts from regular soybeans, on the other hand, did not prompt any signs of allergic response, leading the researchers to conclude that the allergen in the Brazil nuts was in fact transferred to the genetically altered beans. Skin-prick testing conducted on people with Brazil nut allergies confirmed the findings: that is, people allergic to Brazil nuts reacted to extracts from the new soybeans but not to regular beans.

According to protocol

"I view our study as good news," says Steve Taylor,

PhD, one of the University of Nebraska scientists who conducted the research. "Pioneer recognized its responsibility and did something about it."

Indeed, the company did more than it was required to do. Currently, the Food and Drug Administration protocol requires that companies notify the government if a gene from a food that commonly causes allergies is likely to be transferred to another food and then test the new food for allergens. If the tests show that an allergen has indeed been transferred, the company must consult with the FDA to determine, for instance, whether the food must carry a warning label.

In the case of the soybeans, not only did Pioneer carry out the necessary tests to see whether its new soybeans contained allergens, it also decided not to sell them. Even though the beans were designed for use in animal feed, the company did not want to risk accidentally mixing them with regular soybeans. If the new beans inadvertently got into the human food supply, they could potentially cause life-threatening allergic reactions.

Still, some experts believe that the findings highlight the need for stricter federal regulation of genetically engineered foods. What worries them is that the FDA protocol applies only to situations in which companies are dealing with foods *known* to provoke allergies. "The policy doesn't cover anything that isn't a known allergen," notes Marion Nestle, PhD, MPH, of New York University, who wrote an editorial accompanying the study in *The New England Journal of Medicine*.

But Dr. Taylor notes that the chances of developing an allergy-causing food using genes from foods not known to be allergenic are remote. Furthermore, he adds that the great majority of companies shy away from experimenting with genes from foods with known allergens. Why? They don't want to risk running into the same problems and costs that Pioneer encountered.

Alcohol: Spirit of health?

A little alcohol can be good for some people. Is it good for you?

Three years ago, we described the research showing that moderate drinking can protect the heart and help people live longer. Since then, researchers have uncovered evidence of a possibly major benefit: a reduced risk of diabetes. In its new Dietary Guidelines for Americans, released this January, the U.S. Government for the first time acknowledged the potential health benefits of alcohol.

But there's more to the story. New studies indicate that moderate drinking may raise the risk of breast cancer significantly more than previously believed. For that and other reasons, researchers are abandoning their blanket endorsement of moderate drinking; instead they're specifying who stands to gain—and who may actually be harmed.

How alcohol helps

Several large studies, involving a total of more than 600,000 people and lasting up to 12 years, have shown that people who drink moderately—no more than one drink a day for women, two for men—have 20 to 40 percent less risk of developing coronary disease than nondrinkers do. That reduction in risk is comparable to what you might gain from a strict low-fat diet.

Moderate drinking seems to protect the heart in three ways:

■ It boosts HDL. Studies have consistently shown that blood levels of HDL cholesterol (the "good" kind) are 10 to 15 percent higher in moderate drinkers than in nondrinkers. And several intervention trials have confirmed that drinking does raise HDL levels.

■ It inhibits potentially dangerous blood clots. As a result, the risk of heart attack drops significantly in the 24 hours after you take a drink.

■ It may increase the body's response to the hormone insulin. That can lead to decreased secretion of insulin. And lower insulin levels may be good for the heart, since insulin lowers HDL levels and increases both blood pressure and triglycerides, a fat that may raise coronary risk.

An improved insulin response also tends to lower blood-sugar levels. That may explain the latest apparent benefit of alcohol: a reduced risk of developing diabetes. Three large, lengthy studies, two of them published last year, have found that moderate drinkers are less likely to develop the disease than nondrinkers are.

Finally, the anti-clotting effect of moderate drinking increases the risk of hemorrhagic stroke, caused by bleeding in the brain; but it reduces the risk of thrombotic stroke, the more common though less deadly kind, caused by blood clots. The net result: a slight drop in the overall risk of having a stroke, though not of dying from one.

The sobering news

Until recently, research suggested that moderate drinking might marginally increase a woman's risk of breast cancer, by perhaps 10 percent. But two careful studies published last year have caused greater concern. One, a report on some 60,000 Dutch women, found that those who had just one drink a day faced a 30 percent increase in breast-cancer risk. The other, a study that compared some 6600 breast-cancer patients with 9200 other women, linked a single daily drink with a 40 percent increase and two drinks with a 70 percent increase. One possible explanation: Alcohol may boost blood levels of estrogen, which helps fuel the growth of breast cancer.

Other potential risks of moderate drinking include:

■ **Accidents.** A single drink in the average woman or two in the average man can disrupt coordination, cloud judgment, and weaken inhibitions. As a result, the risk of dying from accidents or violence is up to 40 percent higher in moderate drinkers than in abstainers.

■ **Other cancers.** Some research suggests that moderate drinking may slightly increase the likelihood of cancer in regions exposed to high concentrations of alcohol, including the mouth, throat, larynx, esophagus, and liver.

■ **Cirrhosis of the liver.** Several studies have found that moderate drinkers are more likely to die of cirrhosis, or irreversible liver damage, than non-

> ## Alcohol's impact on health depends partly on your gender. But the most important factor is age.

drinkers are. But it's not clear whether those findings are accurate, since cirrhosis patients often misrepresent how much they actually drink.

Longer lives—for some

In theory, the ability of moderate drinking to help prevent coronary disease and possibly diabetes should outweigh the risks. And indeed, the overall death rate is roughly 10 percent lower in moderate drinkers than in nondrinkers.

But that doesn't mean all Americans should start stocking their medicine cabinet with spirits. For one thing, that 10 percent reduction comes from studies

that looked mainly at people who have been drinking for some time. So it minimizes another potentially major risk: that new drinkers won't be able to keep their drinking moderate.

Immoderate drinking can harm rather than protect the heart, by raising blood pressure, weakening the heart muscle, and triggering abnormal cardiac rhythms. Excessive drinking increases the risk of breast cancer even more than moderate drinking does, and it clearly increases the chance of liver damage and of digestive-tract cancers. It can inflame the pancreas and the stomach lining, and increase susceptibility to osteoporosis. And it's the leading cause of deadly mishaps and mayhem.

Equally important, that 10 percent lower death rate is an overall average. That average obscures the fact that moderate drinking may have strikingly different effects in different groups of people.

Alcohol and age

The impact of alcohol on your health depends partly on whether you're a man or a woman. But the most important factor is how old you are.

Younger people. Accidents kill more men under age 40 than heart attacks and diabetes combined; accidents plus breast cancer similarly kill more women under age 50 than heart attacks and diabetes. So the increased risk of accidents and breast cancer due to moderate drinking should nullify or outweigh the reduction in the risk of coronary disease and possibly diabetes in those age groups. One other drawback of such drinking: The earlier you start, the greater your risk both of starting to drink heavily and of eventually developing an alcohol-related disease.

In a 12-year prospective study of 86,000 nurses, Harvard researchers found that women in their 30s who drank moderately died at a *faster* rate than those

---

What'll it be?

Five years ago, sales of red wine surged after Morley Safer announced on 60 Minutes that drinking the beverage protected the heart. Late last year, Safer touted wine again on 60 Minutes, citing a recent Danish study. Wine sales surged again—but wine's scientific stock remains flat.

Red wine and, to a lesser extent, white wine do contain flavonoids, which in theory may help protect the heart in two ways: They fight blood clots and they inhibit oxidation, chemical damage that may promote clogged arteries. In addition, red wine contains resveratrol, which also inhibits clotting. At least eight studies have found that either wine in general or red wine in particular cuts coronary risk or total mortality better than other alcoholic beverages.

But just as many studies have supported liquor or beer. In a recent review of the evidence, Harvard researchers concluded that no particular alcoholic beverage is any better for your health than the others. How you drink, they said, is far more important than what you drink.

The researchers noted that the seemingly superior drink

in many studies was simply the one that people typically drank at mealtime—such as wine in France, beer in Hawaii, or cocktails in mainland America. Further, an Italian study on moderate drinkers linked wine with reduced risk only in those who drank while they ate.

Here are some possible reasons why alcohol may be safer or more healthful when it's consumed with food:

■ People who drink with meals typically consume less alcohol at one sitting than other drinkers do. So they're less likely to get drunk and have accidents. And food slows the absorption of alcohol, reducing that risk even more.

■ Drinking with meals—as opposed to just on social occasions—puts a little alcohol in your blood a lot of the time; that may maximize the benefit, much as time-release capsules maximize the effect of some medications.

■ Drinking with meals may provide the alcohol just when you need its anti-clotting ability the most. That's because the digested fat pouring into the blood after you eat makes it stickier and more likely to clot.

who didn't drink at all. Those in their 40s who drank moderately died at the same rate as the nondrinkers did. While there are no corresponding analyses for younger men, researchers anticipate similar trends.

> # Most middle-aged and older people who drink moderately can relax and enjoy the habit.

▶ *Recommendation:* If you do drink, keep it light. That means a maximum of three drinks a week for premenopausal women, one drink a day for men under 40. (There are at least two reasons for the lower limit in women: They have a far greater breast-cancer risk, of course; and they typically have a smaller volume of fluids in their body to dilute the alcohol and less of the stomach enzyme that breaks the alcohol down.)

Older people. The risk of heart attack rises steadily after menopause in women and after age 40 in men, soon outstripping all the possible risks of moderate drinking. In the Harvard study, the nurses over age 50 who drank moderately had a 12 to 20 percent lower death rate than the nondrinkers did. In theory, moderate drinking should save even more lives in older men than in older women, given a man's generally higher coronary risk and much lower breast-cancer risk.

▶ *Recommendation:* Most middle-aged and older people who drink moderately can relax and enjoy the habit. Moderate drinking means no more than one drink a day if you're a woman, two if you're a man, until your mid-60s or so. After that, gradually reduce the size of your drinks, since the body can no longer handle as much alcohol as before, increasing the chance of accidents, confusion, and insomnia.

Safe to start?

Some older people, particularly those who face an increased risk for coronary heart disease, may wonder if they should start having, say, a glass of wine with dinner to help protect their heart—even if they don't really like the taste of alcoholic beverages. That decision should be made only after discussing the pros and cons thoroughly with your doctor. Don't even think about starting to drink—or even continuing to drink moderately—if you have a family history of alcoholism or depression; a personal history

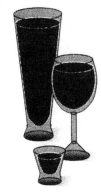

A drink's a drink
One "drink" equals:
- 12 oz. of beer.
- 5 oz. of wine.
- 1½ oz. of 80-proof liquor.

of anxiety, depression, or dependency on a medication or illicit drugs; or the slightest doubt about your own self-control.

Several medical factors can also make even moderate drinking potentially unsafe. Avoid alcohol or at least minimize your intake:

- If you have liver disease, abnormal heart rhythms, a previous hemorrhagic stroke, peptic ulcers, gout, pancreatitis, or high triglyceride levels.

- If you have either chronic insomnia or sleep apnea (spasmodic breathing during sleep).

- If you take certain medications. Alcohol can make certain common drugs dangerous, including antihistamines, aspirin or other nonsteroidal anti-inflammatory drugs such as ibuprofen (*Advil*) or diclofenac (*Voltaren*), nitrates (*ISMO, Nitrostat*), certain painkillers, sleeping pills, and tranquilizers. And alcohol can reduce the effectiveness of other drugs, including anticonvulsants and beta-blockers such as propranolol (*Inderal*) or metoprolol (*Lopressor*).

- If you may be pregnant, or are breast feeding. Some studies suggest that having as little as one drink a day during pregnancy may increase the chance of miscarriage, slightly low birth weight, cognitive and behavioral problems, or minor physical defects. In addition, one study found that breast-fed children of women who drank moderately had poorer motor development than the children of nondrinkers. While none of that evidence is conclusive, it's best to play it safe and avoid alcohol if you're either pregnant or breast feeding.

Of course, you should never drink before driving, boating, operating machinery, or doing anything else that requires good coordination and sharp reflexes.

Summing up

On average, moderate drinking reduces the overall death rate by about 10 percent. But middle-aged and older people may benefit more than that, while younger people may not benefit at all, or may even be harmed. Here's our advice:

- **Women:** Have no more than three drinks a week if you're premenopausal, one drink a day if you're postmenopausal. And don't drink at all if you're pregnant or breast feeding.

- **Men:** Have no more than one drink a day if you're under age 40, two a day if you're over 40.

- **For maximum benefit and minimum risk, drink mainly with meals** (see box, "What'll it be?").

- Don't start to drink for your health's sake unless you've discussed the pros and cons thoroughly with your doctor—and don't start at all if you have any susceptibility to alcoholism.

- Avoid alcohol if you take certain medications, have trouble sleeping, or have liver disease, certain heart problems, or any other medical reason for not drinking. And never drink before driving.

Nutrients

> One cannot think well, love well, sleep well, if one has not dined well.
>
> —Virginia Woolf

Some basic aspects of nutrition have remained relatively unchanged for many years. The list of nutrients is one of these. Even the specific vitamins and minerals have undergone little revision. Nutrients that provide energy are still identified as carbohydrates, lipids, and proteins. Fiber is not a nutrient because it is not essential to life, but it is included in this unit because it clearly performs a significant role in maintaining normal physiological functioning.

Significant concepts about each nutrient, however, have changed, often dramatically. With today's available technology, the turnover in data from nutrition studies is so rapid that information may become obsolete even before it is printed and certainly before it is accepted or acted upon. Nor does the availability of voluminous data mean that theories are proven. Studies and experiments must be replicated, subjected to peer review, refined, and tried again. Conflicts in data, a common occurrence, must be resolved before any actionable conclusions can be reached. And, while epidemiological evidence may indicate a relationship, that does not prove cause and effect. Years may pass and numerous other studies be concluded before any firm recommendations for either normal or therapeutic diets can be supported. Outside the scientific community this is frequently misunderstood, and sometimes every media report is taken as a new breakthrough.

Compounding the problem of formulating recommendations is the fact that differences among human beings are truly remarkable; an average human being simply does not exist. Physiological variations preclude accurate predictions of exact nutrient amounts that cause the negative effects of either deficiency or excess. It is the task of the National Academy of Sciences to establish recommendations that more than cover most people's actual requirements but are not high enough to cause harm. The result is the periodically revised Recommended Dietary Allowances (RDAs). The current 1989 edition is under review and is certain to undergo changes. Available new evidence regarding nutrient need and performance is being seriously considered. Some of the discussion centers upon evidence that higher than RDA amounts of vitamins may have prophylactic effects that minimize chronic diseases and that exceed the traditional roles of preventing deficiencies. Dr. A. E. Harper, of national renown, rebuts this approach: "The . . . critical question is: Are the effects observed physiologic/nutritional or pharmacologic?"

The articles in this unit were selected because they reflect up-to-date thinking about a variety of nutrients that are currently newsworthy or about which we frequently have questions and/or misconceptions. The first article on protein is a good example. Few of us in the United States get too little protein. Even vegetarians, it seems, can easily eat ample amounts that include all of the essential amino acids. Yet many of us grew up with the notion that more protein is always desirable and definitely necessary to increase muscle mass. Experts tell us this isn't so, that too much protein can even be harmful, and that substituting high-carbohydrate foods would often be more beneficial.

Mythology also still abounds regarding the inherent dangers and values of sugar, according to "What's Wrong with Sugar?" Often people are convinced, or at least they suspect, that sugar causes many serious problems, especially hyperactivity, juvenile delinquency, and crime. To date, sugar has been convicted only of causing dental caries. Furthermore, sugar is sugar, whether in the sugar bowl or in fruit juice.

Fats, of course, are another matter. The role of lipids in promoting disease, especially the saturated lipids found in animal products and tropical oils, is quite well established. Still, exact predictions cannot be made regarding individual reactions and tolerances to fat. "The Facts about Fats" discusses the relationship of fat to health (also see related articles in unit 1). Current guidelines set one's fat budget at no more than 30 percent of total calories, although the average intake is closer to 34 percent, according to the National Health and Nutrition Examination Survey (NHANES III) study. Americans are, however, *very* conscious of fat in food and eagerly look for new products with low-fat and no-fat claims. The food industry, eager to exploit marketing opportunities, has responded with hundreds of new products yearly. The single-minded consumer, however, sometimes neglects to note that many of the lower fat items actually have equal or more calories. Nor has America's taste declined for super-premium ice creams and other rich desserts, often to the tune of well over half the kilocalories from fat.

There follows a series of five articles on vitamins, an indication both of the amount of current research and the degree of public interest. The article by Paul Thomas is very significant because it addresses the fallacious philosophical mindset that some of us have regarding vitamins. No doubt vitamins seemed to present "miraculous cures" when they were first discovered as the key to terrible diseases such as pellagra, scurvy, and beri-beri. But vitamins are workhorses, not magic bullets, which go about their everyday jobs of making the body operate smoothly. In large doses they will have pharmacological effects, some of which may be beneficial, but often they are harmful as well. For many reasons, food sources rather than supplement sources are a better choice.

The Vitamin A form found in most supplements, fortified products, and animal foods is an obvious example of the risks associated with excesses. In this case, risks include significantly increased chances of producing a baby with such defects as cleft palate and heart abnormalities. A plant form of Vitamin A, beta-carotene, was originally thought to be protective as an antioxidant against cancer and heart disease. Research trials have been stopped due to evidence that high intakes might actually be *causing* death and cancer rates to increase. Vitamin E research, likewise, has shown some promise in protecting against cardiovascular disease, but significant concerns regarding safety and benefits are evident as well. Where does the truth lie? Nobody yet knows, but the evidence is generally much stronger for the consumption of foods high in antioxidants rather than for supplements. Certainly current knowledge provides strong support for consuming a variety of foods and *at least* the recommended five daily fruit/vegetable servings, something only 10 percent of the U.S. population apparently accomplishes.

Vitamin C, ascorbic acid, is a vitamin that has been newsworthy since the days when Linus Pauling first proclaimed that humans should consume more than three grams daily rather than the mere 60 mg suggested in the RDA table. The article on Vitamin C by Jane Brody should be read for its current discussion on this controversial topic. It is certainly not clear that greater than currently recommended intakes are desirable and advisable for most people. On the other hand, fortification of grain products with folic acid has been mandated by the FDA. Clear evidence that there is a connection between a lack of folic acid and neural tube defects is a good public health reason to ensure that women of childbearing age have adequate intakes at the point of conception.

Whether or not one should take supplementary iron is the topic in "Iron Overkill." On the one hand, we are told that a high iron level in the body may increase heart attack risks because it boosts the action of free radicals. These reports have been generally refuted. On the other hand, there is evidence that women of childbearing age and others have low or nonexistent iron stores. To complicate the picture, there are as many as a million Americans with hemochromatosis, a genetic condition that allows the absorption of too much iron. Once again, we find different responses based on different physiologies.

Evidence that dietary fiber does, indeed, offer disease protection can be supported by a substantial body of research, although few Americans get the recommended amounts. "Fiber" summarizes these findings and offers advice about how to get more in one's diet. Eating more fruits, vegetables, and whole grains is the key.

Much as we would like them, there are few absolutes in the science of nutrition. Perhaps there never will be, for nutrition is an applied rather than a pure science. The present decades are a period of great discovery. For those who marvel at the continued unfolding of the mysteries of human physiology, this is both a confusing and a tremendously exciting era in which to live.

Looking Ahead: Challenge Questions

Are some nutrients more important than others in maintaining health? Support your answer.

What claims are made for vitamins that you know to be false?

Determine the amount of protein you need and the amount you actually get each day. Based on the information in the article on protein, should you make changes? What are they?

How should one decide whether or not to take supplements? Are the issues involving supplements of a single vitamin or mineral any different than for multivitamins?

Should fiber be designated a nutrient? Why or why not?

Determine the percentage of your average daily calories that is contributed by total fat and saturated fat. What did your calculation tell you?

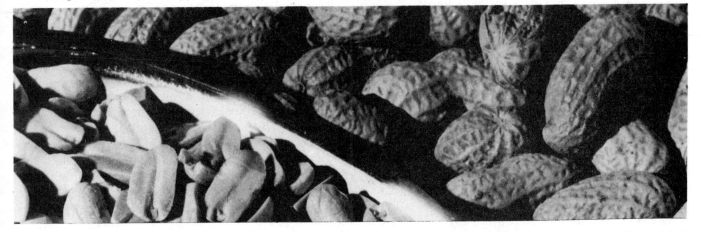

Should you be eating more protein—or less?

Americans have had a love/hate relationship with protein, and the protein pendulum has been swinging like crazy lately. Many of us grew up thinking only good things about protein. Indeed, we can't live without it. But the trouble may be too much of a good thing. Indeed, some researchers have linked a high intake of animal protein to heart disease and other chronic disorders. On the other hand, high-protein weight-loss diets are the craze once again, as they were in the late sixties and early seventies (see box). If all this increasingly contradictory advice about protein makes your head spin, here's the lowdown.

What's the problem with eating lots of protein?

A diet high in protein—especially animal protein—is associated with an increased risk not only of heart disease and some cancers (such as colon and prostate), but also of osteoporosis and kidney damage. *However, it's hard to prove this link, since we seldom eat pure protein.* People who eat lots of animal protein do have higher rates of heart disease and cancers, but their diets also tend to be high in fat and low in antioxidants and fiber, as well as other potentially beneficial substances. Moreover, those who eat lots of animal protein may also be less health-conscious in general and less physically active than others. It may be such factors, rather than protein intake itself, that account for most of the increased risks.

Is protein from plants more healthful?

In carefully controlled studies, animals fed large amounts of isolated animal protein develop higher levels of blood cholesterol (especially LDL, the "bad" kind) than those fed vegetable protein. This suggests that something about the composition of animal protein boosts cholesterol.

People who get their protein from plants have a lower risk of heart disease and are healthier in general. Last year, for instance, a widely publicized analysis of the benefits of soy protein suggested that it helps lower blood cholesterol and is thus good for the heart (though other compounds in soy may be largely responsible, see *Wellness Letter,* November 1995). Vegetarian sources of protein are also preferable because they're usually low in fat and high in fiber and other potentially beneficial sub-

stances. Nevertheless, a few studies have suggested that a very high intake of even plant protein is undesirable, but it's rare for vegetarians to consume such large amounts of protein.

Don't vegetarians have trouble getting enough protein?

Vegetarian diets generally supply more than enough protein. Many grains, legumes, nuts, and seeds are good sources of protein. However, except for soybeans, plant foods contain protein that's incomplete—that is, it has low and sometimes insufficient amounts of one or more of the nine essential amino acids. (Amino acids are protein's building blocks; the essential ones are those the body can't synthesize.) But if vegetarians eat a wide variety of foods each day, they're likely to absorb a full complement of amino acids. They don't need to eat the complementary proteins at the same meal.

What's the link between protein and osteoporosis?

As your protein intake rises, so does the amount of calcium excreted in urine. If you eat lots of protein, this calcium loss may affect the density of your bones and thus may hasten the development of osteoporosis (bone thinning). This notion is still controversial, but was recently bolstered by a 12-year Harvard study of 86,000 nurses. In it, women who ate lots of animal protein (more than 95 grams a day), especially red meat, had 22% more forearm fractures than those consuming less protein. However, the study didn't actually measure the degree of osteoporosis in the women. In addition, it's likely that a high protein intake endangers your bones only if you consume inadequate amounts of calcium. Thus you should continue to consume milk and other dairy products.

If you exercise a lot, don't you need more protein?

Yes and no. You need adequate protein intake to build and repair muscles, but most active Americans, including vegetarians, get more than enough of it. In the old days, in their quest for added protein, athletes were likely to wolf down T-bone steaks or raw eggs. Today they often turn to high-protein powders, drinks, tablets, capsules, and bars. This is unnecessary. Recent studies do suggest that some endurance athletes or serious weight lifters need more protein than the Recommended Dietary Allowance

Reprinted with permission from *University of California at Berkeley Wellness Letter,* June 1996, pp. 4-5. © 1996 by Health Letter Associates.

(RDA, see below), but because of their greater food intake, they get the extra protein with little trouble. Protein supplements or isolated amino acids won't stimulate muscle growth—only exercise, specifically strength training, does. Excess protein is simply broken down in the body and burned for energy or turned into fat. Strength training, like any exercise, requires extra calories, but the bulk of these should come from complex carbohydrates (starches).

What about the elderly?

This is one group that may have a protein shortfall. Several studies have found that the elderly need a little more protein than the RDA, since the body uses protein less efficiently as it ages. Meanwhile about one-quarter of elderly women actually consume less than the RDA, particularly since they tend to eat less food. This shortfall may compromise their health. If you're over 65, keep an eye on your protein intake.

How much protein do you need?

Proteins are constantly being broken down in our bodies. Most of the amino acids are reused, but we must regularly replace those that are lost.

The daily RDA for protein is the amount the average person needs to stay healthy. It's based on age and weight, and usually works out to about 8% of daily calories—that's fairly little, about as much as is consumed in China. The RDA for adults is 0.8 grams of protein for each kilogram (2.2 pounds) of body weight. That adds up to 64 grams (about 2 ounces) of pure protein for a 175-pound man, and 47 grams for a 130-pound woman. To estimate *your* protein requirement, determine your weight in

---

Do you *really* want to lose weight on a high-protein diet?

High-protein, low-carbohydrate (and usually high-fat) diets are back, and with a vengeance. Newspapers, books, and TV shows are offering testimonials from "carbohydrate dropouts" who swear by them. The fact is, there are basically only a handful of crash diets, and this type pops up every decade or two.

The protein craze has been making headlines because of the growing distrust of "established" nutritional wisdom, and specifically a backlash against high-carbohydrate diets. The protein-diet advocates are now blaming the rise in obesity in this country on excessive carbohydrate intake, which they claim causes insulin resistance and thus weight gain in millions. As we reported in May 1995 in our article on the "pasta scare," this argument doesn't hold water. There's no evidence that carbohydrates, especially complex carbohydrates (starches), stimulate appetite and/or lead to more or easier fat storage and weight gain. And if you do cut down on complex carbohydrates such as grains and vegetables, what are your alternatives? Certainly not more fat: the dangers of a high-fat diet are clear. And not more protein: excessive protein intake carries potential health risks, from kidney damage to osteoporosis, as described above.

Carbo bashers, protein pushers

Among the recent protein-diet books are *Protein Power* by Drs. Michael and Mary Eades, *The Carbohydrate Addict's Diet* by Drs. Rachael and Richard Heller, and *The Zone* by Dr. Barry Sears. The most extreme of these diets is Dr. Robert Atkins's *New Diet Revolution,* a rehash of his 1972 book. It claims that a high-protein, high-fat, low-carbohydrate diet not only promotes weight loss, but also reduces cholesterol and blood pressure and lowers the risk of heart disease and cancer.

On the Atkins diet, you get bacon and eggs for breakfast, but no bread, cereal, or orange juice. Lunch may be a bunless bacon cheeseburger with a small salad. You do without bread, rice, pasta, vegetables, and fruit, eating virtually nothing but protein and fat. Dr. Atkins's plan, like all these diets, is actually a low-calorie diet in disguise. He doesn't specify quantities, but there's not much food in the weight-loss phase of the diet, certainly not enough to supply the vitamins and minerals you need (Atkins recommends pills, preferably the "formulas" he

sells). Cut calories and you lose weight—surprise, surprise.

Your body will indeed begin to burn its own fat on this regimen. Actually, you burn fat all the time, but without carbohydrates your body does not burn the fat completely, and thus substances called ketones are formed and released into your bloodstream. At first, this condition, known as ketosis, may make dieting easier, because it often kills the appetite and even causes nausea. Dr. Atkins and the other protein promoters consider this state "normal" and even "benign." Ketosis is indeed the body's normal way to adapt to this abnormal situation, as it would to fasting. However, ketosis will eventually increase blood levels of uric acid—a risk factor for gout and kidney stones in susceptible people. But before that, if you consume inadequate amounts of carbohydrates, other adverse effects can also occur—weakness, diarrhea, dizziness, headaches, to name just a few. No wonder you lose weight.

What about all the diet doctors' "evidence"?

Their evidence is almost all anecdotal. There are no controlled studies showing that high-protein diets are more effective than any other low-calorie diets. Several of the doctors talk a great deal about eicosanoids, hormone-like substances that control countless physiological functions. They claim that a high carbohydrate intake, by boosting insulin levels, produces a dangerous balance of eicosanoids. However, these compounds are still little understood, and diet (except perhaps for certain fats, such as fish oil) probably has only a minor effect on them.

A diet rich in complex carbohydrates remains the best. Fruits, grains, and vegetables, along with low-fat dairy products and small amounts of meats, provide the vitamins, minerals, and fiber you need. Numerous controlled studies have shown that such a diet helps protect against heart disease, diabetes, and various cancers, as well as aiding in weight control. And it's *not* a crash diet, but a way of eating for the rest of your life.

Words to the wise: In the short term, you could lose weight on these high-protein diets, but they could be dangerous, particularly if followed beyond a few weeks. Like all crash diets, they don't work over the long haul. Quick weight loss is easy—keeping the weight off is the hard part.

kilograms by dividing your weight in pounds by 2.2. Then multiply the result by 0.8. For example, a 150-pound person would require $(150 \div 2.2) \times 0.8 = 55$ grams. If you are overweight, you may need less than your result.

Where do those grams of protein come from?

Leading sources of protein are:

■ Meat, chicken, and fish: 6 to 8 grams per ounce.
■ Dairy products: a cup of milk, 8 grams; yogurt, 10 to 13.
■ Eggs: 6 grams each.
■ Grains: 1 slice of bread or half cup of pasta, 3 grams.
■ Beans: 7 grams per half cup (cooked).
■ Nuts: 6 grams per ounce.

Grain products are often overlooked as protein sources—they supply 16 to 20% of the total protein intake in the U.S. Even vegetables contain some protein, albeit smaller amounts (a half cup of broccoli or asparagus has 2 grams).

As you can see, it's hard *not* to get the RDA. For most people, three ounces of lean meat, half a cup of beans, and a cup each of pasta, yogurt, and milk supply more than enough protein for a day. The RDA assumes that you eat a mixed diet of proteins— some from animal sources (high-quality because it offers a complete mix of essential amino acids), some from plant sources (mostly incomplete). Children under 18, along with pregnant or lactating women, need a little more protein per pound of body weight than others.

How much is too much?

Government surveys show that the *average* American man under age 65 consumes 90 to 110 grams of protein per day, and the average woman, 65 to 70 grams—about 50% more than the RDA. There's no evidence that such levels endanger your health, provided the protein isn't accompanied by lots of fat. However, many Americans consume much more than that. A one-pound steak, not unusual fare in restaurants, can supply 100 grams of protein by itself.

The "upper bound" for protein is twice the RDA, according to the National Research Council. Consuming more than that, over the long term, increases the risk of chronic disease and is definitely not recommended. If you eat more than 120 grams of protein a day, cut back. *Most important, try to get more of your protein from plants than from animals.* That way you're likely to get less fat and cholesterol and more of the good things found in grains, beans, and vegetables.

WHAT'S WRONG WITH SUGAR?

Sugar's reputation as a health heavy is much overblown.

Over the years, sugar has been blamed for ills ranging from obesity to hyperactivity—even psychotic rage. Fear of sugar has created an industry devoted to sugar substitutes and has turned *Cokes* into guilt trips. A look at the facts may help put sugar into a more realistic health perspective.

Weight gain: Thin evidence

Sugar is not nutritious. It contributes only "empty" calories to the diet. And those calories can add up. If you drank three 12-ounce cans (160 calories each) of sugar-sweetened soda a day and otherwise maintained your usual diet and exercise habits, you could gain about a pound a week. The desire to avoid extra calories has fed the demand for artificial sweeteners (see box, next page).

But sugar is not the only caloric culprit or even the main one in most sweets. Fat shares the blame. A chocolate eclair, for example, gets 133 calories from fat and only 55 from sugar. Even a chocolate candy bar gets more calories from fat (122) than from sugar (92). And the calories in a cup of vanilla ice cream are just about evenly divided between the two (roughly 130 calories apiece).

Indeed, many overweight people suffer less from a "sweet tooth" than from a "fat tooth." Observational studies have found that overweight people actually eat *less* sugar than thin people—but more dietary fat.

Hyperactivity: No defense

For years, parents and teachers have observed that children "bounce off the walls" after eating sweets. That observation has led to the belief that sugar causes hyperactivity. In adults, the same logic has been taken to its extreme with the now infamous "*Twinkie* defense"—the contention that certain murderers were driven to their violent behavior by sugary junk food. Numerous studies have discredited those notions.

Earlier this year, researchers published in The New England Journal of Medicine the strongest case yet against the alleged link to hyperactivity—findings that were described as "resoundingly negative" by an accompanying editorial. The study involved some 50 children, ages 3 to 10, half of them believed by their parents to be sensitive to sugar. For one week the children and their families ate specially prepared meals high in sugar; during two separate weeks, the same meals were prepared with artificial sweeteners.

The participants weren't told which was which—and they couldn't tell the difference.

At the end of each week, the researchers gathered data on 39 measures of the children's behavior, mood, and thinking ability. They found no sign of hyperactivity after the high-sugar meals. Even the parents who believed their children usually reacted to sugar didn't notice any effect. So if sugary treats make kids bouncy, it's due to the treat, not the sugar.

If anything, sugar may have the opposite effect. Some of the children in that study showed slight improvements in learning tasks and slightly slower times in tests of speed and agility when on the high-sugar diet. The authors interpreted those findings as evidence of a modest *relaxing* influence from sugar, a possibility that has more scientific basis than theories about hyperactivity. As we noted in our May report on foods and performance, at least a half dozen clinical trials suggest that a meal high in carbohydrates such as sugar makes people feel somewhat more relaxed or even sluggish.

Blood sugar: Not so low

Some people believe that sugar triggers symptoms of hypoglycemia, or low blood sugar, such as sweating, trembling, rapid heartbeat, and hunger. But those symptoms are rarely due to sugar.

True, eating lots of sugar can sometimes cause blood-sugar levels to drop a bit. That's because the pancreas responds to a hefty dose of sugar by secreting the hormone insulin, which helps the body's cells draw sugar out of the bloodstream. In a few people, that can push blood-sugar levels below normal. But such drops in blood sugar almost never cause symptoms. The rare exceptions occur in people with a condition called reactive hypoglycemia. For the vast majority of people who believe their symptoms are caused by sugar consumption, there's actually some other cause, such as an overactive thyroid or panic attacks. People who suspect hypoglycemia should have their physician help determine if their symptoms coincide with a drop in blood sugar.

A different sort of hypoglycemia is more common among diabetics. But in those people, hypoglycemia has nothing to do with eating too much sugar. Instead, it happens only when they inject too much insulin (or take too much oral antidiabetic medication), eat too little food, or exercise too much.

SUGAR IS SWEET AND SO ARE SUBSTITUTES

The appeal of artificial sweeteners lies largely in their lack of calories, a benefit that leads dieters to put up with the artificial taste. But research suggests that many would-be dieters sabotage that potential benefit by loading up on other high-calorie treats as a reward for using "diet" products.

Still, artificial sweeteners can help control calories so long as the rest of the diet is under control. And unlike sugar, the artificial sweeteners don't promote cavities or affect blood-sugar levels in diabetics. Here's a rundown of the three artificial sweeteners now on the market and three more on the horizon.

■ **Saccharin** (*Sugar Twin, Sweet 'N Low*), the oldest artificial sweetener, is 300 times sweeter than table sugar. It's used in baked goods, candy, canned fruit, chewing gum, dessert toppings, jams, and soft drinks. (It's also widely used in medications and vitamins.) In 1977, the U.S. Food and Drug Administration proposed banning saccharin because animal studies suggested a cancer risk. Under pressure from soft-drink makers and calorie-conscious consumers, Congress placed a moratorium on the proposed ban and mandated a warning label instead. In 1991, the FDA quietly withdrew its proposal. The warning label remains.

■ **Aspartame** (*Equal, NutraSweet, NatraTaste*), 180 times sweeter than sucrose, is widely used in candy, cereals, frozen desserts, and soft drinks. Although some commercial baked goods contain aspartame, it shouldn't be used for most home

cooking because it's unstable at high temperatures. As one of the most thoroughly tested additives ever approved by the FDA, aspartame appears to be entirely safe—almost: People with the inherited disorder phenylketonuria (PKU), which affects roughly 1 in 15,000 Americans, must limit their intake of the amino acid phenylalanine, a component of aspartame. For that reason, aspartame-containing products bear a warning aimed at people with PKU.

■ **Acesulfame K** (*Sunette, Sweet One*), 200 times sweeter than sucrose, is used in dry beverage mixes, candy, chewing gum, gelatins, and puddings. It's the only sugar substitute that bears no warning label of a possible health hazard.

The following sweeteners are currently seeking FDA approval:

■ **Cyclamate**, 30 times sweeter than table sugar, was widely used as an artificial sweetener in the 1950s and '60s, but was banned in the U.S. as a potential carcinogen in 1970. The manufacturer and a trade association are now urging the FDA to rescind the ban.

■ **Sucralose**, 600 times sweeter than table sugar, has shown no health risks in more than 100 animal and human studies conducted over the past 15 years.

■ **Alitame** is 2000 times sweeter than table sugar. The FDA has requested more studies to bolster the dozen or so supporting the sweetener's safety.

Diabetes: Off the hook

Traditionally, physicians have warned diabetics to avoid or strictly limit sugary foods—not because of resulting low blood-sugar levels, but to control the abnormally *high* blood-sugar levels that characterize the disease and damage the eyes, kidneys, nerves, and circulatory system. Now even that prohibition has been repealed.

Earlier this year, the American Diabetes Association issued revolutionary dietary guidelines based on the contention that sweets are no more upsetting to a diabetic's blood-sugar levels than other carbohydrates such as bread, pasta, and potatoes. The new guidelines call for a balance between carbohydrates and fat, the two main dietary components.

One legacy of the longtime prohibition against sugar in diabetics is the popular belief that sugar somehow *causes* diabetes. It doesn't. The real culprits are problems with the body's production of insulin and its sensitivity to the hormone.

Decay: One charge with teeth

The only real risk from sugar for most people is tooth decay. While fluoride, plastic sealants for children's teeth, and improved oral hygiene have dramatically reduced the incidence of cavities, it's still important to watch what you eat—and when you eat it (see CRH, 4/93).

All carbohydrates—starches as well as sweets—

can be converted into tooth-dissolving acid by the bacteria in dental plaque. Since the simple sugars in sweets are most readily available to the bacteria, they pose a special risk. But starches can be equally harmful if they stick around long enough for their complex carbohydrates to get broken down into simple ones. The most damaging foods seem to be sweet baked goods like cookies and cakes, which cling to the teeth and contain both quick-acting sugars and slower starches. Sugar-sweetened products that dissolve slowly, such as hard candy and throat lozenges, can also prolong the acid attack.

To minimize the cavity risk from sugars, wait for mealtime to consume carbohydrates. That way, other foods will increase saliva production, which neutralizes the acids and helps clear food particles and sugar from the mouth. When you want a snack, choose fruit or raw vegetables instead of a sweet or starchy snack. Although the sugar in fruit can cause cavities, most raw fruits are safe to snack on because they're relatively low in sugar and aren't very sticky. The exceptions are bananas, which are quite high in sugar, and dried fruits, such as dates and raisins, which are both sugary and sticky.

Natural appeal: Artificial argument

Many people believe that sucrose—table sugar—is somehow less healthy than so-called natural sugars, like honey or fruit sugar. Many food companies cash in on that mistaken belief with an array of "naturally sweetened" products ranging from cereals and yogurts to cookies and candies. In some cases, that just boosts the overall sugar content of the food. For example, a bowlful of *Honey Nut Cheerios* contains 11 grams of sugar to plain *Cheerios'* 1 gram.

In any case, sugar is sugar. "Natural" sugars are no more nutritious than sucrose. Like sucrose, natural sweeteners such as honey, brown sugar, and corn syrup contain only calories and nothing else worth measuring. (The one exception is blackstrap mo-lasses, which contains calcium, iron, and some other nutrients.) While fruit juices do contain many nutrients, the tiny amount used in fruit-juice-sweetened products has no significant nutritional value.

Natural sugars provide just as many calories as sucrose and are at least as bad for the teeth. In fact, syrupy sweeteners like honey may be worse because they're sticky. And contrary to what many diabetics have been led to believe, products sweetened with fruit juice have no less an impact on blood-sugar levels than foods sweetened with sucrose.

THE FACTS ABOUT FATS

The three
major dietary
goals still
apply: Eat less,
eat less fat,
and eat less
saturated fat in
particular.
Here's how.

The war on fat seemed to be going so well. Over the past decade Americans ate less beef and more chicken, drank less whole milk and more skim. *Snackwell's*, an upstart line of reduced-fat cookies, last year usurped *Oreos* as the nation's favorite. Taco Bell was moved to develop a new, reduced-fat menu called "Border Lights." Oscar Mayer introduced a no-fat frank. And last year the Government announced that American adults' fat consumption had dropped to 34 percent of calories—a small but significant step down from 36 percent, the level a decade earlier.

Deeper in that Government report, however, was an unsettling piece of news: Americans are eating more *calories* each day—231 more on average—than a decade ago. Moreover, they are getting fatter, suggesting just where those calories are going. Somewhere in the grocery aisles a nation of fat-fighters has taken a wrong turn.

Confusing claims about the relative importance of fat and calories may be partly to blame. Recent TV ads for *Hershey's Syrup*, for example, crow that it contains no fat, and never has. Viewers are left to recall for themselves that the chocolate syrup contains 100 sugary calories per 2-tablespoon serving.

Moreover, consumers have gotten mixed messages about the importance of various types of fat. At different times over the past three decades, fat-watchers have been told to crank up the polyunsaturates, to keep the polys steady but increase monounsaturated fats, to make deep cuts in total fat, and to eat as much fat as they liked as long as it was olive oil.

A healthy diet need not be so complicated. Most Americans have three main dietary problems: They eat too much; they eat too much fat; and, in particular, they eat too much saturated fat. The challenge is to cut down—and, at the same time, to craft a diet that you still enjoy. We'll tell you how to accomplish those sometimes conflicting goals when you shop for groceries, cook at home, and order in a restaurant.

Fat and your health

Focusing on fat alone, nutritionists say, is no more productive than obsessing about vitamins, cholesterol, or sweeteners. As one nutritionist says, "Cutting down on fat isn't a stand-alone strategy."

Weight-loss experts have backed away from their recent assertion that counting grams of fat is more important than counting calories. That strategy worked fine when it was difficult to consume excess calories on a low-fat diet. No more. "Food technologists have changed all that," says psychologist John Foreyt, director of the Baylor College of Medicine's Nutrition Research Clinic, in Houston. For example, now you can buy Sunshine Biscuit's "reduced fat" version of its *Vienna Fingers* cookie, which contains about 40 percent less fat than the original—but just four of those cookies add up to 260 calories. Faced with such low-fat-but-high-calorie products, we've got to go back to counting calories, Foreyt says.

If you're concerned about your diet's contribution to your risk of cancer, several leading epidemiologists now believe that fat intake isn't the whole story. Even the apparent connection between adult fat consumption and breast cancer, loudly heralded a few years ago, is very shaky, several epidemiologists say. Colon cancer appears to be the cancer most strongly influenced by fat, and even that apparent link may really reflect the effects of eating too much red meat and too little fiber. In the long run, many researchers believe, the diet most protective against cancer is one based on fruits, vegetables, grains, and beans—not just because it is likely to be low in fat, but also because it is high in fiber, the protective vitamins and minerals known as antioxidants, and possibly other useful compounds. (See "Taking Vitamins," CONSUMER REPORTS, September 1994.)

What hasn't changed is the strong connection between saturated fats, high blood cholesterol, and heart disease. That link is the main reason people have been urged to pay close attention to both the amount and the types of fats they consume.

The Government now recommends that Americans get no more than 30 percent of their daily calories from fat, with no more than one-third of that fat being saturated.

Nutrition experts we've surveyed say that less fat would be even better. Their advice for an ideal diet: Limit total fat to 20 to 25 percent of calories, with a 7 percent cutoff for saturated fat. (See "Are You Eating Right?," October 1992.)

The Government recommendations mean your daily fat consumption should be no more than 67 grams for a 2000-calorie diet. (At 9 calories per gram of fat, 67 grams equals about 600 calories. Carbohydrates and protein carry 4 calories per gram.) Unfortunately, exceeding the fat limit is as easy as pie. A bologna-and-cheese sandwich with mayonnaise has about 39 grams of fat. A modest half-cup serving of super-premium ice cream packs 18 grams of fat, more than half of it saturated. And a slice of apple pie has 19 grams, almost all in the crust.

Most people have no idea how much of their diet consists of fat. But there is now a simple self-test to see whether your fat intake is too high. To assess your own diet, see "How Much Fat Is in Your Diet?"

Avoiding packaged fats

The new Nutrition Facts labels, required by the U.S. Food and Drug Administration on nearly all packaged foods, have made it much easier to avoid fats in processed foods. You can use the labels to design a low-fat diet that closely meets your daily caloric needs, or you can use the figures as a rough guide.

Precise word definitions, issued by the FDA, also brought order to what had become a free-for-all on food labels. *Low fat* now signifies, in most cases, a product with no more than three grams of fat per serving. A *low saturated fat* product has no more than one gram per serving and gets no more than 15 percent of its calories from saturated fat. And products proclaimed as *fat-free* or *saturated-fat-free* must have less than half a gram of fat, or saturated fat, per serving.

The rules also let companies take credit for removing some fat from foods typically loaded with it, such as microwave popcorn or cheese. A *reduced-fat* product has at least 25 percent less fat than usually found in that food; *light* in fat means a food has half the fat or one-third the calories of its regular counterpart. But those foods can still have lots of fat: Reduced-fat *Better Cheddar* crackers, for example, still contain 6 grams

of fat per serving and get 36 percent of their calories from fat.

Elsewhere in the store:

☐ The FDA's glossary doesn't define such label terms as "thin" or "smart," which suggest good-for-you but can mean just about anything.

☐ Nutrition labels aren't required on fresh products, including meat. As a general guide, the lowest fat and fewest calories are found in skinless chicken breasts, skinless turkey breasts, and pork tenderloin.

☐ "Low fat" is defined differently when it's on a milk carton. Dairies were permitted to keep this term for 2 percent milk, although in this case the product contains more than 4.5 grams of fat per serving.

The types of fat

What we call "fat" is actually a class of molecules called fatty acids—strings of carbon atoms dotted with hydrogen atoms. The hydrogen makes the difference. The "saturated" fat that dominates in butter, lard, and tropical oils is thoroughly saturated with hydrogen atoms, carrying as many as the carbon atoms are chemically able to; the "unsaturated" fats that dominate vegetable oils carry less than a full complement of hydrogen. Saturated fats tend to be hard at room temperature, as well as hard on your heart; unsaturated fats tend to remain liquid at room temperature, and are less harmful to your health.

Are all unsaturated fats equally desirable? Opinions have varied. Early concern about saturated fats first shifted interest to polyunsaturated fats, which predominate in vegetable oils such as safflower, soybean, and corn. Studies had shown that polyunsaturates reduced blood-cholesterol levels when substituted for saturated fat.

Then, in the 1980s, attention shifted to monounsaturated fats, found predominantly in olive and canola oils (the difference between polys and monos, both unsaturated, is the number of hydrogen atoms missing from the string of carbon atoms). A research team from Texas and California reported that monos could lower total blood cholesterol just as well as polyunsaturates. But apparently unlike polys, the monos didn't reduce HDLs, or high-density lipoproteins, blood compounds that reduce heart-attack risk.

That apparent difference enhanced an already good reputation. Mediterranean populations had for generations consumed large quantities

of olive oil, and had very low rates of heart disease. Olive-oil companies couldn't have been happier.

The celebration was premature. Further research couldn't confirm polyunsaturates' effects on HDL. All the nutrition scientists we queried now believe that, at levels commonly found in the diet, monos and polys appear to have the same effects on blood cholesterol. Since a tablespoon of any vegetable oil has 14 grams of fat—in most, only one or two grams are saturated fat—and 125 calories, whichever one you consume should make little difference to your health. (The exceptions, worth avoiding, are the "tropical" vegetable oils—palm, palm kernel, and coconut—with 7 to 12 grams of saturated fat per tablespoon, and cottonseed oil, with 4 grams of saturated fat.)

So when you're picking a cooking oil to use at home, base your selection on taste. When you can, use a flavored oil, such as sesame oil for stir-fries, extra-virgin olive oil for pasta, or walnut oil for a nutty-tasting salad dressing. The distinctive taste lets you use very little and still get the oil's flavor. If you need a bland-tasting oil, you might as well choose one that's especially low in saturated fat; canola oil is the lowest, with safflower oil close behind.

The rise of trans fat

Although food manufacturers have been forced to cut back on saturated fat because of health concerns, they have been reluctant to give up some of its physical properties. So they often use a sort of hybrid. By bubbling hydrogen through vegetable oil, they add some hydrogen to the fatty acids, in a process called hydrogenation. The result—partially hydrogenated vegetable oils—can be used in a semisolid spread like margarine, and is better suited for deep frying than unsaturated fats. Because of the particular chemical configuration they take, some of the fatty acids in hydrogenated oils are known as trans-fatty acids, or trans fats.

Trans fat is what gives margarine, a vegetable-oil product, its butter-like consistency. The familiar texture has helped margarine flourish as an apparently heart-healthy alternative. Trans fat also has become more common in prepared foods such as baked goods and snacks.

But in 1990 Dutch researchers reported that trans fat might raise blood cholesterol, as butter does.

Trans fat's role is not yet entirely

resolved; clinical studies haven't linked trans fats directly to heart attacks. But there's a growing consensus among epidemiologists that, gram for gram, trans fat increases your blood cholesterol nearly as much as saturated fat does. (Two researchers independently told us their calculations suggest trans fat is about three-fourths as bad for you as is saturated fat.)

The bottom line: If you're concerned about your cholesterol level, stick with margarine, but use it sparingly. Butter hasn't gotten any better; it still has 7 grams of saturated fat per tablespoon, more than the combined total of trans and saturated fats in a tablespoon of stick margarine. As a rule, you'll reduce your intake of trans fat if instead of solid margarine you use a soft, tub-style spread that lists water or liquid vegetable oil as first ingredient. (Ingredient lists are ranked by weight.) Even better, try other spreads for your bread. Jam, chutney, and apple butter have no fat at all.

Partially hydrogenated vegetable oils are used in packaged cookies, crackers, and other baked goods to prolong shelf life. But it takes careful label reading to detect its presence (see "Finding the Hidden Trans Fat," below), and often there is no way to find out. Since trans fat has harmful effects similar to saturated fat, we think the Government should require its inclusion on the label.

New ways to cook

You can only cut back on fats and oil so much before you start robbing your usual meals of their familiar flavors and textures—or you start burning them. To create interesting low-fat meals in your kitchen may require experimenting with other techniques and dishes, says Catharine Powers, a nutritionist at the Culinary Institute of America, in Hyde Park, N.Y. "We need to shift from a negative emphasis of taking things out of the diet to thinking creatively about putting things in," she says. Some ways to do that:

☐ **Look beyond fats for flavor.** Cook with fresh herbs, spices, garlic, onion, scallions, flavored vinegars, and high-quality mustard to boost flavor. Instead of sautéing onions, carrots, and other vegetables, "sweat" them in their own juices for a pungent flavor by cooking slowly in a covered pan. Adding a little water, stock, wine, or fruit juice during the process will prevent sticking. When steaming vegetables, chicken, and fish—a good way to preserve nutrients and protect natural juices—use

YOUR FOOD BUDGET

Here's a way to estimate how many calories you can consume each day without gaining or losing weight, and how much fat you can include in your diet.

To calculate your calorie budget, start with your weight in pounds. Multiply it by 10 if you're a woman, by 11 if you're a man. That yields your basal metabolic requirement. Then, decide which of the following four phrases best describes your highest level of regular exercise, and select the corresponding activity factor.

Sedentary 1.40	
Light . . . . .1.60 (housework, cooking, short stroll)	
Moderate .1.70 (brisk swimming or walking)	
Strenuous . . . . .1.85 (heart-pounding exercise)	

Multiply your metabolic requirement by your activity factor to get your approximate daily calorie budget.

To calculate your daily fat allowance, here's a mathematical shortcut: Divide your daily calorie budget by 30. The answer will be the approximate number of grams of fat you can eat according to the Government's recommendations—30 percent of calories from fat; each gram of fat has 9 calories. (Many nutritionists say you really should eat even less fat than that.)

FINDING THE HIDDEN TRANS FAT

The new food labels go a long way toward helping consumers know how much total fat and saturated fat they're eating. But it's difficult or impossible to know how much trans fat a product contains, even though many researchers consider it nearly as villainous as saturated fat. These two guides should help.

Reading between the lines. If the ingredients list includes "partially hydrogenated" oils, the product contains trans fat. How much? The label won't tell you directly. But sometimes you can tell indirectly. If the label gives the amount of other fats—saturated, polyunsaturated, and monounsaturated—add those figures together and subtract them from the amount of total fat. What remains should be the approximate amount of trans fat the product contains. In the example shown here—Reduced Fat Wheat Thins crackers—adding the amounts of those three fats and subtracting them from the total shows about 2 grams, or half the fat in the crackers, unaccounted for. It's probably 2 grams of trans fat.

INGREDIENTS: WHOLE WHEAT FLOUR, ENRICHED WHEAT FLOUR (CONTAINS NIACIN, REDUCED IRON, THIAMINE MONONITRATE [VITAMIN B₁], RIBOFLAVIN [VITAMIN B₂]), VEGETABLE SHORTENING (PARTIALLY HYDROGENATED SOYBEAN OIL), SUGAR, SALT, HIGH FRUCTOSE CORN SYRUP, MALTED BARLEY FLOUR, LEAVENING (CALCIUM PHOSPHATE, BAKING SODA), ANNATTO EXTRACT AND TURMERIC OLEORESIN (VEGETABLE COLORS).

Total Fat 4g	6%
Saturated Fat 0.5g	3%
Polyunsaturated Fat 0g	
Monounsaturated Fat 1.5g	

Relying on the USDA. This new data, just released by the U.S. Department of Agriculture, lists several packaged foods that contain particularly high levels of trans fat—often more trans fat than saturated fat. Each item represents a national brand—which the agency declines to name. In most categories, the trans fat content of the product we've listed is similar to that of other brands, but not always. To give you the full picture, we've provided the number of grams of total fat, saturated fat, and trans fat per standard serving.

	Serving Size	Total fat	Saturated fat	Trans fat
Biscuits refrigerated dough	55g	6.5 g	1.5 g	2.0 g
Cake frosting (chocolate, ready-to-eat)	35	6.5	2.0	1.0
Cheese crackers	30	9.5	2.0	2.0
Chocolate chip cookies	30	8.0	2.0	3.0
Doughnuts sugar or glazed	55	14.0	3.5	4.0
French fries frozen (before cooking)	85	8.5	1.5	3.0
Graham crackers	30	3.0	0.5	2.0
Popcorn, microwave	30	7.5	2.0	2.5
Pound cake	80	16.5	3.5	4.5
Snack crackers	30	7.0	1.0	2.5
Taco shells	30	8.0	1.5	2.5

herbs and spices on the food and in the steaming water. For added taste after cooking, use a pastry brush to thinly paint on a flavored oil such as walnut or basil olive oil.

☐ **Use alternatives for texture.** Most cooks agree there's no substitute for solid shortening in a pie crust, but you can safely pull out one-third of the fat in recipes for cookies and muffins. Replace it with applesauce or banana puree to maintain a creamy texture. Use part-skim ricotta cheese—pureed and blended with nonfat yogurt—for Bavarian pie and chocolate mousse, and you'll never miss the egg yolks and cream. Evaporated skim milk is a fine understudy for cream in cream-based sauces and soups, and buttermilk—low-fat despite its name—can replace cream or whole milk in ranch dressing, pancakes and muffins.

☐ **Seek out new sauces.** Many chefs are turning to fruits, vegetables, and legumes to create purees, relishes, coulis and compotes. Relishes—known as salsa in Mexico, chutneys in India, and sambals in Indonesia and Malaysia—can be hot or cold, chunky or smooth. Add them to rice, pasta, steamed vegetables, or meats.

☐ **Rewrite the recipe.** You can dramatically decrease the fat content of conventional foods by making them with low-fat ingredients. Two examples: pizza made with bobolis, a low-fat tomato sauce, and part-skim shredded mozzarella; tacos made with corn tortillas, fat-free refried beans, and ground turkey breast.

Check out *Cooking Light* and *Eating Well* magazines, available by subscription or on the newsstand. Both contain recipes that aim for a diet with 30 percent or fewer calories from fat. Other resources are the *Good Eating, Good Health Cookbook* and *Catch of the Day*, with unusual recipes for fish, published by Consumer Reports Books. (To order the books, call 515 237-4903.)

Eating out, eating smart

Thanks to the well-publicized efforts of the Center for Science in the Public Interest, a consumer group focused on nutrition issues, Americans have learned that there are fat-laden meals waiting to snare them at Chinese, Mexican, and Italian restaurants. Still, you can order a satisfying, low-fat meal in most restaurants if you know how.

In general, look for items that are broiled, grilled, roasted, baked,

---

TEST YOURSELF

HOW MUCH FAT IS IN YOUR DIET?

How well are you keeping extra fat out of your diet? One way to check is to keep a careful daily record of how many calories and grams of fat you eat. A much simpler way to check your fat consumption is to complete this new quiz, designed by researchers at Seattle's Fred Hutchinson Cancer Research Center, whose studies have found it a fairly accurate way to estimate consumption. The questionnaire also lets you know how well you're doing on five basic fat-cutting strategies recommended by dietitians.

Think about your diet over the past three months and answer each of the following questions with a number from this list. If a question doesn't apply to your diet, leave it blank. (For instance, if you don't eat red meat, don't answer questions 5, 6, and 19—your score is based on the rest of your diet.)

1= Usually/Always 3=Sometimes

2= Often 4= Rarely/Never

QUIZ
In the past three months, when you—

1) ate fish, did you avoid frying it? _____

2) ate chicken, did you avoid frying it? _____

3) ate chicken, did you remove the skin? _____

4) ate spaghetti or noodles, did you eat it plain or with a meatless tomato sauce? _____

5) ate red meat, did you trim all the visible fat? _____

6) ate ground beef, did you choose extra lean? _____

7) ate bread, rolls, or muffins, did you eat them *without* butter or margarine? _____

8) drank milk, was it skim or 1% milk instead of 2% or whole? _____

9) ate cheese, was it a reduced-fat variety? _____

10) ate a frozen dessert, was it sherbet, ice milk, or nonfat yogurt or ice cream? _____

11) ate cooked vegetables, did you eat them *without* adding butter, margarine, salt pork, or bacon fat? _____

12) ate cooked vegetables, did you avoid frying them? _____

13) ate potatoes, were they cooked by a method other than frying? _____

14) ate boiled or baked potatoes, did you eat them *without* butter, margarine, or sour cream? _____

15) ate green salads with dressing, did you use a low-fat or nonfat dressing? _____

16) ate dessert, did you eat only fruit? _____

17) ate a snack, was it raw vegetables? _____

18) ate a snack, was it fresh fruit? _____

19) cooked red meat, did you trim all the fat before cooking? _____

20) used mayonnaise or a mayonnaise-type dressing, was it low-fat or nonfat? _____

SCORING

To estimate the percentage of calories from fat in your diet, transfer the numbers above to the score sheet below. Disregard questions that were left blank. (Note that the items are arranged within five fat-lowering strategies rather than according to their order in the quiz.) Figure your average score for each of the strategies (the total divided by the number of answers you gave). Add up the five averages and divide by five. Then check the chart.

Strategy 1: Avoid frying
Items: 1 _____
   2 _____
   12 _____
   13 _____
Subtotal _____
Average _____

Strategy 2: Modify meat
Item 3 _____
  5 _____
  6 _____
  19 _____
Subtotal _____
Average _____

Strategy 3: Avoid fat as flavoring
Items: 4 _____
   7 _____
   11 _____
   14 _____
Subtotal _____
Average _____

Strategy 4: Substitute low-fat or nonfat versions
Items: 8 _____
   9 _____
   10 _____
   15 _____
   20 _____
Subtotal _____
Average _____

Strategy 5: Replace fatty foods with produce
Items: 16 _____
   17 _____
   18 _____
Subtotal _____
Average _____

Overall score _____
(sum of 5 averages):

Divide overall score by 5 to get overall average: _____

If overall average is...	your % of fats from calories is...
1.0 to 1.5	**under 25%**
1.5 to 2	**25 to 29%**
2 to 2.5	**30 to 34%**
2.5 to 3	**35 to 39%**
3 to 3.5	**40 to 44%**
3.5 to 4	**45% or more**

steamed, or poached. Keep your distance from fried, deep-fried, and "crispy" dishes. Ask for vegetables seasoned with herbs instead of butter, pancakes with fruit or yogurt topping, and a baked potato instead of fries.

Here are some guidelines for specific types of restaurants:

☐ **Fast food.** Our tests of fast foods in the past two years showed that grilled chicken sandwiches, roast beef sandwiches, and salads with low-fat dressings are the best choices nutritionally. Among the lowest in fat were Wendy's *Grilled Chicken*, Arby's *Light Roast Beef Deluxe*, and Arby's *Light Roast Turkey Deluxe*. The basic burgers also scored well in nutrition, but most didn't taste very good; Wendy's *Plain Single* was an exception.

High-fat favorites get slimmer when you hold the mayonnaise-based dressings, skip the cheese, skin the chicken, and go easy on the dipping sauce. At McDonald's,

for instance, you can lunch on a *McGrilled Chicken Classic* (which claims a modest 250 calories and 3 grams of fat), a side salad with Lite Vinaigrette (95 calories and 4 grams of fat), and a vanilla low-fat frozen yogurt cone (120 calories and half a gram of fat). For more examples, see "Can Fast Food Be Good Food?," August 1994.

☐ **Chinese.** Eat as the Chinese do, with small amounts of meat, poultry, and vegetables atop a mound of steamed (not fried) rice. Egg-drop soup, wonton soup, and steamed dumplings make good beginnings; avoid egg rolls, fried noodles, and spare ribs. Select steamed foods with a variety of sauces. Stir-fried dishes are not always low in fat; when you order, ask that less oil than usual be used.

☐ **Mexican.** Request baked or steamed corn tortillas instead of the usual tortilla chips. Similarly, look for baked tortillas rather than fried ones as a basis of tamales, tostadas,

and enchiladas. Use salsa instead of sour cream, guacamole, or cheese. Chicken fajitas are a good choice; ask that they be cooked in little or no oil. Taco Bell's new "Border Light" menu cuts fat by more than 50 percent and reduces calories an average of 20 percent.

☐ **Italian.** The richness of a pasta dish depends on the sauce. Choose a tomato-based (marinara, pomodoro) or clam sauce instead of a cream sauce like Alfredo. Order chicken, meat, or seafood broiled or grilled instead of breaded and fried.

☐ **French.** "Nouvelle" cuisine typically offers sauces featuring meat juices, stocks, and herbs, and is lower in fat than classic French cuisine. Start with consommé or steamed mussels rather than pâté or vichyssoise. Choose light stews such as bouillabaisse or ratatouille, meats with a wine sauce such as bordelaise, or broiled, poached, or steamed fish.

Food for Thought about Dietary Supplements

The surge of public interest in nutrition supplements has been fired by the recently enacted federal regulations governing health claims, which permits the health food industry to make claims about the function of nutrients not permitted for food products. This article provides healthy skepticism about the common rationales for the use of supplements.

PAUL R. THOMAS, Ed.D., R.D.

Paul Thomas, currently a Fellow at the Georgetown Center for Food and Nutrition Policy, Georgetown University, previously served as a staff scientist for the Food and Nutrition Board, Institute of Medicine, National Academy of Sciences. He is a registered dietitian who received an Ed.D. degree in nutrition education from Columbia University. He is an author and editor of several books on contemporary nutrition issues. Correspondence can be directed to him at the Georgetown Center for Food and Nutrition Policy, 3240 Prospect Street, N.W., Washington, DC 20007.

The dietary supplements industry is very healthy. Sales of vitamins, minerals, and other food concentrates are roughly $4 billion per year. Although at least one quarter of American adults swallow these pills, powders, and potions daily,[1] probably the majority of us take them at least occasionally. What are we getting in return?

I've asked myself this question since the 1960s when, as a teenager, I began taking dozens of supplements after reading about their magical powers in *Prevention* and *Let's Live* magazines, and books by Adelle Davis. Surely they would help cure my adolescent acne; I just needed to find the right combination. But my pizza face only improved when I took tetracycline and topical retinoic acid (the drug, not the vitamin) prescribed by a dermatologist. Growing out of adolescence also helped.

My education about dietary supplements became more comprehensive when I discovered the medical library during my college education as a biology ("pre-med") major. I learned that the hype surrounding them in the popular press was rarely supported by studies in the journals. Dietary supplements have benefited me in that they developed my interest in nutrition to the point where I chose to make a career in this discipline. But over time, and despite the growing popularity of supplements even among nutrition professionals, I have gone from being an enthusiastic vitamin promoter to a skeptic.

Most of us would agree that it's best to meet our nutritional needs with food, which means that everyone should eat a healthy, balanced diet. I believe that, short of that, dietary supplements are at best a poor and inadequate substitute. Supplements are appropriate for some people for specific purposes. But should they be taken every day, by everybody? I don't think so, and I make my case with the following eight points.

POINT 1: NO EXPERT BODY OF NUTRITION EXPERTS RECOMMENDS THE ROUTINE USE OF SUPPLEMENTS

A small number of nutritionists support regular supplement use. But no scientific body of nutrition experts recommends that everyone take supplements on a routine basis as dietary insurance or for optimal health. Expert bodies are by nature conservative and unlikely to recommend a practice until the evidence is convincing and perhaps even overwhelming. That's the point, since dietary guidance for most people should be based on strong evidence.

In 1989, the Food and Nutrition Board of the National Academy of Sciences issued a comprehensive review of the relationships between diet and health.[2] The report stated that dietary supplements should be avoided at levels above the Recommended Dietary Allowances (RDAs). Finally, however, a group of nutrition experts was not warning people to stay away from supplements with pronouncements of dire risks from their use.

The recommendation was not to stay away from supplements, but to take them in no more than RDA amounts. The Food and Nutrition Board acknowledged that the long-term potential risks and benefits of supplements had not been adequately studied and called for more research.

> **The Food and Nutrition Board recommends that those who choose supplements limit the dose to levels of the RDA or less.**

The latest pronouncements on supplements are found in the new (4th) edition of *Dietary Guidelines for Americans*, which was released in January.[3] The report states that "diets that meet RDAs are almost certain to ensure intake of enough essential nutrients by most healthy people," and that people with average requirements are likely to have adequate diets even if they don't meet RDAs.

About supplements, the report states: "Daily vitamin and mineral supplements at or below the Recommended Dietary Allowances are considered safe, but are usually not needed by people who eat the variety of foods depicted in the Food Guide Pyramid." It acknowledged, however, that some people might benefit from supplements. These include older people and others with little exposure to sunlight who may need extra vitamin D. Women of childbearing age might reduce the risk of neural-tube defects in their infants with folate-rich foods or folic acid supplements. Pregnant women usually benefit from iron supplements. And vegans, who avoid animal products, might need some nutrients in pill form. The report urges the public not to rely on supplements.

Surveys show that most supplementers take a one-a-day multiple-vitamin-mineral product. But some take large doses of single nutrients or nutrient combinations as self-prescribed medication for disease

or to try to reach a more optimal state of health, the latter fueled most recently by the enthusiasm for antioxidants. The practices of these aggressive supplementers merit some concern.

POINT 2: NUTRITION IS ONLY ONE FACTOR THAT INFLUENCES HEALTH, WELL-BEING, AND RESISTANCE TO DISEASE

The major chronic diseases that prematurely maim and kill most Americans have multiple causes. However, just as the advent of antibiotics and vaccines led many to think that the cure of diseases awaited specific "magic bullets," some proponents of supplements seem to think that these products are nutritional magic bullets for cancer, heart disease, and other maladies.

Health reporter Jane Brody calls us "a nation hungry for simple nutritional solutions to complex health problems."[4] Edward Golub, in his recent book, *The Limits of Medicine*, warns us against "thinking in penicillin mode."[5] It can be easy to do in nutrition because the first identified nutrient-related diseases (eg, scurvy and beriberi) were

> **Some proponents feel that supplements are "magic bullets" for cancer, heart disease, and other maladies.**

caused by dietary deficiencies. Anyone who doesn't get enough of the proper nutrient will eventually succumb to the relevant deficiency disease. No matter how much you exercise, who your parents are, or whether or not you smoke, you will become scorbutic without sufficient vitamin C.

Unfortunately, there is no such simple cause-effect relationship for diseases such as cardiovascular disease, cancer, stroke, and diabetes. Large doses of vitamin E, for example, may or may not influence the risk of developing heart disease. For some people, it may potentially be important. For most, however, it is at best one factor, and probably not a major one.

A primary contributor to chronic disease risk is our genetic heritage. Nutritionist Elizabeth Hiser writes, "Genes have a powerful influence over body size and disease risk, and though diet helps temper unwanted tendencies, *who* you are is often more important than *what* you eat. . . . Because of genetics, diet helps some people a lot, some people a little, and a very few people not at all."[6] Genetic endowment accounts in large measure for why some people get heart disease when young, for example, no matter how well they care for themselves, and why others live long lives even when they violate many of the commandments of healthy living.

Chronic disease risk is also affected by whether or not we exercise, refrain from smoking, avoid drinking to excess, limit exposure to unproductive stressors, and have sufficient rest, relaxation, and fun—and, of course, eating a diet that meets dietary guidelines and the RDAs. In our enthusiasm for supplements, however, we run the risk of reducing the importance of these factors.

One example of "thinking in penicillin mode" is linking calcium with the treatment, and especially prevention, of osteoporosis. However, bone health is influenced by many factors, including smoking, alcohol consumption, exercise, and intake of nutrients such as phosphorus, protein, and boron that affect calcium absorption, utilization, and excretion. In fact, osteoporosis is uncommon in several countries with relatively low calcium intakes.

Social commentator H. L. Mencken said, "For every complicated problem there is a simple solution—and it is wrong."[7] Supplements are not the answer to health and disease for the vast majority of people. Who our parents are, how we live our lives, and the food we put into our mouths several times a day affect our health more profoundly.

POINT 3: FOOD IS MORE THAN THE SUM OF ITS NUTRIENTS

Nutritionists used to think that macro- and micronutrients made a food nutritious and good for health. Other food constituents, such as fiber, were seen as nonessential, and therefore unimportant, since death is not directly associated with fiber deficiency. However, we have learned that, while fiber is not essential in the traditional sense, its presence in the diet makes it much easier to defecate and influences blood cholesterol levels and risk of diseases such as diverticulosis and certain cancers.

> **Supplements are not the answer to health and disease for the vast majority of people.**

Many compounds in food that are not classical nutrients can apparently influence health and risk of disease. Several hundred studies show that heavy fruit and vegetable eaters have approximately half the risk of cancer compared with those who don't eat these foods, but the results are not consistently related to one or several nutrients. New biologically active constituents found mostly in plant foods—phytochemicals (or "phytomins" as *Prevention* magazine calls them)—are being discovered regularly. They include flavonoids, monoterpenes, phenolics, indoles, allylic sulfides, and isothiocyanates. Phy-

> **Even, when and if, phytochemicals are reliably found in supplements, it will never be appropriate to take them in that form rather than from foods that contain them.**

tochemicals became a "hot item" in 1994 when they were the subject of a cover story in *Newsweek* that April.[8] The title: "Better than Vitamins: The Search for the Magic Pill." (There's that word too often linked with supplements: magic! So is "miracle.")

Whole natural foods, to quote *Newsweek*, "harbor a whole ratatouille of compounds that have never seen the inside of a vitamin bottle for the simple reason that scientists have not, until very recently, even known they existed, let alone brewed them into pills." Even when phytochemicals can reliably be found in supplements, it will never be appropriate to swallow pills (or consume specially fortified processed foods) instead of eating recommended amounts of the foods that contain them, such as vegetables, fruits, whole grains, and legumes. To do so would be to inappropriately rely on preliminary science, when the future will bring the discovery of new phytochemicals that have always been available from today's natural foods. Determining whether and how isolated food constituents with biologic activity may improve health, treat disease, or extend life is a daunting task that will occupy researchers for decades or longer.

Scientists continue to learn more about the complexity of foods and the myriad of biologically active constituents they contain that can influence health and disease risk. How ironic, then, that the calls this research generates for renewed efforts to persuade people to eat healthier diets—the tried and true—often seems to be drowned out by the acclaim for dietary supplements.

POINT 4: DEVELOPING RDAs AND OPTIMAL NUTRIENT RECOMMENDATIONS IS VERY DIFFICULT

As a staff scientist with the Food and Nutrition Board, I worked with the subcommittee that developed the most recent (10th) edition of the RDAs. I was surprised to learn that the research base for the RDAs is quite limited. There are not as many studies as one would like to determine minimum and average nutrient requirements for each age-sex group, estimate the population variability in need, and to feel more comfortable about the judgments made to derive nutrient allowances. Setting RDAs is tough work!

Now there is substantial discussion about so-called optimal intakes of nutrients, levels of intake

that might allow people to be healthy and fit for a longer time. Some nutrition scientists believe optimal nutrient intakes will typically exceed RDA levels and may require supplements in some cases to achieve. Still, no one doubts that developing optimal nutrient intakes will be orders of magnitude more complex than developing RDAs.

The optimal intake of any nutrient will probably vary substantially among individuals and even throughout one person's life from infancy to old age. It will probably also depend on the parameter of interest. For example, an optimal intake of a nutrient to reduce the risk of heart disease might not be optimal to decrease cancer risk and might actually increase it. Defining, understanding, and assessing optimal nutrition is becoming one of the most exciting challenges for

> **Developing recommendations for optimal nutrient intakes will be many times more complex than developing RDAs.**

investigators in the nutrition and food sciences.

POINT 5: TAKING SUPPLEMENTS OF SINGLE NUTRIENTS IN LARGE DOSES MAY HAVE DETRIMENTAL EFFECTS ON NUTRITIONAL STATUS AND HEALTH

On April 14, 1994, the *New England Journal of Medicine* published the infamous Finnish study.[9] In this clinical trial, 29,000 male smokers in Finland were randomly divided into four groups, receiving either a placebo, 20 mg beta-carotene (approximately four to five times the amount in five servings of fruits and vegetables), 50 IU of vitamin E (about three to four times average dietary intakes, but still a small dose as a supplement), or both the beta-carotene and vitamin E. After 5 to 8 years, the beta-carotene takers had an 18% *higher* incidence of lung cancer, with hints that this carotenoid might also have raised their risk of heart disease. Vitamin E seemed to reduce the risk of prostate cancer but increased the risk of hemorrhagic stroke.

This study is noteworthy, both because of its surprising findings and the fact that it is one of the few large clinical trials on supplements and disease risk. The majority of studies investigating this relationship are epidemiologic in nature. Clinical trials in which subjects are randomly assigned to treatment or control groups help to identify cause-and-effect relationships. Epidemiologic studies, in contrast, can only identify whether the variables under study are related in some way.

The Finnish study showed that antioxidant nutrients might harm rather than help male smokers, so it has been scrutinized intensely. Blumberg, for example, noted that those with the highest plasma concentrations of vitamin E and beta-

> **Clinical studies help identify cause-and-effect relationships, whereas epidemiologic studies can only identify whether variables are related.**

carotene at the start of the study had the lowest risk of developing lung cancer[10]; therefore, these nutrients may have provided some protection to some smokers. But for those who would suggest that the subjects should not have expected any benefits from supplements, given their deadly habit, two points should be made. First, several epidemiologic studies show that fruit and vegetable consumption reduces the risk of lung cancer in smokers—again, foods (containing beta-carotene and many other carotenoids and phytochemicals), not supplements. Second, dietary supplements are often promoted to smokers and those who are not eating or taking care of themselves as well as they should with claims that the products protect health.

The Center for Science in the Public Interest, a consumer advocacy group that had recommended antioxidants to its readers, changed its position after the Finnish study.[11] "Shelve the beta-carotene," it said, or take no more than about 3 mg per day, the amount found in many multivitamins. It also advised people to "reconsider taking vitamin E." *New York Times* medical writer Nicholas Wade, commenting on the Finnish study, said: "The vitamin supplement industry . . . would like everyone to believe the issue of benefits is settled. . . . For all who assumed the answer was already known, the Finnish trial offers two lessons. One is that science can't be rushed. The other is not to put all your bets on those convenient little bottles: back to broccoli and bicycles."[12]

Time shows the wisdom of Wade's advice. Two large clinical trials were completed in January of this year that further debunk beta-carotene as a magic bullet. After 12 years of taking either 50 mg beta-carotene or a placebo every other day, 22,071 physicians learned that the phytochemical provided no protection against cancer or heart disease. In the second trial, 18,314 men and women at risk for lung cancer due to smoking or exposure to asbestos were given supplements of beta-carotene (30 mg/day), vitamin A (25,000 IU/day), or a placebo. Those receiving the supplements had a *higher* rate of death from lung cancer and heart disease; although the results were not statistically significant, the study was halted. Dr. Richard Klausner, the director of the National Cancer Institute, which financed both trials, concluded, "With clearly no benefit and even a hint of possible harm, I can see no reason that an individual should take beta-carotene."

> **A major concern with supplements is potential toxicity.**

A major concern with supplements is potential toxicity. Fat-soluble vitamins like A and D, which are stored in the body, are obviously harmful in excess, but so are some water-soluble nutrients. Large doses of vitamin B6, for ex-

ample, can produce neuropathy in the arms and legs, leading to partial paralysis. Some people taking tryptophan have developed and died from eosinophilia-myalgia syndrome, a connective tissue disease characterized by high levels of eosinophils, severe muscle pain, and skin and neuromuscular problems. (It is not yet certain whether the syndrome was caused by the tryptophan itself, by a contaminant produced in the manufacturing process, or by the two in combination.) High-dose niacin supplements, especially in the time-released form, have caused liver damage. Large amounts of beta-carotene can be dangerous to alcoholics with liver disorders. And antioxidant nutrients can act as prooxidants under certain conditions, generating cell-damaging free radicals.[13]

Another concern with supplements is the possibility of adverse nutrient interactions. Calcium, for example, affects the absorption of iron and vice versa. Various amino acids compete with each other for absorption from the small intestine and to cross the blood-brain barrier. Large doses of one nutrient or phytochemical can adversely affect

> **Large doses of one nutrient can adversely affect nutritional status in relation to another nutrient.**

nutritional status in relation to another. In one study, for example, very large doses of beta-carotene, 100 mg/day given for 6 days, decreased the concentration of another important carotenoid, lycopene, in the low-density lipoproteins by 12 to 25%.[14] Beta carotene is not the only carotenoid of benefit to health, or perhaps even the most important one. I am reminded of Walter Mertz, the renowned nutrition and trace mineral expert, who was asked if he took beta-carotene as a supplement. He replied he would be "afraid" to take it, not knowing how extra beta-carotene would affect the balance of all the other carotenoids in his body that he obtained from food.

Little information is available to demonstrate that the long-term and possibly lifetime intake of large doses of nutrients is completely safe. Studies on the consequences of large nutrient intakes in humans rarely have a large sample size and go beyond several months. If high levels of iron in the body, for example, really increase the risk of heart disease, as at least one study suggests,[15] the chances are remote that a physician will think that a patient who died of a heart attack possibly did so because of supplemental iron. In other words, nutrient toxicity may be a cause of more illness and death than suspected, because the problems will not be linked (or even thought to have a possible link) to use of supplements.

POINT 6: DIETARY SUPPLEMENTS VARY SUBSTANTIALLY IN QUALITY

Few federal manufacturing and formulation standards exist for supplements, in part because they fall into a regulatory gray area between foods and drugs.[16] A decade ago, investigators discovered that many calcium supplements did not disintegrate or dissolve in the digestive tract; the calcium was simply excreted. These results prompted the development of disintegration and dissolution standards for some types of supplements by the US Pharmacopoeia, the scientific organization that establishes drug standards....

Garlic supplements provide an example of not necessarily getting what you think you paid for. They have become popular because several studies suggest that garlic may help to lower blood cholesterol and reduce the risk of cancers of the breast, colon, and other organs. Attention has focused on two compounds that may be responsible for these effects: allicin and s-allyl cysteine. The Center for Science in the Public Interest analyzed garlic powder and various garlic pills and found major differences by brand in their content of these two compounds.[17] Plain garlic powder was best and least expensive, whereas the most popular brand of garlic supplement contained no allicin (Table 1). Similarly, Consumers Union recently found that ginseng products varied greatly in their content of ginsenosides, the root's supposed active ingredients.[18]

It is difficult to find a comprehensive, one-a-day type of supplement that supplies nutrients at RDA levels. Most products are not well balanced. They contain, for example, many times the recommended amount of inexpensive B vitamins like thiamin and riboflavin but only small amounts of calcium and magnesium, because recommended amounts of these minerals can add substantially to the size of the pill. Some supplements contain superfluous ingredients such as bee pollen, hesperidin complex, and PABA, which do lit-

tle more than boost the price (see Refs. 19 and 20 for good advice on choosing a supplement).

POINT 7: SUPPLEMENTS ARE PROMOTED BY COMMERCIAL AND OTHER FORCES ON THE BASIS OF INCOMPLETE OR PRELIMINARY SCIENCE

I stated earlier that the bulk of evidence linking supplements to reduced risks of heart disease, cancer, and other diseases is epidemiologic in nature, or based on in vitro, mechanistic, or biochemical studies. They show correlations and indicate the possibility of protective effects, but do not prove cause and effect. So we do not know whether most of these suggestive data are of practical importance to people over the long run as they eat good or bad diets, smoke or refrain from smoking, live in polluted or clean environments, and are either exercisers or couch potatoes.

The scientific community tends to blame journalists for distorted reporting about nutrition. True, there are both good and mediocre reporters on the subject. And too often the reporting is bad, incomplete, prepared from press releases, or focused on one study without placing it in perspective—a poor foundation for people to make intelligent decisions.

A recent study illustrates this point. Houn and colleagues examined popular press coverage of research on the association between alcohol consumption and breast

Table 1
Comparison of Garlic Supplements

Name of Supplement	Cost per Tablet* (cents)	Allicin (µg)†	SAC (µg)‡
McCormick Garlic Powder§	6	5,660	590
KAL Beyond Garlic	18	4,800	270
Garlique	33	3,840	130
Garlicin	18	2,165	145
Nature's Way	8	1,530	140
Kwai	11	815	60
Quintessence	9	535	185
Natural Brand (GNC)	10	300	45
P. Leiner (private label)‖	5	115	45
Kyolic¶	11	0	255

© 1995, CSPI. Adapted from Nutrition Action Healthletter (1875 Connecticut Ave., N.W., Suite 300, Washington DC 20009-5728. $24.00 for 10 issues).
* Based on list price when available or average price paid.
† One large clove of fresh garlic supplies about 5,000 µg allicin.
‡ S-allyl cysteine.
§ One third teaspoon.
‖ Product usually carries the name of the drugstore or other chain where it is sold.
¶ The best-selling garlic supplement.

Responsibility for distorted reporting of nutrition rests as much with some nutritional scientists as with the media; many major journals reach reporters before medical professionals.

cancer.[21] Of the 58 published journal papers on this topic over 7 years, only 11 were cited by the press. Three studies published in the *New England Journal of Medicine* and the *Journal of the Medical Association* were featured in more than three quarters of the news stories. And almost two thirds of the stories gave recommendations to women on alcohol consumption based on one study. Reporters ignored the published review articles and editorials that would have provided a better basis for advice. This highlighting of a few studies, which seems to occur in many other nutrition areas, tends to confuse people and lead them to think that a new study will undoubtedly contradict the findings of the previous one. It's the new math of media nutrition coverage: 1+1 = 0. As syndicated columnist Ellen Goodman puts it, "Fresh research has a sell-by date that is shorter than the one on the cereal box."[22]

Responsibility for distorted reporting of nutrition does not rest with the media alone. Increasingly, it involves nutrition scientists. Although they tend not to make exaggerated claims when reporting their work at scientific meetings, some are more bold when they speak to reporters or the public. Sometimes their institution's press office encourages this boldness. As research funds become harder to secure, scientists and their employers are learning that being in the news raises their visibility, which can help to raise money.

Now, major journals like the *New England Journal of Medicine* and *Journal of the American Medical Association* reach reporters before they reach biomedical professionals. And because a growing amount of research is financed by industry, a company might seek publicity about a new finding to enhance the value of its stock or draw attention to itself. A good book on the changing nature of reporting scientific advances is *Selling Science*, by sociologist Dorothy Nelkin.[23]

The dietary supplements industry is busy making bold claims for its products on the labels, in advertising, and in product literature using preliminary science. The 1990 Nutrition Labeling and Education Act, which resulted in the new nutrition labels on packaged foods, allows supplement manufacturers to present the same health claims that are allowed on foods—claims supported by "significant scientific agreement" and preapproved by FDA. Two of the authorized health claims are relevant to supplements: the links between calcium and osteoporosis and between folate and neural tube defects.

However, the Dietary Supplement Health and Education Act passed in 1994 allows the industry to make claims pertaining to the structure and function of a nutrient. For example, a supplement could not claim that it helps cure AIDS, but it might be possible to state that the product "boosts the immune system." The legal basis for a claim is that (1) some substantiation exist, (2) FDA be notified of the claim within 30 days of its presence on the label, and (3) two additional sentences be added to such claims: "This statement has not been evaluated by FDA. This product is not intended to diagnose, treat, cure, or prevent any disease." Along with these so-called "structure-function" claims, a retailer may now provide literature on supplements, although it is supposed to be balanced scientifically and not be misleading. Some members of the dietary supplements industry are fighting even these limitations, arguing that their absolute freedom of speech to provide whatever information they think is appropriate is being threatened.

An advertisement in *Time* magazine last October for Bayer Corporation's One-A-Day Brand Vitamins suggests the growing boldness of claims for even mainstream dietary supplements. The copy states: "It's been all over the news. Findings on folic acid studies were announced recently at a medical conference in Bar Harbor, Maine, suggesting that adequate intake of folic acid may significantly lower elevated homocysteine levels, one of the risk factors for heart attacks and strokes in men. One-A-Day Men's Formula contains 100% of the US RDA of folic acid. Why not start taking your One-A-Day today?"

Public health may benefit from the promotion of supplements by increasing the public's awareness of nutrient, diet, and disease relationships. But I fear the risks outweigh the benefits. The promotional copy typically fails to give information on food-related alternatives to supplements. In addition, the public rarely has the expertise to evaluate the information in the promotion. Furthermore, consumers' expectations of a product's effectiveness may be heightened by the hype and lead to irrational use of the product.

There can be a great difference between *a* truth and *the* truth. A truthful statement may inevitably be misleading. This lesson was made clear in the plethora of ridiculous health claims on foods back in the late 80s and early 90s. Some high-fat products, for example, were truthfully labeled as being cholesterol free, because manufacturers knew many people would think the product was more healthful.

Supplements supplying nutrients at levels beyond what can reasonably be obtained from food should be viewed as nonprescription drugs. High-potency products should not be used without careful thought and perhaps expert help.

POINT 8: FOCUSING ON NUTRIENTS AND SUPPLEMENTS CAN TAKE ATTENTION AND CONVICTION AWAY FROM IMPROVING ONE'S LIFESTYLE

Nationally representative surveys of American adults show that approximately one third are interested in nutrition and think they are on the right track to healthy eating. In contrast, another third couldn't care less about meeting dietary guidelines. Those in the middle third claim they are trying to eat better, but find it difficult.

So, the good news is that two thirds of adult Americans say they care about their nutrition. But the bad news is that perhaps only 5 to 10% of the US population meets dietary recommendations regularly, such as eating five or more servings of fruits and vegetables per day and limiting fat to no more than 30% of calories. Furthermore, obesity is a growing epidemic in this country, now affecting one third of adults and one quarter of children. The irony is that people who eat well are most likely to take supplements, whereas those most likely to benefit from higher nutrient intakes are least likely to take them.

> ### Dietary supplements provide a false sense of security.

My greatest concern about dietary supplements is the false sense of security it provides some people, those who use supplements to an extent as substitutes for a good diet. It is natural for us to want an easier way or, ideally, some magic bullet, to achieve health short of being vigilant or saintly all the time. We're especially likely to cut corners when we are short of time and feeling stressed, such as by choosing foods on the basis of convenience and ease of preparation and by not exercising. Taking a basic supplement as one small part of a health-promoting lifestyle may be reasonable and perhaps even prudent. But taking supplements is a problem for people, probably the majority, who are not making the lifestyle changes they know they should. A recent advertisement by Hoffman-La Roche, Inc. for vitamin E states . . . "Many doctors . . . believe taking supplements or eating fortified foods containing vitamins and minerals is a sound health measure, particularly for people who don't eat a good diet. . . . " Unfortunately, some people use supplements as a deliberate or unconscious excuse for not trying to improve their diets and lifestyles.

A reporter called me some time ago to ask how people could use vitamins to stay healthy. I replied that people should pay more attention to their diets. He told me to be realistic and used himself as an example. He said he leads a very busy life, has little time to shop for food and prepare it, and there are few places near work that serve nutritious lunches. So what supplements would help him cope more productively with his situation? Here is an example where supplements may harm more than help, by being used as a surrogate for tackling the hard things that would really improve his nutritional status, such as preparing lunches the night before, convincing nearby restaurants to offer more nutritious fare, and making sure he eats a very nutritious breakfast and dinner. This reporter was looking for what he acknowledged to be a second-best solution, but taking a supplement will make him even less likely to attempt the best but more difficult solution.

CONCLUDING THOUGHTS

. . . Those who recommend that healthy people supplement their diets with extra vitamins and minerals often call it a form of dietary insurance, as essential to have as car or home insurance. I disagree. When you purchase insurance, the benefits and costs of the policy are detailed and you choose a specific level of protection. The terms of a dietary insurance policy, though,

> ### Concentrating anything in the food chain, be it vitamin C, beta-carotene, salt, or fat, increases the likelihood of mistakes.

can never be known, much less specified. Taking supplements without a clear need is more analogous to playing the lottery. You hope to win some money, and ideally the jackpot, by buying lottery tickets. You won't hurt yourself unless you buy more tickets over time than you can afford, but you are not likely to win anything either, especially the big prize.

Even comprehensive dietary supplements are, at best, poor substitutes for nutrient-rich foods. Foods, about which we know little, are more than the sum of their parts, about which we have some knowledge. Furthermore, it's harder to hurt yourself with foods than with supplements. Concentrating anything in the food chain—be it vitamin C, beta-carotene, salt, or fat—increases the likelihood of mistakes. Nutrients and other nonnutrient substances relevant to health are readily available in familiar and attractive packages called fruits, vegetables, legumes, grains, and animal products. And they come in concentrations and in combinations with which humans have had long cultural familiarity.[29] . . .

REFERENCES

1. Slesinski MJ, Subar AF, Kahle LL. Trends in use of vitamin and mineral supplements in the United States: The 1987 and 1992 National Health Interview Surveys. *J Am Diet Assoc* 1995;95:921–3.
2. National Research Council. *Diet and Health: Implications for Reducing Chronic Disease Risk.* Washington, DC: National Academy Press, 1989.
3. US Department of Agriculture, Department of Health and Human Services. *Nutrition and Your Health: Dietary Guidelines for Americans,* 4th ed. Washington, DC: Government Printing Office, 1995.
4. Brody J. Personal health: Sorting out the benefits of taking extra vitamin E. *New York Times,* July 26, 1995:C8.
5. Golub E. *The Limits of Medicine: How Science Shapes Our Hope for the Cure.* New York: Times Books, 1994.
6. Hiser E. Getting into your genes. *Eating Well* 1995;6(1):48–9.
7. Herbert V, Kasdan TS. Misleading nutrition claims and their gurus. *Nutr Today* 29(3):28–35, 1994.
8. Begley S. Beyond vitamins: The search for the magic pill. *Newsweek,* April 25, 1994:45–9.
9. The Alpha-Tocopherol, Beta-Carotene Cancer Prevention Study Group. The effect of vitamin E and beta carotene on the incidence of lung cancer and other cancers in male smokers. *N Engl J Med* 1994;330:1029–35.
10. Blumberg JB. Considerations of the scientific substantiation for antioxidant vitamins and β-carotene in disease prevention. *Am J Clin Nutr* 1995;62:1521S–1526S.
11. Liebman B. Antioxidants: Surprise, surprise. *Nutr Action Healthletter* 1994;21(5):4.
12. Wade N. Method and madness: Believing in vitamins. *New York Times Magazine,* May 22, 1994:20.
13. Herbert V. The antioxidant supplement myth. *Am J Clin Nutr* 1994;60:157–8.
14. Graziano JM, Johnson EJ, Russell RM, Manson

JE, Stampfer MJ, Ridker PM, Frei B, Hennekens CH, Krinsky NI. Discrimination in absorption or transport of β-carotene isomers after oral supplementation with either all-*trans-* or 9-*cis*-β-carotene. *Am J Clin Nutr* 1995;61:1248–52.

15. McCord JM. Free radicals and prooxidants in health and nutrition. *Food Tech* 1994;48(5):106–11.

16. Anon. Buying vitamins: what's worth the price? *Consumer Rep* 1994;59:565–9.

17. Schardt D, Schmidt S. Garlic: Clove at first sight? *Nutr Action Healthletter* 1995;22(6)3–5.

18. Anon. Herbal roulette. *Consumer Rep* 1995;60:698–705.

19. Anon. A 9-point guide to choosing the right supplement. *Tufts Univ Diet & Nutr Letter* 1993;11(7)3–6.

20. Liebman B, Schardt D. Vitamin smarts. *Nutr Action Healthletter* 1995;22(9):1,6–10.

21. Houn F, Bober MA, Huerta EE, Hursting SD, Lemon S, Weed DL. The association between alcohol and breast cancer: Popular press coverage of research. *Am J Publ Health* 1995;85:1082–6.

22. Goodman E. To swallow or not to swallow. *Liberal Opinion Week*, April 24, 1994.

23. Nelkin D. *Selling Science: How the Press Covers Science and Technology*, revised edition. New York: WH Freeman and Company, 1995.

24. Anon. Many shoppers not yet aware of nutrition facts label. *Food Labeling News* 1995;3(32):21–3.

25. Gussow JD. *A Word on Behalf of Food*. Presentation at the Alumni Advances Conference of the dietetic internship program at Oregon Health Sciences University, Portland, OR, May 1995.

26. Shepherd SK. Nutrition and the consumer: Meeting the challenge of nutrition education in the 1990s. *Food & Consumer News* 1990;62(1):1–3.

27. Goodman E. Food literacy. *Liberal Opinion Week*, December 14, 1992.

28. Stacey M. *Consumed: Why Americans Love, Hate, and Fear Food*. New York: Touchstone Books, 1994.

29. Gussow JD, Thomas PR. *The Nutrition Debate: Sorting Out Some Answers*. Palo Alto, CA: Bull Publishing Co., 1986.

The views expressed in this article are those of the author and do not reflect the position of the Center for Food and Nutrition Policy.

Vitamin A: Pregnancy Hazard?

THE STORY

In an unusual move that underscores the importance of new findings linking vitamin A and birth defects, the editor of the *New England Journal of Medicine* waived the journal's customary rule forbidding researchers to release their data prior to publication.

The report, scheduled to appear in the November 24 *NEJM*, suggests that vitamin A doses as low as four times the recommended dietary allowance (RDA) markedly increase a pregnant woman's chance of having a baby with a cleft palate, heart defects, or other problems. Dr. Kenneth J. Rothman of Boston University presented his group's findings at an October 6 press conference.

Previous studies have implicated vitamin A as a cause of birth defects, but it's been unclear at how low a dose the hazard begins to emerge. To answer this question, the researchers interviewed more than 22,000 women early in pregnancy about their diets and vitamin use, and from this estimated their vitamin A intake. They then compared the rate of birth defects among babies exposed to different amounts of the vitamin.

The RDA for vitamin A in adult women is 2,700 international units (IU). In this study, the risk of birth defects began to increase with daily vitamin A doses of 10,000 IU and above, and roughly quadrupled in women taking 20,000 IU daily. Although these amounts are well above the RDA, supplements containing these or even higher doses in a single capsule are available at grocery and health-food stores and pharmacies. Excessive amounts of foods rich in vitamin A also pose a possible hazard, the researchers noted.

The researchers estimated that one out of every 60 babies born to women taking vitamin A doses above 10,000 IU is "adversely affected" by the vitamin. — *The Editors*

THE PHYSICIAN'S PERSPECTIVE

Sheldon H. Cherry, MD

This study provides compelling evidence that vitamin A doses even moderately above the recommended daily allowance are potentially harmful to a fetus. On the basis of this finding, **I would advise pregnant women and those planning to become pregnant to carefully watch their vitamin A intake – both from vitamin supplements and from foods – and to keep their daily level below 10,000 international units.** At the same time, they should be aware that getting *inadequate* amounts of any vitamin carries its own hazards to the mother and fetus.

Physicians generally hesitate to make health recommendations on the basis of a single study. In this case, it is true that the study's design could have skewed its findings. For instance, the women's vitamin A intake was estimated from their own reports about their diets, which can be unreliable. But because numerous earlier animal and human studies have shown a strong link between this vitamin and birth defects, the latest results are plausible and the recommendation to avoid high vitamin A doses seems prudent. These data, however, will need to be verified by follow-up studies.

The vitamin A referred to in this research should not be confused with beta carotene, a precursor compound that the body converts to vitamin A. There's no reason to be concerned that consuming beta carotene, either in supplements or in foods such as carrots or tomatoes, is harmful in pregnancy.

What women should be careful about is inadvertently consuming potentially harmful amounts of vitamin A either in supplements or by combining doses from several sources. For example, a woman who takes prenatal vitamin supplements, which typically contain 4,000 IU of the vitamin, and regularly eats vitamin-A-rich foods such as liver, fortified cereals, or dairy products could top 10,000 IU. In addition, many over-the-counter multivitamins contain as much as 10,000 IU. In some vitamin A preparations, single pills contain 25,000 IU.

Pregnant women taking a multivitamin supplement or specially formulated prenatal vitamins should be sure to take no more than one pill a day. And I would discourage these women from taking any supplement of pure vitamin A, unless it's specifically prescribed by a doctor.

Finally, because vitamin A is stored in the body — and because a woman may not know she is pregnant during the first few weeks after conception — a woman of childbearing age should be aware of the possible danger of taking larger doses of vitamin A if she is trying to conceive. HN

Dr. Cherry is a professor of obstetrics and gynecology at Mount Sinai School of Medicine and Medical Center. He has written several books for the general public on pregnancy and women's health.

The trials of beta-carotene: Is the verdict in?

It hasn't been glamorous or provocative, and it may have sounded ultra-conservative. But despite the steady stream of news stories and the constant barrage of advertising touting the magic-bullet benefits of vitamins C and E and beta-carotene, we've urged our readers to think twice before popping antioxidant supplements. The best way to get your antioxidants, we've held firmly, is to eat a diet rich in fruits and vegetables.

Of course, it's easy to see why Americans have been spending $40 million annually on beta-carotene supplements alone. After all, vitamin pills, sold over-the-counter, have seemed so harmless.

Yet the National Cancer Institute recently put the brakes on a long-term, $42 million beta-carotene research trial because of findings that the antioxidant might be harming participants. At the same time, another major study concluded that beta-carotene did not improve the health of more than 22,000 men who had been swallowing supplements for a decade.

Did scientists miss the mark? Have the potential benefits of beta-carotene been overblown? Worse still, have people taking beta-carotene supplements been harming themselves?

Circumstantial evidence

Exactly 15 years ago, in March 1981, a group of internationally renowned cancer researchers published a landmark paper that tossed into the scientific arena a theory rife with possibility. They pointed to a number of studies showing that in populations where consumption of fruits and vegetables rich in beta-carotene runs high, the risk of cancer runs low. These findings suggested that beta-carotene may somehow help stall the development of malignant tumors. Evidence of a link between high blood levels of beta-carotene and low cancer rates lent weight to the theory.

Naturally, the idea that beta-carotene might offer protection against cancer was an enticing one. It had been 10 years since Richard Nixon declared the "war on cancer," yet researchers were making little headway in their search for ways to prevent the disease. If an inexpensive, easy-to-swallow, seemingly harmless substance like beta-carotene could solve the problem, it would be a boon to public health.

So scientists embarked on numerous studies, and the results looked promising, especially for lung cancer. Between 1983 and 1993, more than two dozen studies linking beta-carotene to a reduced incidence of lung cancer were published. Overall, the reports consistently indicated anywhere from a 10 to 70 percent drop in the risk of lung cancer in people whose diets were high in beta-carotene.

Deliberations

While the studies were insightful, their conclusions were far from definitive. They mostly showed loose associations: for example, people with high blood levels of beta-carotene tended to have lower rates of cancer than people with lower beta-carotene blood levels. But that doesn't prove that taking beta-carotene pills will reduce cancer risk.

To learn whether the connection is more than a coincidence, a chemoprevention trial is necessary. In this type of study, people are given the substance in question and then followed to see if they are less likely to develop disease than people not given the test substance.

Because cancer can take decades to develop, chemoprevention trials typically last many years. And they often involve thousands of people. The duration and number of participants make for a very high price tag. But given the enormous potential of beta-carotene, the National Cancer Institute began pouring millions of dollars into a number of beta-carotene chemoprevention trials during the mid-1980s.

In 1994, the results came in for one of the first of these studies, the Alpha-Tocopherol, Beta-Carotene Cancer Prevention Trial—the ATBC Trial, for short. The news was disturbing. After more than 29,000 male smokers in Finland took supplements of either vitamin E, beta-carotene, or a "dummy" placebo pill daily for five to eight years, 18 percent more cases of lung cancer and 8 percent more overall deaths occurred in the beta-carotene group than in the other groups. Because these results countered those of earlier studies, however, scientists chalked them up to a possible statistical fluke and punctuated them with a large question mark.

Then in January of this year, an independent watchdog committee monitoring a similar, ongoing study called the Beta Carotene and Retinol Efficacy Trial

(CARET) noticed the same trend. After an average of four years, 28 percent more cases of lung cancer and 17 percent more overall deaths had occurred in the group taking beta-carotene. Because it looked as if beta-carotene wasn't helping and may actually have been *harming* participants, the trial was halted in January.

Simultaneously, yet another eyebrow-raising announcement was made about the Physicians' Health Study, a 12-year look by Harvard researchers at more than 22,000 male physicians. Again, beta-carotene came up short, apparently conferring no protection against cancer or heart disease.

Rush to judgment?

On the face of it, the newly released results suggest that millions of consumers who have been taking beta-carotene pills may have been hurting themselves—or at least wasting their time. But experts maintain that even in light of the negative findings, the beta-carotene case is not closed.

Consider that the ATBC trial involved only male smokers. And CARET included only smokers, former smokers, and workers exposed to asbestos. Scientists suspect that something about long-term exposure to cigarette smoke or asbestos in combination with beta-carotene supplements may promote lung cancer. It might be that some component of cigarette smoke interacts with beta-carotene to generate particularly harmful by-products in the body, according to Norman Krinsky, PhD, a beta-carotene expert at the Tufts University School of Medicine. But at this point, he says, "We know zilch about what these by-products might be," and more research is required to pinpoint them.

Another unanswered question is why study after study has revealed a significant association between diets rich in beta-carotene and a reduced risk of lung cancer, but the major supplement trials have "failed." Again, possibilities abound. Maybe beta-carotene "works" only in the presence of some other substance in fruits and vegetables, like chlorophyll. Or perhaps it's not beta-carotene at all, but some other substance in produce that confers protection against cancer.

Back in the 1980s, when interest in beta-carotene took off, it was the only member of a group of substances called carotenoids that scientists had singled

---

Beta-carotene and beyond

Time was when nutritionists viewed beta-carotene and other members of the carotenoid family as nothing more than vitamin A precursors, that is, substances that were converted into vitamin A in the body. Today we know of more than 500 different carotenoids, many of which appear to function as much more than just vitamin A precursors.

Scientists have only begun to scratch the surface to learn about how these substances work in the body. Preliminary research suggests that two carotenoids—lutein and zeaxanthin—protect the eyes against age-related macular degeneration, which afflicts one in three people over age 75. Another carotenoid, lycopene, may help stave off prostate cancer.

Despite the potential of carotenoids, food composition tables currently used by nutritionists still lump beta-carotene and its relatives together under vitamin A, making it difficult to identify good sources of particular carotenoids. Fortunately, the U.S. Department of Agriculture and the National Cancer Institute have begun putting together the first carotenoid database, from which the following chart is derived.

Note that there is no recommended dietary allowance for the various carotenoids. The table however, highlights good sources of carotenoids and underscores the benefits of eating a wide variety of produce. It also helps you see what you're missing if you rely on supplements alone rather than eating fruits and vegetables.

	Beta-Carotene (micrograms)*	Lutein & Zeaxanthin (micrograms)	Lycopene (micrograms)
½ cup cooked broccoli	1,014	1,404	0
½ cup Brussels sprouts	374	1,014	0
1 medium raw carrot	5,688	187	0
½ medium pink grapefruit	1,611	0	4,135
½ cup cooked kale	3,055	14,235	0
1 medium peach	86	12	0
1 cup raw spinach	2,296	5,712	0
1 medium tomato	640	123	3,813
¾ cup tomato juice	1,638	0	15,616

*A microgram is a thousandth of a milligram. Amounts are averages taken from a number of samples and should be viewed as estimates rather than hard-and-fast values.

out as a possible disease fighter. And because beta-carotene was available in pill form, it was a convenient substance to test in large-scale trials. During the past few years, however, scientists have come up with more and more research suggesting that beta-carotene is just one of many members of the carotenoid family that may fight disease.

For example, researchers now suspect that the carotenoids called lutein and zeaxanthin, found in spinach, kale, and broccoli, help protect against an eye condition called age-related macular degeneration, which ranks as the leading cause of irreversible blindness among older adults. And in December, Harvard University researchers published a study linking diets rich in another carotenoid named lycopene, found primarily in tomatoes, with a decreased risk of prostate cancer. Because beta-carotene is found along with other carotenoids in fruits and vegetables, it may serve as a marker of fruit and vegetable consumption but not be the ingredient that is staving off disease (see box).

The trials continue

Another reason experts say the jury is still out on beta-carotene concerns the design of the studies that have been concluded or stopped thus far. The Physicians' Health Study was a primary prevention trial aimed at determining if beta-carotene helps prevent cancer or heart disease in a healthy population. The ATBC trial and CARET were both *secondary* prevention trials, which were designed to see whether beta-carotene helps prevent cancer in high-risk groups like smokers or people exposed to asbestos. But if beta-carotene supplements were tested in, say, a secondary prevention study of a large group of men at high risk for a disease other than lung cancer, the outcome might be different. What's more, all three trials involved only men; beta-carotene may behave differently in women.

Because so many questions remain, some of the trials on beta-carotene are continuing despite the latest round of negative findings. One is a secondary prevention trial called the Women's Antioxidant and Cardiovascular Study, designed to evaluate the effect of vitamin E, vitamin C, and beta-carotene in some 8,000 women at high risk for heart disease. Besides acting as an antioxidant, beta-carotene is thought to help relax the artery walls, making them more flexible and less likely to become blocked.

"We haven't seen any evidence of harm from beta-carotene in these women, and there's good reason to believe beta-carotene may benefit them," says JoAnn Manson, MD, a Harvard researcher who is spearheading the trial. "But we're going to be monitoring the interim results very closely."

Vitamin E

Promising, but don't take its reputation to heart yet

From newspapers to magazines to television, vitamin E is being touted as the newest weapon against cardiovascular disease.

But if you're ready to say "Give me an E," hold on. Despite some promising reports, researchers haven't proven vitamin E's benefits.

The bottom line? Vitamin E shows promise in the fight against cardiovascular disease, but the final chapter isn't written.

Slowing down oxidation

Scientists discovered vitamin E in 1922. Also called alpha-tocopherol (al-fuh-to-KOF-ur-ol), vitamin E is necessary for normal function of the nervous system and red blood cell formation. It also protects cell membranes from damage through oxidation.

Dietary sources of vitamin E include green, leafy vegetables and oils, nuts and wheat germ.

One of vitamin E's first commercial uses was to retard food spoilage. This may help you understand its possible role in preventing heart attacks.

Picture a stick of butter. After sitting out a few days, it no longer tastes fresh. The reason? Fatty acids in it turn rancid when exposed to oxygen. This process is oxidation.

When oxidation occurs, fatty acids undergo chemical changes. In foods, that results in different smells or tastes. Vitamin E can slow this process. That's why it's known as an antioxidant.

Fatty acids are also found in your blood, along with low-density lipoproteins (LDL), commonly referred to as "bad cholesterol." Oxidation causes changes in these, too. The changes may enable cells in your arteries to more easily absorb fatty acids and LDL. Over time, this process could cause plaque buildup

and blockage of your arteries. Vitamin E may reduce cardiovascular disease by slowing oxidation.

Promising early studies

Two studies reported in 1993 in the *New England Journal of Medicine* enhanced vitamin E's reputation. In them, researchers reported that vitamin E appeared to reduce your risk of cardiovascular disease by about 40 percent.

Other studies have also indicated that vitamin E may provide protection against cardiovascular disease. One such study involved coronary artery bypass surgery. Patients taking 100 international units (IU) of vitamin E daily had less artery blockage two years after the surgery than those who didn't take vitamin E.

In addition, British researchers reported in March that taking vitamin E appears to reduce your risk of heart attack by 75 percent if you already have cardiovascular disease. But, their study found vitamin E had no impact on the overall death rate from cardiovascular disease. U.S. doctors question the findings.

The other side of the story

The news about vitamin E is certainly promising. But should you be taking supplements? Here are things to keep in mind:

■ *Large doses* — Most studies involved doses much larger than the U.S. Recommended Dietary Allowance (RDA). Often, the dose was 400 IU or more a day. In comparison, the RDA is only 12 IU for women and 15 IU for men.

Supplements are the only way to ingest as much vitamin E as used in studies. Even food sources "rich" in vitamin E contain only small quantities. To get your RDA from broccoli alone, you'd have to eat almost five pounds. From butter alone, you'd have to eat half a pound.

At doses used in these studies, vitamin E becomes a drug, not a nutrient. According to the World Health Organization, you may take up to 1,080 IU daily with no side effects. But more than that can trigger health problems.

■ *Potential side effects* — Side effects can include gastrointestinal complaints. And bleeding can occur if you are taking blood-thinning medications such as warfarin (Coumadin, Panwarfin).

■ *Antioxidant concerns* — Researchers were initially very optimistic about the role of another antioxidant, beta carotene, in fighting cancer and cardiovascular disease. But more recent National Cancer Institute (NCI) studies have found that too much beta carotene can do you more harm than good.

In January, researchers reported that beta carotene may increase your risk of lung cancer if you smoke. Also in January, another NCI study reported that beta carotene provides no protection against cancer and cardiovascular disease.

Study still needed

Initial reports of vitamin E's role in fighting cardiovascular disease appear promising. However, research is incomplete. More study is needed to establish the safety and benefits of vitamin E and other antioxidants.

At RDA levels, vitamin E remains an important part of your diet. Someday, it might be a potent weapon against cardiovascular disease. But until its benefits are proven, you should consult your doctor before taking its reputation to heart.

Vitamin C: Is Anyone Right On Dose?

JANE E. BRODY

HOW much vitamin C is enough? Is it the 60 milligrams a day—the amount in half a cup of fresh orange juice—that is the current Recommended Dietary Allowance (R.D.A.), the 30 to 40 milligrams that some nutritional biochemists think it should be, the hundreds of milligrams that millions of Americans now take as a daily supplement or the thousands of milligrams that Dr. Linus Pauling believed would protect against serious illnesses, including cancer?

A new study says 200 milligrams a day is optimal.

A detailed new federally sponsored study, by far the most comprehensively done to date, says none of the above. The study, directed by Dr. Mark Levine and published today in The Proceedings of the National Academy of Sciences, found that the "optimal" daily intake of vitamin C was more like 200 milligrams, although only about 10 milligrams are needed to prevent vitamin C deficiency.

More than 1,000 milligrams a day of vitamin C may even be hazardous.

The researchers, at the National Institutes of Health, also concluded that daily doses above 400 milligrams "have no evident value" and that amounts of 1,000 milligrams (1 gram) or more, which many people now take as daily supplements or on occasion to prevent or treat illness, could be hazardous. Beyond a dose of about 400 milligrams, the study showed, the body's ability to absorb vitamin C sharply declines and excess vitamin is excreted.

Megadoses of vitamin C are said to do nothing in healthy people.

Unlike previous studies used to establish recommended amounts, this one looked beyond the levels needed to prevent scurvy.

"This means Linus Pauling was all wrong, at least with respect to healthy people," Dr. Levine remarked in an interview. "He had the best of intentions, but he did not have the science to support his hypothesis." Dr. Levine said that "in healthy people, megadoses are doing nothing and may do harm, and in sick people, I don't think they will be helpful either."

Industry sources estimate that 30 to 40 percent of Americans now take vitamin C supplements, and that about 1 in 5 supplement users take more than 1,000 milligrams a day.

Although the 200-milligram level is more than three times the currently recommended amount, it is a level that can still be readily obtained from foods, especially if one follows the latest Federal advice to eat five or more servings a day of fruits and vegetables. For example, one would exceed the 200-milligram level by consuming four ounces of orange juice, half a cup of cooked broccoli, one baked potato and one kiwi fruit.

But the most recent national survey indicated that less than a third of Americans consumed five or more servings of fruits and vegetables a day. This suggests that unless significant improvements are made in people's eating habits, it would be necessary to take supplements or fortify commonly eaten foods with vitamin C for most of the population to consume 200 milligrams each day.

Dr. Adrianne Bendich, assistant director of human nutrition research at Hoffman-La Roche, a major manufacturer of bulk vitamin C, said a recent review she had conducted of dozens of well-designed studies of vitamin C showed that even at daily doses of a 1,000 milligrams or more, no adverse effects had been reported in otherwise healthy people. Dr. Bendich said she saw "no problem with raising the current R.D.A." The R.D.A.'s are established by the academy's Food and Nutrition Board as safe and desirable levels of intake by healthy people to prevent nutritional deficiencies.

Martin Hirsch, public policy director for Hoffman-La Roche, said the company "welcomes publication of new data that support a shift from thinking about the R.D.A.'s as a means of preventing nutritional deficiency to viewing them as a way to promote optimal health."

But other nutrition scientists who served on the last R.D.A. committee challenged the study's conclusions that 200 milligrams of vitamin C, also known as ascorbic acid or ascorbate, are necessary or desirable. Dr. Victor Herbert, a nutrition researcher at the Bronx Veterans Affairs Medical Center who generally disputes the need for supplements, called the study's conclusions "fraudulent." He noted that the study had excluded people with health conditions, like a family history of kidney stones or a tendency to accumulate iron, which could be worsened by taking amounts of vitamin C beyond the current R.D.A. He said that even consuming 200 milligrams a day could be harmful to as many as one-third of Americans. For example, he said, 12 percent of Americans have iron overload and could be made worse by this amount of vitamin C.

A study does not suggest dosages for children or ill adults.

Dr. Levine said he had excluded people with various illnesses because he did not want to risk harming anyone with the high doses used in part of the study. He also said that the findings strictly applied "only to young, healthy men," and he noted, "We don't know what will happen to sick people, women, the elderly or children." A similar study is under way in young, healthy women.

Dr. John N. Hathcock, director for nutritional and regulatory science at the Council for Responsible Nutrition, a[n] organization supported by the supplement industry, agreed that "you can't say from this study that 200 milligrams of vitamin C is safe or harmful for people with conditions that were excluded." But, he added, "If a person has such a condition, that person should be under the care of a physician and should take his or her advice regarding vitamin C intake."

Dr. James Allen Olson, a biochemist at Iowa State University in Ames who, like Dr. Herbert, served on the committee that established the current R.D.A.'s, questioned the study's assumption that because the 200-milligram dose was best absorbed and utilized by body tissues, that this would mean that it was the most desirable amount.

But Dr. John Erdman Jr., a nutritional scientist at the University of Illinois who is a member of the academy's Food and Nutrition Board, said the group was already considering a change in the basic concept of the R.D.A. "to consider outcomes that would go beyond just the prevention of deficiency diseases." For vitamin C, for example, such outcomes might include "enhancing the immune response," he said. He added that the new study provided "the kind of data the R.D.A. committee would look at very strongly." He said the committee "would have to decide whether saturation of cells with vitamin C was a necessary and a desirable goal."

The study, sponsored by the National Institute of Diabetes and Digestive and Kidney Diseases in Bethesda, Md., analyzed the biochemical effects of various amounts of vitamin C administered to seven healthy young men who lived in a hospital ward for four to six months. Nutrient requirement studies, which are very costly and time-consuming, are typically done on small numbers of participants. Although most researchers would prefer that the studies be larger, their exacting nature can yield meaningful results, unlike clinical and epidemiological studies that require many participants to achieve statistical significance.

The men's blood levels of vitamin C were first depleted by placing the men on a daily diet that contained less than five milligrams of this essential nutrient. Then, while continuing their vitamin C-deficient diet, the men were given seven different doses of the vitamin to determine which level was best absorbed and would result in peak amounts in the blood and tissues. The doses studied, which were administered sequentially, were 30, 60, 100, 200, 400, 1,000 and 2,500 milligrams a day.

The team of 11 researchers determined which doses were fully absorbed, which produced "saturation levels" in blood plasma, white blood cells and other tissues and which resulted in excretion of vitamin C or its metabolic products in the stool and urine. The white blood cells, a vital component of the immune system, were saturated at a dose of 100 milligrams a day. That is, beyond this dose no more vitamin C was absorbed by the cells. The blood plasma was nearly saturated by a dose of 200 milligrams and fully saturated at 1,000 milligrams, the researchers found.

But beyond 100 milligrams, the volunteers began to excrete some vitamin C in their urine, indicating that the body was not using all that it absorbed. Absorption levels through the gut also declined as dosages were increased beyond 200 milligrams. At 500 milligrams, less than three-fourths of the vitamin C administered to the volunteers was absorbed, and at 1,250 milligrams, less than half was absorbed, Dr. Levine said.

At 1,000 milligrams or more, the urine was found to contain oxalate, a breakdown product of vitamin C that in some people can result in the formation of kidney stones. A second substance, urate, which results from the breakdown of nucleic acids, the building blocks of genes, also accumulated in urine at these high doses, Dr. Levine reported. An endocrinologist by training, Dr. Levine is chief of the molecular and clinical nutrition section at the Federal institute.

"It looks as if the body is very tightly regulated with respect to vitamin C," Dr. Levine said. "It seems to be saying 'enough is enough.' Beyond 200 milligrams, the cells don't fill up any more, plasma fills up very little, absorption goes down and excretion goes up."

Dr. Levine said there was no "absolute proof" that it was best to be saturated with vitamin C. "Our study doesn't prove that 200 milligrams a day will prevent heart disease, cancer or infectious illnesses," he said. But he added that he and his colleagues were impressed by the fact that many pieces of evidence "converge on 200 milligrams as the right dose," including the amount that people get from diets rich in fruits and vegetables, how much is absorbed by the body, the dose that results in saturation of cells and blood, the amount that may be toxic and the amount that is consumed by people who are relatively protected against various serious diseases.

Dr. Levine said: "The current R.D.A. for vitamin C is based on flawed studies and that its very concept—to prevent scurvy—is outmoded. We should be basing our recommendation on what is best for the population, not just to prevent a deficiency disease."

Special report: iron overkill

Eat foods rich in iron—that advice has been a cornerstone of modern nutrition. Indeed, millions of Americans, including up to 10% of women aged 20 to 50, have an iron deficiency. That's why a Finnish study made headlines in 1992 when it raised fears about iron by suggesting that a high level of the mineral in the body increases the risk of a heart attack. At the time, we concluded that the study raised more questions than it answered. Still, some people started avoiding iron—or at least stopped trying to get enough of it. Since then, many studies, of a variety of types, have looked at the iron question. Most have disputed the results of the Finnish study, but have received far less media attention. Iron deserves another look.

Casting iron as a villain

The theory linking high levels of stored iron (usually measured as ferritin) in the body with coronary artery disease (CAD) was first proposed in 1981. According to it, many factors that alter the risk for heart attacks can be explained by their effect on the body's iron levels. For instance, young women may be at lower cardiac risk because their menstrual blood loss keeps their iron stores low; thus after menopause, women's iron stores rise, as does their CAD risk. Similarly, aspirin may protect the heart by causing slight gastrointestinal bleeding, thereby reducing iron stores. However, as we previously concluded, there's little or no evidence to support these iron-based explanations.

The 1992 study found that among men from eastern Finland (where the average ferritin level and death rate from heart attacks are among the highest in the world), those with higher levels of ferritin were twice as likely to have a heart attack as men with lower levels. The Finnish researchers theorized that iron triggers CAD by increasing the formation of free radicals. These highly reactive substances in turn oxidize "bad" (LDL) cholesterol, making it sticky and thus likelier to block coronary arteries. Some researchers suggest that by boosting free radicals, iron overload may also increase the risk of cancer.

Ironing out the differences

Here's a sampling of the studies since then. Two studies, one from Iceland, the other from Harvard, followed subjects over time and found no relation between ferritin and CAD. Another study from Harvard found that rather than iron per se, only iron from animal sources, primarily red meat, increased the risk of heart attack in men. In that case, iron may be a marker for meat intake, and the meat's saturated fat (or some other component) could be part of the problem. Another way to gauge the body's iron status is to measure transferrin, a protein that shuttles iron around the body. Three studies that looked at this in men and women found no link to heart disease; one actually found higher levels of stored iron to be *protective* against CAD. In five case-control studies, in which people with CAD were compared with healthy "controls," only one found a link between iron levels and heart disease. And two studies looking at autopsies found no relationship between very high iron stores and CAD.

The iron you eat

Nearly all the studies have focused on iron stored in the body, not the amount of iron people eat. It has long been known that there is little correlation between the two: the body doesn't simply store away extra iron from foods. Only a little dietary iron is absorbed by the body. The absorption process is affected not only by the amount of iron you eat, but also by its sources (for instance, the "heme" iron in meat is best absorbed), the composition of your meals, genetic factors, and your body's needs (if your iron stores are low or you have greater needs because of rapid growth or pregnancy, for instance, you absorb more iron through the intestinal tract). Thus an iron-rich diet by itself won't necessarily lead to iron overload. And cutting down on the iron you eat may not significantly reduce the amount of iron stored in your body, especially if you are genetically predisposed to over-absorb iron.

The genetic issue: hemochromatosis

There is no dispute that some people *do* need to worry about iron overload: more than one million Americans have a hereditary disorder known as hemochromatosis, which causes them to absorb too much iron. When untreated, this can lead to weakness, headaches, and joint pain, and eventually diabetes, arthritis, cirrhosis of the liver, or heart disorders (but *not* heart attacks). Many more people carry only one gene for hemochromatosis (it takes two genes to develop the full-blown disorder), and may also accumulate higher-than-average stores of iron, but it's not known if this affects their health.

There is no test for the hemochromatosis gene, since it has not been identified. But if you develop symptoms that may be related to the disease or have a family history of it, simple blood tests can help diagnose it.

What to do

While the average American's consumption of iron has increased over the decades, his risk of heart attack has *fallen substantially*, not risen. Since most of the evidence doesn't support the link between iron and CAD, continue to eat the foods that supply your daily requirement of iron. Iron remains an extremely important mineral, essential for the formation of hemoglobin, which carries oxygen in red blood cells, and many other physiological functions. Initially there are no symptoms when the body's iron stores are depleted. But as the iron supply to the bone marrow dwindles, so does the marrow's ability to produce healthy red blood cells. Eventually this can result in iron-deficiency anemia, characterized by weakness, paleness, shortness of breath, and an increased susceptibility to infection.

Meat, poultry, fish, eggs, beans, enriched pasta and breads, fortified cereals, and nuts are all good iron sources. Cooking in iron pots adds iron to foods. Consuming foods rich in vitamin C, as well as small amounts of meats, boosts the absorption of iron from vegetarian sources. Though the iron in meat is best absorbed, strict vegetarians usually have no trouble consuming enough iron.

Even if you consume a balanced diet, you may not be getting adequate iron if you are in one of these groups:

✓ **Menstruating women,** especially those who bleed heavily, since blood losses increase iron needs.

✓ **Pregnant women.** Iron needs increase because of the demands of the fetus and placenta.

✓ **Dieters,** especially premenopausal women. The less you eat, the less likely you are to get enough iron.

✓ **Long-distance runners and other endurance athletes,** especially women and/or vegetarians, tend to have a higher incidence of iron deficiency, which, if severe, can impair performance. This iron shortfall has been attributed to a variety of reasons, including the increased elimination of iron during prolonged, especially high-impact, exercise.

✓ **Infants, children, and adolescents.** Youngsters need a high iron intake because of their rapid growth; deficiencies may adversely affect their learning capacity.

If you fall into one of these groups, you may need iron supplements. *But before taking them, consult your doctor, who, unless you're pregnant, should first determine if you are iron-deficient.* If you have hemochromatosis, prolonged consumption of iron pills can damage the liver, pancreas, and heart, and even be fatal. Since they consume enough iron, most men do not need iron pills, nor do most postmenopausal women. On the whole, eating more iron-rich foods is usually a better solution.

In the near future: *Doctors will probably screen patients routinely for iron overload by a blood test that will be part of regular physical exams. The test would be done once in a lifetime, preferably in early adulthood. Those thus found to be at risk for hemochromatosis will be advised to donate blood periodically to lower their iron stores, and told to avoid iron supplements.*

Fiber

Why you may need more, and good ways to get it

Remember oat bran? Back in the late 1980s, this source of dietary fiber became a national craze following reports that it significantly lowered cholesterol.

When oat bran didn't turn out to be the wonder product researchers had hoped, interest in high-fiber foods nose-dived. But studies continue to show there are health benefits to a high-fiber diet. And slowly, fiber is regaining favor.

Are you getting enough? If you're like most Americans, probably not.

Tough stuff

Your mother or grandmother may have called it "roughage" or "bulk." Dietary fiber is largely plant cell material that resists digestion. It moves unaltered through your stomach and small intestine and into your colon. There, some forms of fiber are fermented by bacteria. Others pass through unchanged.

The kinds of dietary fiber are:

■ *Insoluble* — This fiber doesn't dissolve in water and moves through your digestive system quickly. It's found mainly in vegetables, wheat bran and whole-grain breads and cereals.

■ *Soluble* — This forms a gel-like material in water. You can find it in generous quantities in oats, legumes (beans and peas) and fruits.

Benefits of bulking up

Dietary fiber is probably best known for its ability to prevent or relieve constipation. Insoluble fiber stimulates movement of your intestinal muscles, increases stool bulk and makes your stools softer and easier to pass.

But a high-fiber diet can also reduce your risk for many other health conditions, including:

■ *Gastrointestinal disorders* — Avoiding constipation reduces your risk of developing swollen anal tissues (hemorrhoids). A high-fiber diet also reduces pressure on colon walls. That can lessen your risk for diverticulosis (pouches that protrude through weak spots in your colon) and irritable bowel syndrome (muscle spasms in the walls of your bowel or stomach).

■ *Elevated cholesterol* — Scientists believe that soluble fiber binds with certain digestive acids made from cholesterol in your liver, and then escorts the acids away in stool. In response, your liver draws cholesterol from your blood to make more acids. That lowers your blood cholesterol.

However, fiber's cholesterol-lowering effects are modest. According to most studies, the average reduction in low-density lipoprotein (LDL or "bad") cholesterol is 3 to 7 percent after changing from a low- to high-fiber diet.

■ *Diabetes* — Soluble fiber slows absorption of blood sugar (glucose) from your small intestine, making sugar levels easier to control. In addition, high-fiber foods tend to be low in calories.

■ *Cancer* — A number of studies have linked a high-fiber diet to a reduced risk of colon cancer. Insoluble fiber speeds movement of digested food through your intestines. This may reduce the amount of time your colon is exposed to cancer-promoting substances formed during digestion. But it's not clear yet whether other ingredients in fibrous foods, or fiber alone, help protect you against cancer.

A high-fiber diet is also usually lower in fat, which may decrease cancer risk.

Ten easy ways you can fill up on dietary fiber

To increase the amount of fiber in your diet:

- Have an orange or grapefruit instead of juice for breakfast.
- Top your yogurt with fresh raspberries.
- Eat whole-wheat bread rather than white bread.
- Add raw bean or soybean sprouts to your sandwich.
- Munch on a carrot, apple (skin on) or pear.
- Choose bran flakes over corn flakes.
- Include beans in soups and vegetable salads.
- Substitute long-grain brown rice for white rice.
- Top your casseroles with a whole-grain cereal, such as shredded wheat.
- Eat the skin on your baked potato.

■ *Obesity* — Because fibrous foods are high in bulk, they require more chewing time. This gives your body time to register when you're no longer hungry, so you don't over-eat. The gel formed by soluble fiber also makes a meal feel larger and linger longer, so you stay full longer. Most high-fiber foods are also low in calories and fat.

■ *Hypertension* — In two observational studies, participants who ate the most fiber were less likely to develop high blood pressure than those who ate the least. However, clinical trials have failed to confirm a similar benefit.

Boosting your fiber intake

Americans typically consume 10 to 15 grams of fiber a day. Dietary guidelines recommend that you eat 20 to 35 grams.

The best way to boost your fiber intake is to eat a variety of fiber-rich foods. Instead of adding only bran cereals to your diet, include fruits, vegetables and legumes.

Products with the words "good source of fiber" or "contains fiber" provide 2.5 to 4.9 grams of fiber per serving. Foods labeled "high" or "rich" in fiber have at least 5 grams.

When buying breads or grains, look for the words "whole-wheat," "whole-grain" or "whole oats," or check to see if whole-wheat flour is listed as the first ingredient. Refined flour contains little fiber because processing removes the outer, fiber-rich layer of bran.

But be careful to increase your fiber intake gradually. That will give your stomach and intestines time to adjust to the dietary change. It will also minimize problems such as diarrhea, bloating or gas that can result when you eat too much fiber.

You should also drink more water than usual — an additional two or more 8-ounce glasses daily. Fiber attracts water to your intestines. Without the additional water, it could become constipating.

Food better than supplements

The best way to get your fiber is from food rather than commercial fiber supplements (Metamucil, Fibercon, Effer-syllium and others). Supplements don't provide the nutrients found in high-fiber foods. In addition, they cost more.

Fiber supplements are generally recommended if you're bothered by constipation but have trouble eating whole grains, beans and other high-fiber foods. Most supplements come in powder form that you mix with water and drink. But some are also available as biscuits, wafers, tablets or granules.

Through the Life Span: Diet and Disease

Food improperly taken, not only produces diseases, but affords those that are already engendered both matter and sustenance; so that, let the father of disease be what it may, intemperance is its mother.

—Richard E. Burton

When someone says, "You are what you eat," is it literally true? The parents of students who read this book may remember Adelle Davis, sometimes called the high priestess of nutrition. Among other things, she claimed that aging would not occur on the days one eats right. All of us know that this is not literally true, but scientists are constantly adding support to the belief that what we eat does affect what we are in both direct and indirect ways. Harry Golden provides an illustration from World War II (*Only in America*, Cleveland, Ohio: World Publishing Company, 1958, p. 308):

> When the Nazis took Denmark they requisitioned everything the Danes produced. The Danes, as you know, are famous dairy farmers and the Nazis took all their butter, animal fats, cheese, and allied products for their own armies. During that period the Danes were forced to lead an austere life and lived mostly on black bread and fish. What they have found out since is that during that austere period the incidence of degenerative diseases went way down—the Danes lived longer—but when the Danes got their butter, cheese, and animal fats back, the health chart went back to "normal" with a tremendous increase in stomach, heart, blood, and vein diseases. It is all a matter of diet, and I should hang my head in shame, being as fat as I am, and with no fewer than eleven thousand stories yet to write.

It is commonly agreed that a good, balanced diet throughout life will help us all reach our genetic potentials and avoid premature aging, disease, and untimely death. Studies of other populations, as in the quote above, often provide clues to diet/disease connections. Researchers must interpret them cautiously, however, as such studies cannot prove all-inclusive cause-and-effect relationships; sometimes the results even appear contradictory.

Many popular admonitions about what to eat or avoid eating have led to a good food/bad food philosophy. High-fat foods are bad for us and will cause unwanted weight gain, but carrots and spinach are good for us. A thoughtful person may realize that no food is inherently good or bad, that it is the quantity eaten that is problematic or beneficial. Thus, moderation is a key concept.

Add variety in what is eaten, and one is well on the way to a good diet.

The articles in this unit were selected because they concern the health of specific groups of people. Much is known and much is yet to be learned about the particular needs of various ethnic, age, and gender groups. Children cannot be viewed as little adults, nor does an adult's physiology remain static while aging. Males and females do not necessarily respond in the same way, and variations of significance can also be found among minority groups and between minority groups and whites. In all cases, knowledge and commitment can help the consumer to avoid the health and dietary pitfalls of either omission or commission.

The first article in this unit discusses the specific challenges related to nutrition/diet and improving the health status of various ethnic groups. Our nation's population is rapidly becoming more diverse, with 25 percent now of African, Hispanic, Asian/Pacific or Native American heritage. Health statistics show that minority groups generally have higher morbidity and mortality rates than do whites due to chronic diseases such as obesity, hypertension, and adult-onset diabetes mellitus. It follows that public health measures to reduce the incidence of these diseases must take cultural uniqueness as well as socioeconomic status into account.

Babies are the expressions of their parents' hopes and dreams, a fulfillment of themselves. Parents want their children's first experiences with the breast or the bottle to provide the very best start possible. Certainly a bottle-fed baby can be nurtured physically and emotionally, and no mother should be made to feel guilty if that is the method she chooses. At the same time, there is ample evidence that human milk provides the perfect nourishment as well as the ideal environment for bonding. No other method can transfer protection against early childhood diseases and be safe from contamination. The essay "Breast-Feeding Best Bet for Babies" identifies the issues that parents should consider very carefully before deciding whether to breast- or bottle-feed their baby.

Parents know that infancy is gone before one thinks about it, and toddlers become preschoolers. Eating habits are established early and in ways that sometimes leave parents mystified. Junior notices that Dad repeatedly passes the broccoli or the carrots without taking any and decides that real men don't eat vegetables. He discovers that certain behaviors are guaranteed to produce promises of treats from Mom. In a general sense, children seem to understand the concepts of healthful eating, but they also think their favorite foods aren't good for them and that healthful foods don't taste good. Like their parents, taste is a primary motivator in food choice. The article "Kids Just Want to Have Fun" talks about the roles that are appropriate for both parent and child in establishing food habits and some of the traps that can be avoided if the parent is knowledgeable and alert.

And then, suddenly, the teenage years arrive! As children, youngsters exerted enormous influence over how the food dollar was spent, often making choices and preparing meals without any parental input. Now, as teens, they are becoming even more independent of parents but decidedly influenced by their peers. Preoccupation with weight and appearance may be evident, often to the extremes of heavy dieting and nutrient deficiencies. Some will become so obsessed that they will join the ranks of those with eating disorders. The teen years will require plenty of nutrients including calcium to support a 45 percent increase in skeletal growth. Read the article "Teens at Risk" for a discussion of teen nutrient needs and dilemmas.

Life moves on, slipping eventfully and uneventfully through a few decades, and the 50th birthday is celebrated, with the golden years just beyond. Typically, we have gained weight, probably more than is currently considered healthy. And, as we reach our sixties and seventies, more and more of us will be dealing with high blood pressure, coronary disease, diabetes, arthritis, and other conditions that cause varying degrees of disability. Since these conditions have a connection to what we eat, lifestyle change becomes inevitable. An article on osteoporosis deals with one of the significant health threats to the elderly, although some people have it before age 50, and all of us have influenced the health of our bones well before that. While this article includes the value of hormone replacement, a thorough understanding of this issue should include reading the article entitled "Estrogen Replacement: More Important than Ever" from *Consumer Reports on Health*, November 1995. Many questions remain about proper nutrition for older people and whether diet can ward off aging, conserve brain function, and help maintain independence. Science is working on the answers.

It is not clear how many of us are vegetarians. In the past it has been reported that about 5 percent of the population claim to be vegetarian, a large increase over the past 15 years. However, this number may be exaggerated, and certainly far fewer are vegans who eat no animal products. Others consume no red meat but may add eggs or milk. Many choose some form of vegetarianism because of the health benefits, including better control over weight, blood pressure, and heart disease. Still others have religious or ethical beliefs that preclude the consumption of animal products. Vegan diets must be carefully planned to ensure adequate protein, iron and calcium, and vitamin B12. It could be argued, however,

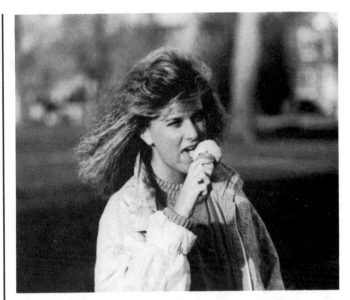

that nonvegetarians should plan just as carefully. Separating the health benefits of a vegetarian diet from those of other lifestyle changes that usually accompany the diet is sometimes difficult. The final article speaks to these issues.

One should remember that there is still much we do not know about nutrition, and that even within age, gender, and ethnic groups, people are physiologically different. Connections between food/nutrition and health can be found in other units in this book. Unit 1 has several articles with information on the benefits of chemicals other than nutrients in food. Articles on vitamins and other nutrients are found in unit 2, and unit 6 discusses information leading to harmful dietary practices. The reader might also review articles in previous *Annual Editions: Nutrition* and in reliable periodicals to fully appreciate the extent of the information—and the confusion—surrounding nutrition.

Looking Ahead: Challenge Questions

Pretend that you are planning research projects relative to nutrition and your age group. Rank by order of importance your top three priorities and defend them.

What changes should you make in your daily diet to conform to the best current knowledge about your nutrient needs?

Think back to your childhood and the influences that affected your eating patterns and attitudes. Plan what you will handle the same way and what you will change if and when you are a parent.

Based on information in the article "Boning Up on Osteoporosis," list the issues to be considered. How would you decide?

Compare the content of infant formula to that of human milk and cow's milk. What are the primary differences and what are the advantages of each?

NUTRITIONAL IMPLICATIONS OF ETHNIC AND CULTURAL DIVERSITY

ETHNIC AND CULTURAL DIVERSITY OF THE U.S. POPULATION

Ethnic minorities comprise nearly 25% of the United States population (1). The four major ethnic minorities include African Americans (12.1%), Hispanic (Latino) Americans (9%), Asian and Pacific Islander Americans (2.9%), and Native Americans and Alaskan Natives (0.8%) (1). These populations differ in many respects, not only from each other, but also from the non-Hispanic white population in the U.S. (1–5). Many major chronic diseases are more common among U.S. ethnic minority populations than among whites (2,3,6–10).

Because eating patterns relate to health risks and are culturally-influenced, diet and nutritional factors may contribute to health status differences between ethnic minorities and whites (3,6). Many aspects of daily living including food preferences and beliefs about the relationship of food to health are influenced by culture (11–13). Culture influences not only what, but also when, where, and how much food is eaten, and how it is obtained, prepared, distributed, and consumed (11,14). Individuals' health perceptions, for example, those related to body weight, are affected by culture (8–10,15).

Because the U.S. population is becoming more ethnically and culturally diverse, individuals in ethnic minority populations may have distinct blends of cultural perspectives and food habits (11,12,14). Acculturation, or the process of adopting or borrowing traits from another culture, may either improve or worsen some dietary practices (11,12).

Percent Distribution of Racial/Ethnic Groups in the United States

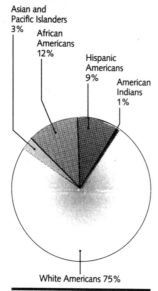

Asian and Pacific Islanders 3%
African Americans 12%
Hispanic Americans 9%
American Indians 1%
White Americans 75%

Source: U.S. Census Bureau

Ethnic minority groups in the U.S. suffer disproportionately from major chronic diseases.

As a result of the growth of ethnic and cultural diversity in the U.S., it is critical that health professionals be aware of how culture influences food behaviors and attitudes, especially those related to health status (16). This *Digest* reviews recent findings regarding dietary patterns and diet-related health problems of ethnic minority populations, with emphasis on the impact of culture. Implications for nutrition intervention and education are also discussed.

NUTRITIONAL IMPLICATIONS OF ETHNIC AND CULTURAL DIVERSITY

African Americans (blacks). The African American (black) population currently constitutes the nation's largest ethnic minority group (1,17). This population is heterogenous and includes several groups with different cultural backgrounds (1,5,13). Although genetics and socioeconomic factors (e.g., high rates of poverty and unemployment) affect the black population's health status, cultural patterns also contribute to blacks' morbidity and mortality from several diet-related diseases (6,17).

Compared to white Americans, blacks are at increased risk of obesity, hypertension, Type II diabetes, cardiovascular disease, and certain cancers (1,6,10,17,18). Differences in risk factor profiles, some of which are culturally-mediated, explain differences in health status between blacks and whites.

Obesity is a serious health problem for blacks, particularly black women (10,15). Data from the most recent National Health and Nutrition Examination Survey (NHANES) III, Phase I (1988–1991) indicate that black women have the highest prevalence of obesity (49.2%) among ethnic and gender subgroups (19). The prevalence of obesity is nearly twice as high for black as for white women (10,16). In addition to their higher rate of obesity, black women are also more likely to have abdominal or upper body obesity which is associated with increased risk of Type II diabetes mellitus, hypertension, and plasma lipid abnormalities (1,16,20).

A combination of genetic, developmental, and environmental factors may contribute to the high prevalence of obesity in black women (8). Preliminary findings from NHANES III indicate that black females consume a slightly higher percentage of energy from fat (35.5%) than do white (33.8%) or Mexican-American (33.7%) females (21). Black women also exhibit lower motivation to manage their weight than white women (8,10,15). Cultural acceptance is thought to be at the core of black women's less intense weight control efforts (7–10,15,22). Black women appear to be more satisfied with their weight than white women (7–10,15, 16,20,22,23).

Hypertension or high blood pressure is also a major health problem for blacks (1,17,24–26). African Americans have a higher prevalence of hypertension (32.4%) than either whites (23.3%) or Mexican Americans (22.6%) (24). Mechanisms that predispose blacks to hypertension may be operative early in life (26,27). Blacks also appear to suffer more from the health consequences of hypertension (e.g., renal damage) than whites (26).

Both genetic and environmental factors contribute to the higher prevalence of hypertension among black individuals (25,26). Among environmental factors, obesity, particularly abdominal or upper body obesity, in black women may contribute to their increased risk for hypertension compared to white women (6,18,26).

Both normotensive and hypertensive black individuals display higher sodium sensitivity and lower plasma renin levels than whites (25,26,28,29). Although blacks do not necessarily consume more sodium than whites,

To improve the effectiveness of weight control programs for African American women, interventions need to be culturally appropriate.

sodium intake for both blacks and whites exceeds recommended intakes (30). Because many blacks are sodium sensitive, they tend to experience a greater increase in blood pressure in response to a given amount of sodium intake than do whites, many of whom are sodium resistant. Cultural preferences for salt and salt-cured foods (6) also may contribute to the higher incidence of elevated blood pressure among African Americans.

A low potassium intake is another dietary factor which may contribute to the increased prevalence of high blood pressure among blacks (26,31,32). Blacks usually consume and excrete less potassium and their blood pressure tends to be higher than whites (30,32). Increasing blacks' intake of potassium (e.g., as found in fruits, vegetables, dairy foods) has been demonstrated to increase plasma renin levels and lower blood pressure (31,32).

The lower calcium intake of blacks (584 mg/day) compared to whites (742 mg/day) (30) may predispose salt sensitive blacks to hypertension (26). Studies have demonstrated that increasing calcium intake reduces blood pressure in salt sensitive hypertensives with low plasma renin activity and ionized calcium levels (29,32,33). Black-white differences in calcium and potassium intake may reflect socioeconomic and cultural differences (25). For blacks who are at risk of hypertension, increasing intake of foods rich in calcium, potassium, and other minerals (e.g., dairy foods), moderately reducing salt intake, and maintaining a healthy weight are recommended (26).

Hypertension and, importantly, overall and upper body obesity contribute to increased coronary heart disease morbidity and mortality in blacks (9,34–36). Psychosocial (e.g., stress, poverty) and cultural factors may also contribute to blacks' higher risk of heart disease (36).

Type II diabetes is an independent cardiovascular disease risk factor that is substantially more prevalent in black than in white individuals (36). Moreover, complications from diabetes generally are more severe for blacks and other ethnic minority populations than for whites (9). Obesity is strongly associated with Type II diabetes. Many cultural factors that influence obesity therefore also affect diabetes.

Compared to whites, blacks are at lower risk for osteoporosis (9,37,38). Nevertheless, a substantial number of black women develop this disease (37,38) and osteoporosis-related disabilities and mortality are higher for black than for white women (38).

Black-white differences in osteoporotic disease and fracture rates may be explained in part by differences in peak bone mineral mass (38–40). Blacks' greater peak bone mass may help protect them from osteoporotic fractures (9,38–40). Genetic differences in calcium metabolism (including vitamin D) and the higher incidence of obesity in blacks than in whites may explain why blacks are at reduced risk of osteoporosis than whites (9,38,41,42).

Milk and milk products are the major dietary source of calcium and vitamin D in U.S. diets (33). Data indicate that black individuals in the U.S. consume fewer servings of milk a week than whites and Hispanics (43). However, whether this lower consumption is due to perceived or actual lactose intolerance and/or cultural factors is unknown. For individuals who have difficulty digesting lactose or milk's sugar, consuming smaller quantities of milk more frequently can maximize milk intake and minimize symptoms (33). Also, other dairy foods such as cheese, yogurt with active cultures, and lactose reduced or lactose free dairy foods are well tolerated by lactose intolerant individuals (33).

The incidence of osteoporosis in blacks is anticipated to rise with the aging of the population (44). In addition, recent findings indicate that some older blacks are at risk of vitamin D deficiency (45). For these reasons, it is important that blacks consume the recommended number of daily servings of milk and other dairy foods, along with other calcium-containing foods that may be traditionally consumed (e.g., dark, leafy green vegetables).

The dietary intake and health status of Hispanic Americans vary widely and are influenced by socioeconomic status, the indigenous culture, and the degree of acculturation.

Hispanic (Latino) Americans.

The Hispanic American population is the second largest ethnic minority in the U.S. and is projected to outnumber the black population by the early 21st century (1,5,17,46–48). Hispanic Americans are a heterogenous mixture of cultures and ethnicity. The majority of these individuals are Mexican Americans (62.3%), with Puerto Ricans (11.1%), Cuban Americans (4.9%), South and Central Americans (13.8%), and others (7.6%) comprising the remainder (1).

Cultural attitudes influence the dietary intake and health status of Hispanic Americans (48). Many Hispanic Americans believe that life events (e.g., disease) are beyond one's control (48). This cultural attitude may jeopardize their willingness to make lifestyle changes to improve health (48). The "hot-cold" theory of disease and its treatment is another common theme. According to this philosophy, foods, herbs, illnesses, and bodily states are symbolically characterized as either "hot" or "cold." A "hot" illness is treated with a "cold" food/medication, and vice versa (48). Believers in this philosophy may unnecessarily restrict certain foods from their diets. Length of U.S. residence also influences dietary patterns and food intake of Hispanic Americans (49–52). With acculturation, dietary intake and health status worsen for many Hispanic Americans (49,50,52).

There are some similarities as well as notable differences in the types and frequency of foods consumed among different groups of Hispanic Americans (48,52–54). For example, tortillas, corn, dried beans, chili peppers, and tomatoes are staple foods of a traditional Mexican American diet, whereas rice and legumes are staples of a traditional Puerto Rican diet (48,53). Dairy products, in particular whole milk and cheese, are an important source of dietary calcium for Hispanic Americans (42,54).

With respect to diet-related health risks, a significant proportion of Hispanic American adults are obese, with the highest percentage occurring in Mexican American females (42.3%) and the lowest (38.2%) occurring in Cuban

American females (1,3,8,10,19,48). Obesity not only is high among Hispanic Americans, but its prevalence appears to be increasing (3). Moreover, Hispanic Americans have a predominance of upper body or centralized adiposity which increases their risk of diabetes mellitus, cardiovascular disease, and gallbladder disease (8,48). Genetics and several environmental factors (e.g., high calorie intake, low physical activity) as well as cultural factors contribute to obesity in Hispanic Americans.

Type II diabetes is approximately three times more common in Hispanic Americans than in non-Hispanic whites (3,10, 46,48,52). Mexican Americans have the highest prevalance of this disease, followed by Puerto Ricans, and to a lesser extent Cuban Americans (52). Rates of diabetes in Hispanic Americans have increased dramatically in recent years (3). Researchers project that obesity and a sedentary lifestyle contribute to the rising incidence of this disease (3,10,48).

Hispanic Americans exhibit a lower risk for hypertension and osteoporosis than whites (1,37,42,44,46). Hispanic Americans' relatively higher protection against these diseases may be due to a variety of genetic, biological, and cultural factors (44).

Calcium intake is similar for Hispanic Americans and non-Hispanic whites and is lower for females than for males (30). Although milk and milk products are the main dietary source of calcium for Hispanics, calcium sources vary among Hispanic ethnic groups (42). Cultural factors and regional availability influence milk intake (55).

Asian and Pacific Islanders. The Asian/Pacific American population is the nation's third largest ethnic minority and the fastest growing (1,17). Asian/Pacific Americans are characterized by their diversity (1,5,13,17). This population includes Chinese, Japanese, Korean, Filipino, and numerous Southeast Asian (e.g., Vietnamese, Cambodians) Americans and represents a variety of cultures, languages, socioeconomic levels, and educational backgrounds (1).

The ethnic and cultural diversity of the U.S. population presents a major challenge for nutrition and other health professionals.

The dietary intake and health status of Asian Pacific populations are varied and influenced by the cultural heritage of the specific subgroup (14,56). In many Asian cultures, just as in the Hispanic culture, the search for equilibrium or balance is important to health (14,56). Acculturation is another determinant of the dietary intake and health status of Asian/Pacific Americans (57,58). Some traditional Asian foods are good sources of calcium. However, because most Asians are unfamiliar with or unaccustomed to the taste of dairy foods, their overall intake of calcium tends to be low, especially for older adults (57,58).

Information regarding the health status or risk of nutrition-related diseases among Asian/Pacific Americans is limited (59). Nevertheless, some recent findings indicate that the Asian/Pacific American population is at increased risk for several chronic diseases, in part due to acculturation (59). An example is the increase in obesity among native Hawaiians with length of exposure to Western culture (59).

Native Americans. Although Native Americans represent less than 1% of the total U.S. population, they are an extremely diverse population which includes American Indians and Alaska Natives (Eskimos, Aleuts) (1,5,13,17).

Little is known regarding the food habits and dietary intakes of American Indians as a result of the exclusion of Native Americans living on reservations from national surveys, including the most recent NHANES III (60). Nevertheless, studies of small groups have identified nutritional excesses and shortcomings (60).

Obesity and diabetes are major health problems for Native Americans (1,3,10, 17,60,61). Not only is the prevalence of obesity high and rising, but this disease is an important risk factor for Type II diabetes, hypertension, cardiovascular disease, and gallbladder disease which are prevalent among Native Americans (10,62). The Pima Indians in particular have high rates of obesity and diabetes (6,63,64).

A variety of factors, genetic and environmental (e.g., diet, sedentary lifestyle), are implicated in the development of obesity in Native Americans. Cultural, social, and economic circumstances have decreased Native Americans' use of indigenous foods (e.g., vegetables, grains) and increased their intake of convenience foods, many of which are high in energy and low in essential nutrients (10,60). Although it has been speculated that a cultural acceptance of overweight may contribute to the high prevalence of obesity in Native Americans, findings of a recent study fail to support this assumption (65).

IMPLICATIONS FOR NUTRITION EDUCATION

It is clear that dietary patterns and risk of specific diseases are tied to an individual's ethnic and cultural background (13,48,52,66). Nutrition interventions, including nutrition education programs and materials, must be culturally sensitive to different groups. Cross-cultural counseling skills are also essential for health professionals working with individuals whose traditions, values, and beliefs differ from their own (66). Several resources are available to help dietitians and health professionals meet the challenge of serving the increasing number of clients with different ethnic and cultural backgrounds (12,14,67–69).

REFERENCES

1. National Heart, Lung, and Blood Institute, National Institutes of Health. Fact sheets on Black Americans, Hispanic Americans, Asian/Pacific Islanders, and American Indians. May 1992.

2. National Center for Health Statistics. *Health, United States, 1993.* Hyattsville, MD: Public Health Service, 1994.

3. McGinnis, J.M., and P.R. Lee. JAMA 273: 1123, 1995.

4. Kumanyika, S. J. Nutr. Educ. 22: 89, 1990.

5. Newman, J.M. *Melting Pot. An Annotated Bibliography and Guide to Food and Nutrition Information for Ethnic Groups in America.* 2nd ed. New York: Garland Publ. Inc., 1993.

6. Kumanyika, S.K. Ann. Epidemiol. 3: 154, 1993.

7. Kumanyika, S. Ann. N.Y. Acad. Sci. 699: 81, 1993.

8. Kumanyika, S.K. Obesity Res. 2(2): 166, 1994.

9. Kumanyika, S. J. Am. Diet. Assoc. 95: 299, 1995.

10. Ernst, N.D., and W.R. Harlan. Am. J. Clin. Nutr. 53(6): 1507S, 1991.

11. Terry, R.D. J. Am. Diet. Assoc. 94(5): 501, 1994.

12. Gonzalez, V.M., J.T. Gonzalez, V. Freeman, et. al. *Health Promotion In Diverse Cultural Communities.* Palo Alto, CA: Health Promotion Resource Center, Stanford Center for Research in Disease Prevention, 1991.

13. Kittler, P.G., and K. Sucher. *Food and Culture in America. A Nutrition Handbook.* New York: Van Nostrand Reinhold, 1989.

14. Eliades, D.C., and C.W. Suitor. *Celebrating Diversity: Approaching Families Through Their Food.* Arlington, VA: National Center for Education in Maternal and Child Health, 1994.

15. Kumanyika, S.K., C. Morssink, and T. Agurs. Ethn. Dis. 2: 166, 1992.

16. Melnyk, M.G., and E. Weinstein. J. Am. Diet. Assoc. 94: 536, 1994.

17. U.S. Department of Health and Human Services, Public Health Service. *Healthy People 2000. National Health Promotion and Disease Prevention Objectives.* DHHS Publ. No. (PHS) 91-50213. Washington, DC: U.S. Government Printing Office, 1991, pp. 31–43.

18. Lenfant, C. Circulation 90(4): 1613, 1994.

19. Kuczmarski, R.J., K.M. Flegal, S.M. Campbell, et. al. JAMA 272: 205, 1994.

20. Allison, D.B., B.S. Kanders, G.D. Osage, et. al. J. Nutr. Educ. 27: 18, 1995.

21. McDowell, M.A., R.R. Briefel, K. Alaimo, et. al. Energy and macronutrient intakes of persons ages 2 months and over in the United States: Third National Health and Nutrition Examination Survey, Phase 1, 1988–91. Advance data from Vital and Health Statistics; No. 255. Hyattsville, Maryland: National Center for Health Statistics, 1994.

22. Kumanyika, S., J.F. Wilson, and M. Guilford-Davenport. J. Am. Diet. Assoc. 93: 416, 1993.

23. Food Marketing Institute and PREVENTION Magazine. *Shopping For Health, 1993. A Food Marketing Institute PREVENTION Magazine Report on Diet, Nutrition and Ethnic Foods.* Washington, DC: Food Marketing Institute, 1993.

24. Burt, V.L., P. Whelton, E.J. Roccella, et. al. Hypertension 25: 305, 1995.

25. Grim, C.E., J.P. Henry, and H. Myers. In: *Hypertension: Pathophysiology, Diagnosis, and Management.* Second Edition. J.H. Laragh and B.M. Brenner (Eds). New York: Raven Press, Ltd., 1995, pp. 171–207.

26. Kaplan, N.M. The Lancet 344: 450, 1994.

27. Manatunga, A.K., J.J. Jones, and J.H. Pratt. Hypertension 22: 84, 1993.

28. Sowers, J.R., M.B. Zemel, P. Zemel, et. al. Hypertension 12: 485, 1988.

29. Zemel, P., S. Gualdoni, and J.R. Sowers. Am. J. Hypertens. 1: 146S, 1988.

30. Alaimo, K., M.A. McDowell, R.R. Briefel, et. al. Dietary intake of vitamins, minerals, and fiber of persons ages 2 months and over in the United States: Third National Health and Nutrition Examination Survey, Phase 1, 1988–91. Advance Data from Vital and Health Statistics; No. 258. Hyattsville, Maryland: National Center for Health Statistics, 1994.

31. Matlou, S., G. Isles, A. Higgs, et. al. J. Hypertens. 4: 61, 1986.

32. Langford, H.G., W.C. Cushman, and H. Hsu. Am. J. Hypertens. 4: 399, 1991.

33. Miller, G.D., J.K. Jarvis, and L.D. McBean. *Handbook of Dairy Foods and Nutrition.* Boca Raton, FL: CRC Press, Inc., 1995.

34. Morrison, J.A., G. Payne, B.A. Barton, et. al. Am. J. Public Health 84: 1761, 1994.

35. Burke, G.L., P.J. Savage, T.A. Manolio, et. al. Am. J. Public Health 82: 1621, 1992.

36. Kumanyika, S., and L.L. Adams-Campbell. In: *Cardiovascular Diseases in Blacks.* E. Saunders and A. Brest (Eds). Philadelphia: F.A. Davis Co.

Cardiovascular Clin. 21(3): 47–73, 1991.

37. Looker, A.C., C.C. Johnston, Jr., H.W. Wahner, et. al. J. Bone Min. Res. 10(5): 796, 1995.

38. Grisso, J.A., J.L. Kelsey, B.L. Strom, et. al. N. Engl. J. Med. 330: 1555, 1994.

39. Gasperino, J.A., J. Wang, R.N. Pierson, Jr., et. al. Metabolism 44(1): 30, 1995.

40. Nelson, D.A., G. Jacobsen, D.A. Barondess, et. al. J. Bone Miner. Res. 10(5): 782, 1995.

41. Abrams, S.A., K.O. O'Brien, L.K. Liang, et. al. J. Bone Miner. Res. 10(5): 829, 1995.

42. Looker, A.C., C.M. Loria, M.D. Carroll, et. al. J. Am. Diet. Assoc. 93: 1274, 1993.

43. Patterson, B.H., L.C. Harlan, G. Block, et. al. Nutr. Cancer 23: 105, 1995.

44. Villa, M.L. J. Bone Miner. Res. 9(9): 1329, 1994.

45. Perry, H.M., D.K. Miller, J.E. Morley, et. al. J. Am. Geriatr. Soc. 41: 612, 1993.

46. Stern, M.P. Ethn. Dis. 3(1): 7, 1993.

47. Policy and Research, National Coalition of Hispanic Health and Human Services Organizations (COSSMHO). Am. J. Health Promot. 9(4): 300, 1995.

48. Sanjur, D. *Hispanic Foodways, Nutrition, and Health.* Needham Heights, MA: Simon & Schuster Co., 1995.

49. American Medical Association, Council on Scientific Affairs. JAMA 265: 248, 1991.

50. Chavez, N., L. Sha, V. Persky, et. al. J. Nutr. Educ. 26: 79, 1994.

51. Guendelman, S., and B. Abrams. Am. J. Public Health 85: 20, 1995.

52. Romero-Gwynn, E., D. Gwynn, L. Grivetti, et. al. Nutr. Today 28(4): 6, 1993.

53. Kuczmarski, M.F., R.J. Kuczmarski, and M. Najjar. Nutr. Today 30(1): 30, 1995.

54. Block, G., J.C. Norris, R.M. Mandel, et. al. J. Am. Diet. Assoc. 95: 195, 1995.

55. Rosado, J.L., C. Gonzalez, M.E. Valencia, et. al. J. Nutr. 124: 1052, 1994.

56. Frye, B.A. Am. J. Health Promot. 9(4): 269, 1995.

57. Kim, K.K., E.S. Yu, W.T. Liu, et. al. J. Am. Diet. Assoc. 93: 1416, 1993.

58. Schultz, J.D., A.A. Spindler, and R.V. Josephson. J. Nutr. Educ. 26: 266, 1994.

59. Chen, M.S., Jr., and B.L. Hawks. Am. J. Health Promot. 9(4): 261, 1995.

60. Brown, A.C., and B. Brenton. J. Am. Diet. Assoc. 94: 517, 1994.

61. Jackson, M.Y. J. Am. Diet. Assoc. 93: 1136, 1993.

62. Alpert, J.S., R. Goldberg, I.S. Ockene, et. al. Cardiology 78: 3, 1991.

63. Warne, D.K., D.R. McCance, M.A. Charles, et. al. Diabetes Care 18(4): 435, 1995.

64. Hanson, R.L., D.R. McCance, L.T.H. Jacobsson, et. al. J. Clin. Epidemiol. 48(7): 903, 1995.

65. Story, M., F.R. Hauck, B.A. Broussard, et. al. Arch. Pediatr. Adoles. Med. 148: 567, 1994.

66. Sucher, K.P., and P.G. Kittler. J. Am. Diet. Assoc. 91: 297, 1991.

67. Diabetes Care and Education, Dietetic Practice Group of The American Dietetic Association. *Ethnic And Regional Food Practices. A Series.* Chicago, IL: The American Dietetic Association, 1989–1994.

68. National Dairy Council. *Guía Para La Buena Alimentacion (Spanish version of the "Guide to Good Eating").* Rosemont, IL: National Dairy Council, 1993.

69. U.S. Department of Agriculture, U.S. Department of Health and Human Services. *Cross-Cultural Counseling. A Guide for Nutrition and Health Counselors.* Washington, DC: U.S. Government Printing Office, May 1990.

Breast-Feeding Best Bet For Babies

Rebecca D. Williams
Rebecca D. Williams is a writer in Oak Ridge, Tenn.

New parents want to give their babies the very best. When it comes to nutrition, the best first food for babies is breast milk.

More than two decades of research have established that breast milk is perfectly suited to nourish infants and protect them from illness. Breast-fed infants have lower rates of hospital admissions, ear infections, diarrhea, rashes, allergies, and other medical problems than bottle-fed babies.

"There are 4,000 species of mammals, and they all make a different milk. Human milk is made for human infants and it meets all their specific nutrient needs," says Ruth Lawrence, M.D., professor of pediatrics and obstetrics at the University of Rochester School of Medicine in Rochester, N.Y., and spokeswoman for the American Academy of Pediatrics.

The academy recommends that babies be breast-fed for six to 12 months. The only acceptable alternative to breast milk is infant formula. Solid foods can be introduced when the baby is 4 to 6 months old, but a baby should drink breast milk or formula, not cow's milk, for a full year.

"There aren't any rules about when to stop breast-feeding," says Lawrence. "As long as the baby is eating age-appropriate solid foods, a mother may nurse a couple of years if she wishes. A baby needs breast milk for the first year of life, and then as long as desired after that."

In 1993, 55.9 percent of American mothers breast-fed their babies in the hospital. Only 19 percent were still breast-feeding when their babies were 6 months old. Government and private health experts are working to raise those numbers.

The U.S. Food and Drug Administration is conducting a study on infant feeding practices as part of its ongoing goal to improve nutrition in the United States. The study is looking at how long mothers breast-feed and how they introduce formula or other foods.

Health experts say increased breast-feeding rates would save consumers money, spent both on infant formula and in health-care dollars. It could save lives as well.

"We've known for years that the death rates in Third World countries are lower among breast-fed babies," says Lawrence. "Breast-fed babies are healthier and have fewer infections than formula-fed babies."

Human Milk for Human Infants

The primary benefit of breast milk is nutritional. Human milk contains just the right amount of fatty acids, lactose, water, and amino acids for human digestion, brain development, and growth.

Cow's milk contains a different type of protein than breast milk. This is good for calves, but human infants can have difficulty digesting it. Bottle-fed infants tend to be fatter than breast-fed infants, but not necessarily healthier.

Breast-fed babies have fewer illnesses because human milk transfers to the infant a mother's antibodies to disease.

About 80 percent of the cells in breast milk are macrophages, cells that kill bacteria, fungi and viruses. Breast-fed babies are protected, in varying degrees, from a number of illnesses, including pneumonia, botulism, bronchitis, staphylococcal infections, influenza, ear infections, and German measles. Furthermore, mothers produce antibodies to whatever disease is present in their environment, making their milk custom-designed to fight the diseases their babies are exposed to as well.

A breast-fed baby's digestive tract contains large amounts of *Lactobacillus bifidus,* beneficial bacteria that prevent the growth of harmful organisms. Human milk straight from the breast is always sterile, never contaminated by polluted water or dirty bottles, which can also lead to diarrhea in the infant.

Human milk contains at least 100 ingredients not found in formula. No babies are allergic to their mother's milk, although they may have a reaction to something the mother eats. If she eliminates it from her diet, the problem resolves itself.

Sucking at the breast promotes good jaw development as well. It's harder work to get milk out of a breast than a bottle, and the exercise strengthens the jaws and encourages the growth of straight, healthy teeth. The baby at the breast also can control the flow of milk by sucking and stopping. With a bottle, the baby must constantly suck or react to the pressure of the nipple placed in the mouth.

Nursing may have psychological benefits for the infant as well, creating an

From *FDA Consumer,* October 1995, pp. 19-23. Reprinted by permission of *FDA Consumer,* the magazine of the U.S. Food and Drug Administration.

The Lactating Breast

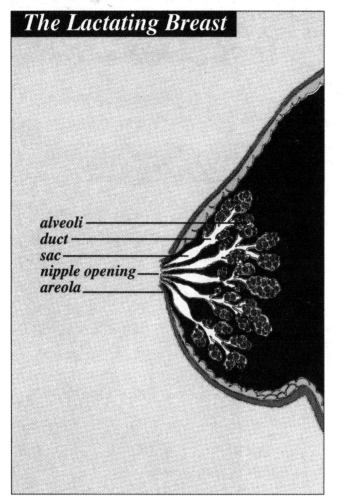

alveoli
duct
sac
nipple opening
areola

When the baby sucks, a hormone called oxytoxin starts the milk flowing from the alveoli, through the ducts (milk canals) into the sacs (milk pools) behind the areola, and finally into the baby's mouth.

early attachment between mother and child. At birth, infants see only 12 to 15 inches, the distance between a nursing baby and its mother's face. Studies have found that infants as young as 1 week prefer the smell of their own mother's milk. When nursing pads soaked with breast milk are placed in their cribs, they turn their faces toward the one that smells familiar.

Many psychologists believe the nursing baby enjoys a sense of security from the warmth and presence of the mother, especially when there's skin-to-skin contact during feeding. Parents of bottle-fed babies may be tempted to prop bottles in the baby's mouth, with no human contact during feeding. But a nursing mother must cuddle her infant closely many times during the day. Nursing becomes more than a way to feed a baby; it's a source of warmth and comfort.

Benefits to Mothers

Breast-feeding is good for new moth-ers as well as for their babies. There are no bottles to sterilize and no formula to buy, measure and mix. It may be easier for a nursing mother to lose the pounds of pregnancy as well, since nursing uses up extra calories. Lactation also stimulates the uterus to contract back to its original size.

A nursing mother is forced to get needed rest. She must sit down, put her feet up, and relax every few hours to nurse. Nursing at night is easy as well. No one has to stumble to the refrigerator for a bottle and warm it while the baby cries. If she's lying down, a mother can doze while she nurses.

Nursing is also nature's contraceptive—although not a very reliable one. Frequent nursing suppresses ovulation, making it less likely for a nursing mother to menstruate, ovulate, or get pregnant. There are no guarantees, however. Mothers who don't want more children right away should use contraception even while nursing. Hormone injections and implants are safe during

nursing, as are all barrier methods of birth control. The labeling on birth control pills says if possible another form of contraception should be used until the baby is weaned.

Breast-feeding is economical also. Even though a nursing mother works up a big appetite and consumes extra calories, the extra food for her is less expensive than buying formula for the baby. Nursing saves money while providing the best nourishment possible.

When Formula's Necessary

There are very few medical reasons why a mother shouldn't breast-feed, according to Lawrence.

Most common illnesses, such as colds, flu, skin infections, or diarrhea, cannot be passed through breast milk. In fact, if a mother has an illness, her breast milk will contain antibodies to it that will help protect her baby from those same illnesses.

A few viruses can pass through breast milk, however. HIV, the virus that causes AIDS, is one of them. Women who are HIV positive should not breast-feed.

A few other illnesses—such as herpes, hepatitis, and beta streptococcus infections—can also be transmitted through breast milk. But that doesn't always mean a mother with those diseases shouldn't breast-feed, Lawrence says.

"Each case must be evaluated on an individual basis with the woman's doctor," she says.

Breast cancer is not passed through breast milk. Women who have had breast cancer can usually breast-feed from the unaffected breast. There is some concern that the hormones produced during pregnancy and lactation may trigger a recurrence of cancer, but so far this has not been proven. Studies have shown, however, that breast-feeding a child reduces a woman's chance of developing breast cancer later.

Silicone breast implants usually do not interfere with a woman's ability to nurse, but if the implants leak, there is some concern that the silicone may harm the baby. Some small studies have suggested a link between breast-feeding with implants and later development of problems with the child's esophagus.

Tips for Breast-Feeding Success

It's helpful for a woman who wants to breast-feed to learn as much about it as possible before delivery, while she is not exhausted from caring for an infant around-the-clock. The following tips can help foster successful nursing:

• *Get an early start:* Nursing should begin within an hour after delivery if possible, when an infant is awake and the sucking instinct is strong. Even though the mother won't be producing milk yet, her breasts contain colostrum, a thin fluid that contains antibodies to disease.

• *Proper positioning:* The baby's mouth should be wide open, with the nipple as far back into his or her mouth as possible. This minimizes soreness for the mother. A nurse, midwife, or other knowledgeable person can help her find a comfortable nursing position.

• *Nurse on demand:* Newborns need to nurse frequently, at least every two hours, and not on any strict schedule. This will stimulate the mother's breasts to produce plenty of milk. Later, the baby can settle into a more predictable routine. But because breast milk is more easily digested than formula, breast-fed babies often eat more frequently than bottle-fed babies.

• *No supplements:* Nursing babies don't need sugar water or formula supplements. These may interfere with their appetite for nursing, which can lead to a diminished milk supply. The more the baby nurses, the more milk the mother will produce.

• *Delay artificial nipples:* It's best to wait a week or two before introducing a pacifier, so that the baby doesn't get confused. Artificial nipples require a different sucking action than real ones.

Sucking at a bottle could also confuse some babies in the early days. They, too, are learning how to breast-feed.

• *Air dry:* In the early postpartum period or until her nipples toughen, the mother should air dry them after each nursing to prevent them from cracking, which can lead to infection. If her nipples do crack, the mother can coat them with breast milk or other natural moisturizers to help them heal. Vitamin E oil and lanolin are commonly used, although some babies may have allergic reactions to them. Proper positioning at the breast can help prevent sore nipples. If the mother's very sore, the baby may not have the nipple far enough back in his or her mouth.

• *Watch for infection:* Symptoms of breast infection include fever and painful lumps and redness in the breast. These require immediate medical attention.

• *Expect engorgement:* A new mother usually produces lots of milk, making her breasts big, hard and painful for a few days. To relieve this engorgement, she should feed the baby frequently and on demand until her body adjusts and produces only what the baby needs. In the meantime, the mother can take over-the-counter pain relievers, apply warm, wet compresses to her breasts, and take warm baths to relieve the pain.

• *Eat right, get rest:* To produce plenty of good milk, the nursing mother needs a balanced diet that includes 500 extra calories a day and six to eight glasses of fluid. She should also rest as much as possible to prevent breast infections, which are aggravated by fatigue.

—*R.D.W.*

Further studies are needed in this area. But if a woman with implants wants to breast-feed, she should first discuss the potential benefits and risks with her child's doctor.

Possible Problems

For all its health benefits, breast-feeding does have some disadvantages. In the early weeks, it can be painful. A woman's nipples may become sore or cracked. She may experience engorgement more than a bottle-feeding mother, when the breasts become so full of milk they're hard and painful. Some nursing women also develop clogged milk ducts, which can lead to mastitis, a painful infection of the breast. While most nursing problems can be solved with home remedies, mastitis requires prompt medical care.

Another possible disadvantage of nursing is that it affects a woman's entire lifestyle. A nursing mother with baby-in-tow must wear clothes that enable her to nurse anywhere, or she'll have to find a private place to undress. She should eat a balanced diet and she might need to avoid foods that irritate the baby. She also shouldn't smoke, which can cause vomiting, diarrhea and restlessness in the baby, as well as decreased milk production.

Women who plan to go back to work soon after birth will have to plan carefully if they want to breast-feed. If her job allows, a new mother can pump her breast milk several times during the day and refrigerate or freeze it for the baby to take in a bottle later. Or, some women alternate nursing at night and on weekends with daytime bottles of formula.

In either case, a nursing mother is physically tied to her baby more than a bottle-feeding mother. The baby needs her for nourishment, and she needs to nurse regularly to avoid getting uncomfortably full breasts. But instead of feeling it's a chore, nursing mothers often cite this close relationship as one of the greatest joys of nursing. Besides, nursing mothers can get away between feedings if they need a break.

Finally, some women just don't feel comfortable with the idea of nursing. They don't want to handle their breasts, or they want to think of them as sexual, not functional. They may be concerned about modesty and the possibility of having to nurse in public. They may want a break from child care to let someone else feed the baby, especially in the wee hours of the morning.

If a woman is unsure whether she wants to nurse, she can try it for a few weeks and switch if she doesn't

Medicines And Nursing Mothers

Most medications have not been tested in nursing women, so no one knows exactly how a given drug will affect a breast-fed child. Since very few problems have been reported, however, most over-the-counter and prescription drugs, taken in moderation and only when necessary, are considered safe.

Even mothers who must take daily medication for conditions such as epilepsy, diabetes, or high blood pressure can usually breast-feed. They should first check with the child's pediatrician, however. To minimize the baby's exposure, the mother can take the drug just after nursing or before the child sleeps. In the January 1994 issue of *Pediatrics*, the American Academy of Pediatrics included the following in a list of drugs that are usually compatible with breast-feeding:

- acetaminophen
- many antibiotics
- antiepileptics (although one, Primidone, should be given with caution)
- most antihistamines
- alcohol in moderation (large amounts of alcohol can cause drowsiness, weakness, and abnormal weight gain in an infant)
- most antihypertensives
- aspirin (should be used with caution)
- caffeine (moderate amounts in drinks or food)
- codeine
- decongestants
- ibuprofen
- insulin
- quinine
- thyroid medications

Drugs That Are NOT Safe While Nursing

Some drugs can be taken by a nursing mother if she stops breast-feeding for a few days or weeks. She can pump her milk and discard it during this time to keep up her supply, while the baby drinks previously frozen milk or formula.

Radioactive drugs used for some diagnostic tests like Gallium–69, Iodine–125, Iodine–131, or Technetium–99m can be taken if the woman stops nursing temporarily.

Drugs that should never be taken while breast-feeding include:

Bromocriptine (Parlodel): A drug for Parkinson's disease, it also decreases a woman's milk supply.

Most Chemotherapy Drugs for Cancer: Since they kill cells in the mother's body, they may harm the baby as well.

Ergotamine (for migraine headaches): Causes vomiting, diarrhea, convulsions in infants.

Lithium (for manic-depressive illness): Excreted in human milk.

Methotrexate (for arthritis): Can suppress the baby's immune system.

Drugs of Abuse: Some drugs, such as cocaine and PCP, can intoxicate the baby. Others, such as amphetamines, heroin and marijuana, can cause a variety of symptoms, including irritability, poor sleeping patterns, tremors, and vomiting. Babies become addicted to these drugs.

Tobacco Smoke: Nursing mothers should avoid smoking. Nicotine can cause vomiting, diarrhea and restlessness for the baby, as well as decreased milk production for the mother. Maternal smoking or passive smoke may increase the risk of sudden infant death syndrome (SIDS) and may increase respiratory and ear infections.

like it. It's very difficult to switch to breast-feeding after bottle-feeding is begun.

If she plans to breast-feed, a new mother should learn as much as possible about it before the baby is born. Obstetricians, pediatricians, childbirth instructors, nurses, and midwives can all offer information about nursing. But perhaps the best ongoing support for a nursing mother is someone who has successfully nursed a baby.

La Leche League, a national support organization for nursing mothers, has chapters in many cities that meet regularly to discuss breast-feeding problems and offer support.

"We encourage mothers to come to La Leche League before their babies are born," says Mary Lofton, a league spokeswoman. "On-the-job training is hard to do. It's so important to learn how to breast-feed beforehand to avoid problems."

Most La Leche League chapters allow women to come to a few meetings without charge. League leaders offer advice by phone as well. To find a convenient La Leche League chapter, call (1-800) LA-LECHE

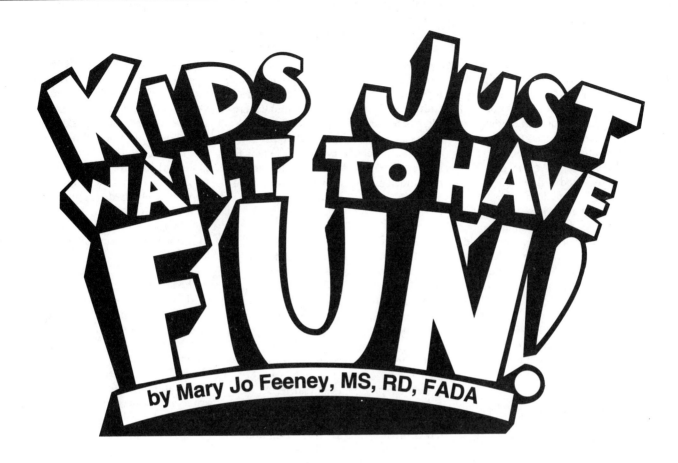

KIDS JUST WANT TO HAVE FUN!

by Mary Jo Feeney, MS, RD, FADA

There have been dramatic changes in families' lifestyles that have affected what, where and with whom children eat. Parents, once the primary teachers of sound food choices, now compete with all the eating situations children encounter both inside and outside the home. Kids just want to have fun, though, so the challenge is to make good nutrition fun for them.

Over four million children enter the marketplace yearly, many of them cruising supermarket aisles deciding on their own what foods they will eat:

✗ Children influence close to $300 billion in purchases made yearly by parents and caregivers — much of which is for food;

✗ The average 10-year-old makes about 250 purchases a year without his or her parents;

✗ In one study, over half of 4th and 5th graders report preparing their own breakfasts, lunches and dinners;

✗ Children see about three hours a week of food advertisements on television;

✗ Most children under six cannot tell the difference between a program and an advertisement;

✗ The more hours children watch television the more they request, buy and eat the advertised foods.

In addition to these outside influences on food choices, studies show that kids already have adopted some adult attitudes and patterns about eating and physical activity. Kids, like adults:

✗ Rate taste as the reason for choosing foods to eat;

✗ Agree that a balanced diet and physical activity are very important for good health even if they are not involved in regular physical activity;

✗ Think their favorite foods are not good for them; and

✗ Think foods that are good for them do not taste good.

Kids, though, are more than just "little adults." Children have their own special nutrient needs. They are on a journey to develop habits that can help them reach their optimal physical health. The "best" diet for children to delay or offset adult chronic disease is not clearly defined — there is just too little information on this relationship. There are answers, however, to the common questions parents and caregivers ask as they help children along their journey to an enjoyable and healthful life:

1. What and how much should my child eat?
2. How much influence should I have (or can I have) over what my child eats?
3. How can eating be fun in a time-pressured world?

Food Guide Basics

Use the Food Guide Pyramid as the basis for food selection for your entire family, including your child. Kids are beginning to understand the value of variety, balance and moderation. Studies show that they like eating different types of foods and they agree that eating smaller amounts of many foods is better than eating huge amounts of a few foods. Offer a variety of foods and compare

From *Positively Pasta*, Winter 1996, pp. 4-5. Reprinted by permission of *Positively Pasta*, the newsletter on pasta published by the National Pasta Association.

what your child eats to the Food Guide Pyramid.

Look for balance over time. A child who eats poorly for one or two days often balances out food choices over the next several days. Studies show that children eat less servings from the fruit, vegetable and grain groups, so use snacks from these food groups to round out what a child might overlook during the day.

Children often want to eat a certain favorite food every chance they get. If the food is from the Food Guide Pyramid, and if the food fixation does not last too long, do not be overly concerned. Introduce new foods and encourage your child to try at least one bite. If your child does not like the food, re-introduce it again sometime later. Keep trying even after your child turns up his or her nose two or three times. Children sometimes need to taste a new food eight to 10 times before they learn to accept it.

Tablespoons to Quarts

Because children have high energy needs and fill up fast, be sure the foods you offer are "nutrient-dense" — foods from the Food Guide Pyramid. Snacks and mini-meals of smaller portions can help relieve a child's hunger and contribute important nutrients. Although an adult's stomach can hold a quart or more, an infant's stomach might only hold the equivalent of two tablespoons of food. An easy guide to minimum serving sizes for children is one measuring tablespoon of cooked food for each year of a child's age. For instance, one-quarter cup cooked pasta would be an appropriate serving for a four-year old (four tablespoons is one-quarter cup). As children get older, they can follow the portion sizes of the Food Guide Pyramid, such as one-half cup cooked pasta, or one medium piece of fruit.

When and Where, But Probably Not What

Children tend to copy the positive and negative habits of their peers and other family members. Studies show that parents who cannot control their own eating (that is, they do not stop eating when they no longer are hungry) have children who have problems controlling the amount they eat. Children eat more food some days than others.

Resist micro-managing food choices and amounts. There is evidence that children know the difference between feeling hungry and full, and can regulate their own food intake. A child may not understand that he or she needs a piece of fruit, for example, but may know how much fruit he or she wants to eat. Child expert Ellyn Satter says that parents or caregivers are responsible for what the child is offered to eat and the setting in which food is offered. Kids, though, determine how much and what they eat from those foods.

Just Move It

Government studies indicate that more children today are heavier than their 1960s counterparts, due in part to changing eating patterns and decreased physical activity. An obese child is more likely than a child of normal weight to become an obese adult— with the risk of developing chronic health problems including heart disease and some types of cancer.

Obesity is the result of a variety of habits and actions, not just eating. Food, then, is not the single solution to curtailing weight. Overweight children benefit when less emphasis is placed on eating and more emphasis is placed on keeping physically active while enjoying a variety of nutritious foods. Ironically, or maybe coincidentally, the increase in the number of overweight children and adolescents is similar to that seen in adults, suggesting that perhaps family patterns of eating and activity need improvement. Because children look for role models, if you lead a fairly sedentary life, your child may do likewise.

Children can expend boundless energy in just having fun, flying kites, jumping rope, skating, rollerblading, running. Kids can even combine physical activity with earning money, such as a pet walking service. Playing for fun hopefully turns into playing for keeps—keeping the habit of physical activity into adulthood when staying fit is important for health. A family that plays together helps everyone stay fit. Think of fitness in terms of daily activity patterns: walking rather than riding to the corner convenience store; taking the stairs rather than elevators in buildings. A couple of times during the week, put activities in high gear and rev up the body-machine

aerobically: walk briskly with your child as he or she rides a bike.

Nourishing More than the Body

Many children do not eat three meals a day. According to a recent survey of children 9 to 15, about half skip breakfast, a quarter skip lunch and about a fifth of children skip dinner. Another study of 4th and 8th graders discovered that breakfast skipping was a big problem, and that the number of children skipping breakfast increased with age. Hungry children can do poorly in school if they have to focus on their stomach rather than learning.

Family meals can offer a breather in the storm of busy lives, a chance to sit down, to share and to pass along traditions that children can carry through life. In such an atmosphere, sometimes nutrition just "happens" without much ado. Around the table, children learn about what, how, how much, and when to eat. Meals often are more balanced when eaten with family and friends.

Bring out the Curious Eater in Your Child

Curious eaters are made rather than born. A child who sees someone he or she looks up to (a parent/adult) eating a variety of foods may be inclined to do likewise. Also, if a child is involved in preparing the food, the child is more likely to eat it. These activities can be very simple, such as tossing a salad, putting fruit in a basket centerpiece that is enjoyed as a dessert, opening packages of pasta, or helping to add vegetables to the pasta sauce.

There are many ways to spark interest in food when it is linked to everyday events and activities. The goal is for your child to play and move a little more and find joy and excitement in eating good food. Share any of these experiences with your child so that food becomes a part of his or her life.

✘ Children think food comes from packages. Show your child fresh food in different forms. For example, fresh tomatoes, canned tomatoes, tomato juice, dried tomatoes, tomato sauce;

✘ Visit a farmer's market so your child can see not only the food but the people who grow the food;

✘ Check out library books that explain how foods are made or grown;

✘ Use food and cooking to teach other skills, such as counting (peas in a pod) or math (4 cups in a quart);

✘ Tie in school assignments to food and celebrations whenever possible. For instance, children can plant spring gardens in pots and watch food grow from seed to harvest;

✘ Have your child draw a food calendar, make decorations for the table, even personalize "menus" for when you have friends for dinner;

✘ Computer programs and electronic media also provide opportunities for learning. Visit the NPA's World Wide Web site at http://www.ilovepasta.org and learn fun facts about pasta;

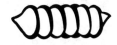

✘ Take advantage of community programs for kid cooks. Supermarkets often sponsor tours, food tastings and demonstrations. Some restaurants team chefs with kids and some hotels have special kid-developed menus;

✘ Talk with your child about your favorite foods, recipes and how eating well and staying active make you feel good;

✘ Talk about the foods available to your family today that were not available when you were a child.

TEENS AT RISK: NUTRITION ISSUES FOR THE '90s

INTRODUCTION

Adolescence is the period of transition between the onset of puberty and adulthood (i.e., 10 to 21 years of age). With the exception of infancy, more changes take place during adolescence than at any other time of life (1,2). During the teenage years, dramatic physiological developments increase the demand for energy and other nutrients. At the same time, psychosocial changes such as growing independence, the need for peer acceptance, concern about appearance and weight, and other attitudes and behaviors affect food choices, food habits, and nutritional status. Many of the attitudes and behaviors formed during adolescence persist into adulthood (1).

Adequate nutrition during the teenage years helps adolescents reach their growth potential and optimal health, as well as reduce the risk of adult chronic diseases. Unfortunately, health, especially long-term health, is not a priority for many teens. This *Digest* addresses the vulnerability of teens to nutrition-related problems imposed by various physiological and psychosocial changes. A discussion of calcium serves to illustrate how both physiological and psychosocial factors during adolescence can increase risk for disease later in life. This *Digest* also reviews how weight-related issues (obesity, dieting, eating disorders), participation in competitive sports, and pregnancy can place some teens at risk.

GENERAL ISSUES IN ADOLESCENT NUTRITION

Physiological Development.
During adolescence, puberty and the simultaneous growth spurt is characterized by rapid increases in height and weight

The physiological and psychosocial changes that occur during adolescence can profoundly affect teens' nutrient needs, nutritional status, and long-term health.

and changes in body composition (i.e., lean body mass and fat distribution). The growth spurt, or period of maximum growth, typically occurs in American female adolescents between the ages of 10 and 13 years and two years later in male adolescents. However, the timing, intensity, and duration of the growth spurt vary among individuals (3). Distinct gender differences in body composition emerge during adolescence. Girls deposit relatively more total body fat, while boys gain proportionately more lean body tissue and skeletal mass. Approximately 15% of adult height, 50% of adult body weight, and 45% of adult skeletal mass is gained during adolescence (3).

Gender and individual differences in the timing and intensity of the growth spurt and changes in body composition have important implications for the nutritional needs of adolescents (3). For example, at the peak of the growth spurt, nutrient needs may be greater than during early or late adolescence (3). Physiological growth or maturational age is a better indicator of teens' nutritional needs than chronologic age. However, for practicality, the Recommended Dietary Allowances (RDAs) are based on chronologic rather than maturational age for teens 11–14, 15–18, and 19–24 years (4).

Psychosocial Changes.
Along with the physical growth of puberty, adolescents undergo profound psychosocial changes that potentially impact their nutritional status. Teens' growing independence often leads to a disregard of family dietary patterns, eating away from home, especially at fast food establishments, and snacking. At the same time, teens often are uncomfortable with their rapidly changing bodies,

From *Dairy Council Digest*, May/June 1996, pp. 4-5. © 1996 by the National Dairy Council. Reprinted by permission.

are overly concerned about their appearance, especially their weight, and are influenced by the media and peer acceptance. Teens' food choices are strongly influenced by friends, group conformity, and the media (3).

The majority of U.S. adolescents eat at least one snack a day, with a range of one to seven daily (5,6). Whether or not intake of snacks compromises teens' nutritional status depends on the choice of foods selected as snacks and on the overall diet. While snacks can help meet teens' high energy and nutrient needs, problems occur when non-nutritious foods are substituted for nutritious foods. Teens' increased social life and busy schedules, as well as dieting, may cause them to skip meals. For many teens, opportunities abound to buy foods of minimal nutritional value from vending machines, fast food restaurants, and concessions at sporting events (7,8).

Adolescents' drive to express their own identity and to be independent leads to experimentation. Food is often used to express this individualization. According to one study, teens associated so-called "junk foods" with independence or freedom from the family and "healthy foods" with family meals and being home (9). Eating patterns such as vegetarianism may be adopted by teens as a means to express their identity, independence, concern about various social and environmental issues, and/or a desire to be thin (3).

Quality of Teens' Diets. The quality of adolescents' diets varies widely among individuals. Nevertheless, national surveys reveal that teens' diets overall tend to be high in total fat, saturated fat, cholesterol, sodium, and sugar (10,11). In contrast, teens often consume lower than recommended amounts of dietary fiber, folate, vitamins A, E, and B_6, iron, calcium, zinc, and magnesium (11–13). Adolescent females are more likely than their male counterparts to consume low intakes of essential vitamins and minerals (10,12).

CALCIUM NUTRITURE

Calcium is particularly problematic for teens, especially females (14,15). Physiologi-

The low calcium intake of many adolescent girls adversely affects peak bone mass and increases the risk of osteoporosis in later years. For healthy bones throughout life, teenage girls need to consume more calcium-rich foods.

cally, adolescence is a period of high calcium demands. The RDA for calcium increases from 800 mg/day during childhood to 1,200 mg/day for teenagers (and young adults) aged 11 to 24 years (4). However, there is substantial scientific evidence that calcium intakes greater than the current RDA for teens, specifically in the range of 1,200 to 1,500 mg/day, are necessary to ensure genetically determined peak bone mass (14–21). Maximizing peak bone mass at skeletal maturity (i.e., by age 30) is considered to be the best protection against age-related bone loss and subsequent fracture risk (19,21). Retrospective studies indicate a positive association between adequate intake of calcium or milk (i.e., a major source of calcium) during the teen years and bone mineral density in adulthood (22–24).

In addition to the dramatic increase in skeletal mass, there are other physiological explanations for the finding that adolescents require calcium in levels that exceed the RDAs. The current RDA for calcium for teenagers assumes that 40% of the calcium consumed is absorbed (5). Yet, recent studies indicate that teens absorb 26 to 34% of calcium intake (25,26). This lower percentage of calcium absorption by teens supports a higher calcium intake. Also, teens' high dietary intake of sodium, which increases urinary calcium excretion, may increase their need for dietary calcium (27).

Paradoxically, at the time of maximal calcium needs, calcium intakes of adolescent girls fall short of even the RDA (5,12). According to the United States Department of Agriculture's Continuing Survey of Food Intakes by Individuals, 1989–91, 12 to 19 year old males consumed an average of 1,145 mg calcium/day, an amount close to the RDA of 1,200 mg/day (5). In contrast, females 12 to 19 years of age consumed 797 mg calcium/day or 66% of their RDA (5).

A variety of psychosocial factors affect teens' calcium intake. Skipping meals, increased snacking on high energy, low nutrient foods, eating foods away from home, especially at fast food establishments, peer influence, concern about body weight, and dieting can all potentially compromise teens' calcium intake (3,28). Adolescent females' low calcium intake may be explained in part by the substitution of soft drinks for calcium-rich milk (5,29,30).

Weight preoccupation may influence adolescent girls' calcium intake. If teenage girls perceive high calcium foods such as dairy foods to be fattening, they may not consume these foods. However, recent research demonstrates that weight conscious teens can include dairy foods in their diets to help meet calcium needs without increasing body weight (20) or that are consistent with their desire to lose weight (31).

Dairy foods are particularly advantageous for bone health (32). According to a recent review, when dairy foods were used to increase teens' low calcium intake by 700 mg/day, bone mineral accretion improved up to 10% (20,32). In contrast, when 300 to 700 mg calcium was provided by calcium supplements, teens' bone mineral increased only between 1 and 5% (32). The additional increase in bone mineral density achieved by consuming dairy foods may be explained by other bone beneficial nutrients supplied by these foods (32). The advantage of consuming calcium-rich foods such as dairy foods to protect bone is recognized in the newly released *Dietary Guidelines for Americans* (33). This federal government document recommends that teenage girls consume "more calcium-rich foods to get the calcium needed for healthy bones throughout life" (33).

TEENS AT HIGH RISK

Obese Adolescents. Obesity among teens is a significant public health problem with serious medical and social consequences (34). In 1988–91, 21% of adolescents 12 through 17 years of age weighed more than the 85th percentile for their height and age, an increase of over 5% from 1976 to 1980 (34). Overweight during adolescence is associated with increased risk of morbidity and mortality in adulthood (35,36). In addition, overweight teens may suffer adverse social and economic consequences including feelings of isolation, rejection, low self-esteem, and poor body image (37).

Both food intake, particularly the

Teens need to be encouraged to develop healthy attitudes about their weight and body image and adopt patterns of eating and exercise conducive to health.

increased availability of energy-dense foods in the U.S. food supply, and sedentary lifestyles are thought to contribute to the rise in obesity among teens. Teens' participation in school-based physical education classes has declined over the past decade (38,39) and is substantially below the goals set in *Healthy People 2000* (40). Adolescents' opportunities to exercise both in and out of school have decreased for a variety of reasons (34,41). These include changes in school curricula, safety concerns, parents' work schedules, television viewing, and the availability of video and computer games (34,41).

Because restricting dietary intake may interfere with adolescents' growth and development, health professionals emphasize increasing teens' physical activity to achieve and maintain a healthy weight (33,42,43). All Americans, including adolescents, are encouraged to participate in 30 minutes or more of moderate physical activity on most, and preferably, all days of the week and to balance food intake with physical activity (33). Criteria are available to screen adolescents for overweight (44). Because of the complexities associated with adolescents' growth and development, the frequency of eating disorders in this population, and the potential for physiological and psychosocial harm associated with overweight, the development of separate body weight guidelines for adolescents (and children) is recommended (45).

Dieting Teens. During adolescence, both females and males become preoccupied with and sensitive about their appearance, especially their body weight (39,46). The high prevalence or dissatisfaction with body weight or shape among teens, coupled with the cultural pressure to be thin and society's stigma of obesity, lead many teens to adopt weight-loss regimes (46). According to nationwide surveys, at least one-quarter of adolescents consider themselves to be overweight (46,47). Female adolescents are more likely than their male counterparts to identify themselves as overweight (31, 39,47). Nationwide, over 40% of adolescents, especially females, are attempting to lose weight (39). The majority of teen dieters are not overweight (31,48).

Many teens adopt unhealthy weight control behaviors, including crash diets, fasting, use of diuretics, laxatives, and diet pills, binge eating, and self-induced vomiting (39,46,49). Frequent dieting among teens is associated with other unhealthy and risk-taking behaviors such as greater alcohol intake and tobacco use (50).

Relatively little is known regarding the long-term health impact of frequent dieting by adolescents. However, excessive dieting and weight preoccupation may contribute to clinical eating disorders (51). Other potential harmful consequences include poor eating habits and inadequate intake of nutrients (e.g., calcium, iron), fatigue, anxiety, constipation, poor concentration, and impaired performance in school (51). Thus, dieting during adolescence is not necessarily harmless.

Teens with Eating Disorders.

Eating disorders such as anorexia nervosa and bulimia nervosa place teens at high risk of nutrition-related morbidity and mortality (52–54). Anorexia nervosa, or voluntary self-starvation, occurs among 0.48% of girls 15 to 19 years of age, while bulimia nervosa, or episodes of binge eating and purging, affects 1 to 5% of teens (53). Diagnostic criteria for these eating disorders are provided by the American Psychiatric Association (55). Eating disorders affect both male and female adolescents, but are more common among females (56).

The cause of eating disorders is complex and involves biological, psychosocial, and familial factors (52–54). Preoccupation with thinness and body shape manifested by restrictive eating is often associated with the onset of eating disorders in vulnerable adolescents (52,57).

Adolescents with anorexia nervosa experience a dramatic weight loss, have an intense fear of gaining weight despite being underweight, are preoccupied with food, and have abnormal food intake patterns (52). Physiological complications of anorexia nervosa include stunted growth, delayed or interrupted puberty,

Teen athletes and pregnant teens may be at nutritional risk because of their high nutrient requirements and poor eating habits.

hypotension, and cardiac arrhythmias (53). Bone loss is a serious consequence of anorexia nervosa (58–61). Because these teens may not attain their genetically determined peak bone mass, they are at risk of osteoporosis later in life (53). In bulimia nervosa, problems are related to the recurrent episodes of binge eating followed by attempts to minimize the effects of overeating (e.g., self-induced vomiting, abuse of laxatives or diuretics, fasting, and exercise) (52–55).

A multidisciplinary team approach to address the medical and psychological aspects of eating disorders in teens is recommended (52,53). More emphasis needs to be placed on prevention of eating disorders (51).

Teen Athletes.

Teens involved in competitive sports may have high energy requirements compared to their sedentary counterparts (1,3). Failure to meet energy needs can compromise intake of essential vitamins and minerals (e.g., vitamin B_6, folic acid, calcium, iron, zinc) and athletic performance (1).

Teen athletes such as wrestlers may adopt unhealthy weight control practices to qualify for a certain weight class (62, 63). Food restriction, fasting, vomiting, use of laxatives and/or diuretics, fluid deprivation, and induced sweating are examples of weight-cutting measures taken by adolescent wrestlers to gain a competitive edge (62,63). These practices may compromise teens' nutrient intakes, health status, and athletic performance (63). Also, frequent cycles of rapid weight reduction and regain may make future weight control more difficult (63). Adolescent wrestlers, as well as teens who participate in sports such as gymnastics or running that emphasize thinness, are at risk for suboptimal nutrient intakes and eating disorders (e.g., anorexia nervosa and bulimia nervosa) (62). Female adolescent athletes may be at risk of low bone density (64). Intake of a nutritionally balanced diet containing a variety of foods in moderation and adequate training are the keys to becoming a successful adolescent athlete (1).

Pregnant Teens. One out of 10 teens ages 15 to 19 years old in the U.S. become pregnant each year (65,66). Teenage mothers are more likely than adult mothers to deliver preterm or low birth weight infants.

Reasons for teenagers' generally poor pregnancy outcomes are complex and involve biologic (i.e., physical immaturity) and sociodemographic factors. The low socioeconomic status of many pregnant teens is a strong predictor of low birth weight infants (65,66).

Data regarding the nutrient needs of pregnant teens are limited. However, in general, pregnant adolescents who have not completed their own growth require more energy and nutrients than older pregnant teens or adults (65–67). Energy, iron, folate, and calcium are often low in pregnant teens' diets (65). Adequate calcium intake is particularly important to maximize peak bone mass in pregnant adolescents whose bone mass is still increasing (66). Further, consuming sufficient calcium during pregnancy may protect teens against pregnancy-induced hypertensive disorders (68).

Many teens grow and develop normally. However, the physiological and psychosocial changes that take place during adolescence potentially can place teens at nutritional risk. Teens need to understand how their lifestyle affects both their current and future health.

REFERENCES

1. Rickert, V.I. (Ed.). *Adolescent Nutrition Assessment and Management.* New York, Chapman & Hall, 1996.

2. Friedman, S.B., M. Fisher, and S.K. Schonberg. *Comprehensive Adolescent Health Care.* St. Louis, Missouri: Quality Medical Publ., Inc., 1992.

3. Gong, E.J., and F.P. Heald. In: *Modern Nutrition in Health and Disease.* 8th ed. M.E. Shils, J.A. Olson, and M. Shike (Eds). Philadelphia, PA: Lea & Febiger, 1994, pp. 759–769.

4. National Academy of Sciences, National Research Council, Food and Nutrition Board. *Recommended Dietary Allowances,* 10th ed. Washington, DC: National Academy Press, 1989.

5. Tippett, K.S., S.J. Mickle, J.D. Goldman, et. al. *Food and Nutrient Intakes by Individuals in the United States, 1 Day, 1989–91. Continuing Survey of Food Intakes by Individuals 1989–91.* Nationwide Food Surveys Rep. No. 91-2, September 1995, 263 pp.

6. Dausch, J.G., M. Story, C. Dresser, et. al. Am. J. Health Promot. 10(2): 85, 1995.

7. Schuster, K. Food Management 30: 62, 1995.

8. Story, M., M. Hayes, and B. Kalina. J. Am. Diet. Assoc. 96: 123, 1996.

9. Chapman, G., and H. Maclean. J. Nutr. Educ. 25: 108, 1993.

10. McDowell, M.A., R.R. Briefel, K. Alaimo, et. al. *Energy and Macronutrient Intakes of Persons Ages 2 Months and Over in the United States: Third National Health and Nutrition Examination Survey, Phase 1, 1988–91.* Advance Data from Vital and Health Statistics; No. 255. Hyattsville, MD: National Center for Health Statistics, 1994.

11. Devaney, B.L., A.R. Gordon, and J.A. Burghardt. Am. J. Clin. Nutr. 61(suppl): 2055, 1995.

12. Alaimo, K., M.A. McDowell, R.R. Briefel, et. al. *Dietary Intakes of Vitamins, Minerals, and Fiber of Persons Ages 2 Months and Over in the United States: Third National Health and Nutrition Examination Survey, Phase 1, 1988–91.* Advance Data from Vital and Health Statistics; No. 258. Hyattsville, MD: National Center for Health Statistics, 1994.

13. Williams, C.L., J. Dwyer, C. Agostoni, et. al. Pediatrics 96(5): 1023s, 1995.

14. Matkovic, V., and R.P. Heaney. Am. J. Clin. Nutr. 55: 992, 1992.

15. Matkovic, V., and J.I. Ilich. Nutr. Res. 51: 171, 1993.

16. Johnston, C.C., Jr., J.Z. Miller, C.W. Slemenda, et. al. N. Engl. J. Med. 327: 82, 1992.

17. Lloyd, T., M.B. Andon, N. Rollings, et. al. JAMA 270: 841, 1992.

18. Johnston, C.C., and C. W. Slemenda. Osteoporosis Int. 4(suppl 1): 43, 1994.

19. Optimal Calcium Intake. NIH Consensus Statement. June 6–8; 12(4): 1–31, 1994.

20. Chan, G.M., K. Hoffman, and M. McMurry. J. Pediatr. 126: 551, 1995.

21. Fassler, A.-L.C., and J.-P. Bonjour. Ped. Clin. N. Am. 42(4): 811, 1995.

22. Nieves, J.W., A.L. Golden, E. Siris, et. al. Am. J. Epidemiol. 141: 342, 1995.

23. Soroko, S., T.L. Holbrook, S. Edelstein, et. al. Am. J. Public Health 84: 1319, 1994.

24. Murphy, S., K.T. Khaw, H. May, et. al. Br. Med. J. 308: 939, 1994.

25. Abrams, S.A., and J.E. Stuff. Am. J. Clin. Nutr. 60: 739, 1994.

26. Weaver, C.M., B.R. Martin, K.L. Plawecki, et. al. Am. J. Clin. Nutr. 61: 577, 1995.

27. Matkovic, V., J.Z. Ilich, M.B. Andon, et. al. Am. J. Clin. Nutr. 62: 417, 1995.

28. Barr, S.I. J. Am. Diet. Assoc. 94: 260, 1994.

29. Guenther, P.M. J. Am. Diet. Assoc. 86: 493, 1986.

30. Wyshak, G., and R.E. Frisch. J. Adolesc. Health 15(3): 210, 1994.

31. Barr, S.I. J. Adolesc. Health 16: 458, 1995.

32. Kerstetter, J.E., and K. Insogna. Nutr. Rev. 53(11): 328, 1995.

33. U.S. Department of Agriculture and U.S. Department of Health and Human Services. *Nutrition and Your Health: Dietary Guidelines for Americans.* Home and Garden Bulletin No. 232. Washington, DC: U.S. Government Printing Office, December 1995.

34. Troiano, R.P., K.M. Flegal, R.J. Kuczmarski, et. al. Arch. Pediatr. Adolesc. Med. 149: 1085, 1995.

35. Must, A., P.F. Jacques, G.E. Dallal, et. al. N. Engl. J. Med. 327: 1350, 1992.

36. Rocchini, A. Pediatr. Ann. 21: 235, 1992.

37. Gortmaker, S., A. Must, J. Perrin, et. al. N. Engl. J. Med. 329: 1008, 1993.

38. Heath, G.W., M. Pratt, C.W. Warren, et. al. Arch. Pediatr. Adolesc. Med. 148: 1131, 1994.

39. Kann, L., C.W. Warren, W.A. Harris, et. al. J. Sch. Health 65(5): 163, 1995. (Morbidity & Mortality Weekly Report 44:1, 1995)

40. U.S. Department of Health and Human Services. *Healthy People 2000: National Health Promotion and Disease Prevention Objectives.* Public Health Service. Washington, DC: U.S. Government Printing Office, 1990.

41. American Academy of Pediatrics, Committee on Communications. Pediatrics 96(4): 786, 1995.

42. Sallis, J.F., and K. Patrick. Pediatr. Exerc. Sci. 6: 302, 1994.

43. National Institutes of Health. Consensus Development Conference Statement. *Physical Activity and Cardiovascular Health.* December 18–20, 1995.

44. Himes, J.H., and W.H. Dietz. Am. J. Clin. Nutr. 59(2): 307, 1994.

45. AIN Healthy Weight Steering Committee. J. Nutr. 124: 2240, 1994.

46. Story, M., K. Rosenwinkel, J.H. Himes, et. al. Am. J. Dis. Child. 145: 994, 1991.

47. Felts, W.M., A.V. Parrillo, T. Chenier, et. al. J. Adol. Health 18: 20, 1996.

48. Emmons, L. J. Am. Diet. Assoc. 94: 725, 1994.

49. Story, M., S.A. French, M.D. Resnick, et. al. Int. J. Eating Disorders 18(2): 173, 1995.

50. French, S.A., M. Story, B. Downes, et. al. Am. J. Public Health 85: 695, 1995.

51. Neumark-Sztainer, D. J. Sch. Health 66(2): 64, 1996.

52. The American Dietetic Association. J. Am. Diet. Assoc. 94(8): 902, 1994.

53. Fisher, M., N.H. Golden, D.K. Katzman, et. al. J. Adolesc. Health 16: 420, 1995.

54. Kriepe, R.E., N.H. Golden, D.K. Katzman, et. al. J. Adolesc. Health 16: 476, 1995.

55. American Psychiatric Association. *Diagnostic and Statistical Manual of Mental Disorders.* 4th ed. Washington, DC: American Psychiatric Association, 1994.

56. Siegel, J.H., D. Hardoff, N.H. Golden, et. al. J. Adolesc. Health 16: 448, 1995.

57. Killen, J.D., C.B. Taylor, C. Hayward, et. al. Int. J. Eating Disorders 16: 227, 1994.

58. La Ban, M.M., J.C. Wilkins, A.H. Sackeyfio, et. al. Arch. Phys. Med. Rehabil. 76: 884, 1995.

59. Abrams, S., T. Silbert, N. Estaban, et. al. J. Pediatr. 123: 326, 1993.

60. Bachrach, L.K., D. Guido, D. Katzman, et. al. Pediatrics 86: 440, 1990.

61. Hergenroeder, A.C. J. Pediatr. 126: 683, 1995.

62. Oppliger, R.A., G.L. Landry, S.W. Foster, et. al. Pediatrics 91: 826, 1993.

63. Marquart, L.F., and J. Sobal. J. Adolesc. Health 15: 410, 1994.

64. Baer, J.T., J. Taper, F.G. Gwazdauskas, et. al. J. Sports Med. Phys. Fitness 32: 51, 1992.

65. The American Dietetic Association. J. Am. Diet. Assoc. 94(4): 449, 1994.

66. Story, M., and I. Alton. Nutr. Today 30(4): 142, 1995.

67. Gutierrez, Y., and J. King. Pediatr. Ann. 22: 99, 1993.

68. Guillermo, C., L. Duley, J.M. Belizan, et. al. Br. J. Obstet. Gynecol. 101: 753, 1994.

BONING UP ON
OSTEOPOROSIS

Consider an insidious condition that drains away bone—the hardest, most durable substance in the body. It happens slowly, over years, so that often neither doctor nor patient is aware of weakening bones until one snaps unexpectedly. Unfortunately, this isn't science fiction. It's why osteoporosis is called the silent thief.

Carolyn J. Strange

Carolyn J. Strange is a science and medical writer living in Northern California.

There is no cure for osteoporosis, but the onset can be delayed and the severity diminished.

And it steals more than bone. It's the primary cause of hip fracture, which can lead to permanent disability, loss of independence, and sometimes even death. Collapsing spinal vertebrae can produce stooped posture and a "dowager's hump." Lives collapse too. The chronic pain and anxiety that accompany a frail frame make people curtail meaningful activities, because the simplest things can cause broken bones: Stepping off a curb. A sneeze. Bending to pick up something. A hug. "Don't touch Mom, she might break" is the sad joke in many families.

Osteoporosis leads to 1.5 million fractures, or breaks, per year, mostly in the hip, spine and wrist, and costs $10 billion annually, according to the National Osteoporosis Foundation. It threatens 25 million Americans, mostly older women, but older men get it too. One in three women past 50 will suffer a vertebral fracture, according to the foundation. These numbers are predicted to rise as the population ages.

Osteoporosis, which means "porous bones," is a condition of excessive skeletal fragility resulting in bones that break easily. A combination of genetic,

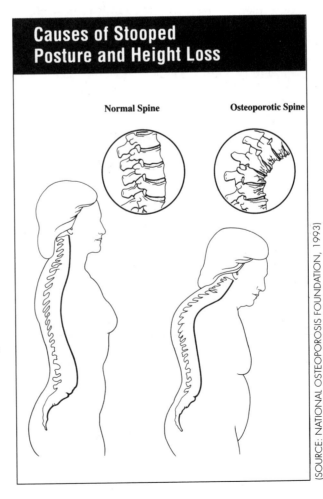

Causes of Stooped Posture and Height Loss

Normal Spine   Osteoporotic Spine

(SOURCE: NATIONAL OSTEOPOROSIS FOUNDATION, 1993)

The spine is made up of a series of small connected bones called vertebrae (left). Healed vertebral fractures become compressed (flattened) or may mend in a wedge shape. Over time, multiple fractures of the spine can result in stooped posture, a loss of height, and continual pain (right).

dietary, hormonal, age-related, and lifestyle factors all contribute to this condition.

Changing attitudes and improving technology are brightening the outlook for people with osteoporosis. Nowadays, many women live 30 years or more—

sponds to the pull of muscles and gravity, repairs itself, and constantly renews itself.

Besides protecting internal organs and allowing us to move about, bone is also involved in the body's handling of minerals. Of the 2 to 4 pounds of cal-

count, but in our skeletal "account" we can deposit bone only during our first three decades. After that, all we can do is try to postpone and minimize the steady withdrawals. Osteoporosis is the bankruptcy that occurs when too little bone is formed during youth, or too

Osteoporosis leads to 1.5 million fractures, or breaks, per year, mostly in the hip, spine and wrist.

perhaps a quarter to a third of their lives—after menopause. Improving the quality of those years has become an important health-care goal. Although some bone loss is expected as people age, osteoporosis is no longer viewed as an inevitable consequence of aging. Diagnosis and treatment need no longer wait until bones break.

There is no cure for osteoporosis, and it can't be prevented outright, but the onset can be delayed, and the severity diminished. Most important, early intervention can prevent devastating fractures. The Food and Drug Administration has revised labeling on foods and supplements to provide valuable information about the level of nutrients that help build and maintain strong bones. FDA has also approved a wide variety of products to help diagnose and treat osteoporosis, including several just last year.

Bone Life

Bone consists of a matrix of fibers of the tough protein collagen, hardened with calcium, phosphorus and other minerals. Two types of architecture give bones strength. Surrounding every bone is a tough, dense rind of cortical bone. Inside is spongy-looking trabecular bone. Its interconnecting structure provides much of the strength of healthy bone, but is especially vulnerable to osteoporosis.

"We tend to think of the skeleton as an inert erector set that holds us up and doesn't do much else. That's not true," says Karl. L. Insogna, M.D., director of the Bone Center at Yale School of Medicine, New Haven, Conn. Every bit as dynamic as other tissues, bone re-

cium in the body, nearly 99 percent is in the teeth and skeleton. The remainder plays a critical role in blood clotting, nerve transmission, muscle contraction (including heartbeat), and other functions. The body keeps the blood level of calcium within a narrow range. When needed, bones release calcium.

A complex interplay of many hormones balances the activity of the two types of cells—osteoclasts and osteoblasts—responsible for the continuous turnover process called remodeling. Osteoclasts break down bone, and osteoblasts build it. In youth, bone building prevails. Bone mass peaks by about age 30, then bone breakdown outpaces formation, and density declines.

The skeleton is like a retirement ac-

much is lost later, or both.

"You've got to get as much bone as you can and not lose it," Insogna says. "The most important risk factor for osteoporosis is a low bone mass."

"The upper limit of bone mass that you can acquire is genetically determined," says Mona S. Calvo, Ph.D., in FDA's Office of Special Nutritionals. "But even though you may be programmed for high bone mass, other factors can influence how much bone you end up with," she says. (See "Reducing Your Risk.") For instance, men tend to build greater bone mass, which is partly why more women face osteoporosis.

But there's another reason. With the decline of the female hormone estrogen at menopause, usually around age 50,

To Learn More

For more information, contact:
• National Osteoporosis Foundation, 1150 17th St., N.W., Suite 500, Washington, DC 20036; (202) 223-2226; World Wide Web: *http://www.nof.org/*. For locations of your nearest bone density testing sites, call (800) 464-6700.
• Osteoporosis and Related Bone Diseases National Resource Center (ORBD-NRC); (800) 624-BONE; TDD: (202) 223-0344.
• Older Women's League (OWL), 666 11th St., N.W., Suite 700, Washington, DC 20001; (202) 783-6686.
• North American Menopause Society, c/o University Hospitals of Cleveland, Department of Obstetrics and Gynecology, 11100 Euclid Ave., Suite 7024, Cleveland, OH 44106; (216) 844-8748; World Wide Web: *http://www.menopause.org/*.
• American Association of Retired Persons (AARP), 601 E St., N.W., Washington, DC 20049; (202) 434-2277; World Wide Web: *http://www.aarp.org/*.

bone breakdown markedly increases. For several years, women lose bone two to four times faster than they did before menopause. The rate usually slows down again, but some women may continue to lose bone rapidly. By age 65, some women have lost half their skeletal mass. Because the changes at menopause increase a woman's risk, many physicians feel it's a good time to measure a woman's bone density, especially if she has other risk factors for osteoporosis.

"The best way to gauge a woman's risk for osteoporotic fracture is to measure her bone mass," says Insogna.

Routine x-rays can't detect osteoporosis until it's quite advanced, but other radiological methods can. FDA has approved several kinds of devices that use various methods to estimate bone density. Most require far less radiation than a chest x-ray. Doctors consider a patient's medical history and risk factors in deciding who should have a bone density test. The method used is often determined by the equipment available locally. Readings are compared to a standard for the patient's age, sex and body size. Different parts of the skeleton may be measured, and low density at any site is worrisome.

Bone density tests are useful for confirming a diagnosis of osteoporosis if a person has already had a suspicious fracture, or for detecting low bone density so that preventative steps can be taken.

"There's a profound relationship between bone mass and risk of fracture," says Robert Recker, M.D., director of the Osteoporosis Research Center at Creighton University, Omaha, Neb.

Readings repeated at intervals of a year or more can determine the rate of bone loss and help monitor treatment effectiveness. However, estimates are not necessarily comparable between machine types because they use different measurement methods, cautions Joseph Arnaudo, in the Center for Devices and Radiological Health. "You always want to go back to the same machine, if you can," he says.

Another new test provides an indicator of bone breakdown. Last year, FDA approved a simple, noninvasive biochemical test that detects in a urine sample a specific component of bone breakdown, called NTx. Clinical labs can get results in about 2 hours. The NTx test, marketed as Osteomark, can help physicians monitor treatment and identify fast losers of bone for more aggressive treatment, but the test may not be used to diagnose osteoporosis.

Expanding Treatment Options

Physicians and patients now have endocrine drug products in FDA's Center for Drug Evaluation and Research.

Before last year, the only choices were the hormones estrogen and calcitonin. While enthusiasm for new weapons against osteoporosis is warranted, one of the old ones is still the top choice.

"Estrogen remains the first thing that women should consider," says Insogna, because the hormone not only helps prevent osteoporosis, but also protects against heart disease.

Last fall, FDA approved the first nonhormonal treatment for osteoporosis.

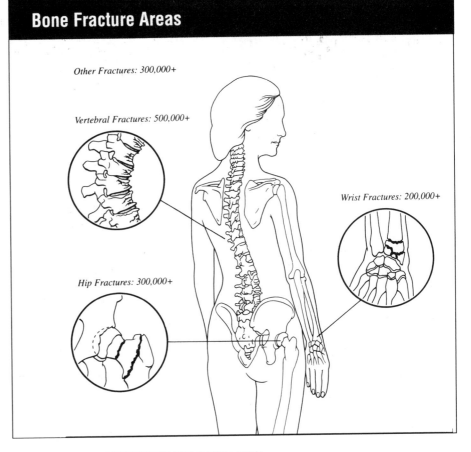

Bone Fracture Areas

Other Fractures: 300,000+

Vertebral Fractures: 500,000+

Wrist Fractures: 200,000+

Hip Fractures: 300,000+

(SOURCE: NATIONAL OSTEOPOROSIS FOUNDATION, 1993)

more treatment options than ever. Under FDA guidelines, drugs to treat osteoporosis must be shown to preserve or increase bone mass and maintain bone quality in order to reduce the risk of fractures. "We want to be sure that the bone is normal or stronger than it was," says Gloria Troendle, M.D., deputy director of the division of metabolism and

Each year, osteoporosis leads to 1.5 million bone fractures, including more than 500,000 vertebral fractures, 300,000 hip fractures, 200,000 wrist fractures, and 300,000 fractures of other bones.

"If you think about what's missing at menopause, it's the hormones," says Paula Stern, Ph.D., a pharmacologist at Northwestern University Medical School, Chicago, Ill.

Estrogen replacement therapy is the best prevention for the drop in bone mass at menopause, and there are more ways to take it than ever. But it's not for everyone. Because estrogen increases the risk of certain cancers and other diseases, taking it may not be appropriate, or it may be given in combination with another female hormone, progesterone, which can also cause undesirable side effects. A woman and her doctor need to carefully weigh the risks and benefits. According to the National Osteoporosis Foundation, a woman's risk of developing a hip fracture is equal to her combined risk of developing breast, uterine and ovarian cancer.

Women who can't or don't want to take hormones—some 30 to 50 percent—have other treatment avenues. Last summer, calcitonin treatment became much easier when FDA approved a nasal spray. Calcitonin, one of the hormones responsible for regulating the level of calcium in the blood, inhibits osteoclasts, the bone dissolvers. The drug, marketed as Miacalcin, is a potent, synthetic version of the hormone, and has been shown to slow and reverse bone loss. The stomach quickly destroys the drug, so before the spray was available, calcitonin had to be injected every day or two.

Last fall, FDA also approved the first nonhormonal treatment for osteoporosis. Alendronate, marketed as Fosamax, falls within a class of drugs called bisphosphonates, which hinder bone breakdown remodeling sites by inhibiting osteoclast activity. In clinical trials lasting three years, alendronate increased the bone mass as much as 8 percent and reduced fractures as much as 30 to 40 percent, depending on skeletal site. Lengthier studies are ongoing.

"Since it's so free of side effects it's a very welcome addition to the armamentarium. But the truth is, we still need a better treatment," says Recker. "We need a drug that will build back bone major league."

"All the drugs approved so far are

Calcium and vitamin D supplements are an integral part of all treatments for osteoporosis

Calcium (Ac)Counts

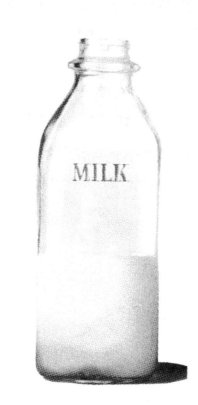

Your skeletal calcium bank has to last through old age. Frequent deposits to this retirement account should begin in youth and be maintained throughout life to help minimize withdrawals. Most women get much less calcium than they need—as little as half.

Nutritionists recommend meeting your calcium needs with foods naturally rich in calcium. Adequate calcium intake in childhood and young adulthood is critical to achieving peak adult bone mass, yet many adolescent girls replace milk with nutrient-poor beverages like soda pop. "Bone health requires a lot of nutrients and you're likely to get most of them in dairy products," says Connie Weaver, Ph.D., who heads the department of food and nutrition at Purdue

University, Indiana. "They're a huge package rather than just a single nutrient." With so many low-fat and nonfat dairy products available, it's easy to make dairy foods part of a healthy diet. People who have trouble digesting milk can look for products treated to reduce lactose. A serving of milk or yogurt contains about 350 milligrams (mg) of calcium. Fortified products have even more.

"People who don't consume dairy foods can meet their calcium needs with foods that are fortified with calcium, such as orange juice, or with calcium supplements," says Mona S. Calvo, Ph.D., in FDA's Office of Special Nutritionals. Other good sources of calcium are broccoli and dark-green leafy vegetables like kale, tofu (if made with calcium), canned fish (eaten with bones), and fortified bread and cereal products.

Nutrition labels can help you identify calcium-rich foods. But keep in mind that the label value is a guideline based on a FDA's Daily Value for calcium, which is 1,000 mg, and your calcium needs may be greater, Calvo says.

What about too much calcium? As much as 2,000 mg per day seems to be safe for most people, but those at risk for kidney stones should discuss calcium with their doctors. Calcium is critical, but even a high intake won't fully protect you against bone loss caused by estrogen deficiency, physical inactivity, alcohol abuse, smoking, or medical disorders and treatments.

—C.J.S.

things that just stop bone turnover. They're not really stimulating more bone production," says Troendle.

Bone mass increases because even though osteoclasts can't start new remodeling sites, osteoblasts continue filling in existing cavities. Increases in bone mass are most pronounced in the first year or two after treatment begins, then taper off. Any gain is helpful, even if it doesn't continue, because increases in bone mass help reduce fracture risk. But experts would like to encourage even greater gains.

Fluoride, known for fighting dental cavities, stimulates bone building, but early studies in osteoporosis patients found that the structure of the new bone was abnormal and weaker than normal bone. Gastrointestinal side effects were also a problem. Investigators are working to find a formulation and dosage regimen that will result in building normal bone.

Drugs Not Enough

Calcium and vitamin D supplements are an integral part of all treatments for osteoporosis. Everyone should make sure they get enough of these two nutrients, but especially those at risk for osteoporosis. Attention to diet and exercise are important not only for treatment, but also for prevention.

"If you go to the doctor and get a prescription, and that's all you do, you're probably not going to be helped very much," Recker says. His prevention clinic is staffed by a physical therapist, a nutritionist, and a nurse, who help people increase their physical activity, improve their diets, and make their homes safer by reducing the risk of falling. "Those three people do more to help the patients than I do with my prescription pad," Recker says.

Calcium intake is critical, and those who need it the most—younger women and girls—don't get enough. (See "Calcium (Ac)Counts.") But calcium alone can't build bone. Without vitamin D, calcium isn't sufficiently absorbed. Most people get enough vitamin D because skin produces it in sunlight. But people confined indoors who have a poor diet—which includes many older

Americans—or who live in northern latitudes in winter may be deficient.

A lifelong habit of weightbearing exercise, such as walking or biking, also helps build and maintain strong bone. The greatest benefit for older people is that physical fitness reduces the risk of fracture, because better balance, muscle strength, and agility make falls less

likely. Exercise also provides many other life-enhancing psychological and cardiovascular benefits. Increased activity can aid nutrition, too, because it boosts appetite, which is often reduced in older people. The biggest reason older people don't get enough calcium, Recker says, is that they simply don't eat much.

"The truth is, you don't have to do

Reducing Your Risk

A host of factors can affect your chances of developing osteoporosis. The good news is that you control some of them. Even though you can't change your genes, you can still lower your risk with attention to certain lifestyle changes. The younger you start, and the longer you keep it up, the better. Here's what you can do for yourself:

• Be sure you get enough calcium and vitamin D.

• Engage in regular physical activity, such as walking.

• Don't smoke.

• If you drink alcohol, do so in moderation.

A sedentary lifestyle, smoking, excessive drinking, and low calcium intake all increase risk. Although coffee has been suspected as a risk factor, studies so far are inconclusive.

Other factors are beyond your control. Being aware of them can provide extra motivation to help yourself in the ways you are able, and aids you and your doctor in health-care decisions. These risk factors are:

• being female: Women have a five times greater risk than men.

• thin, small-boned frame

• broken bones or stooped posture in older family members, especially women, which suggest a family history of osteoporosis

• early estrogen deficiency in women who experience menopause before age 45, either naturally or resulting from surgical removal of the ovaries

• estrogen deficiency due to abnormal absence of menstruation (as may accompany eating disorders)

• ethnic heritage: White and Asian women are at highest risk; African-American and Hispanic women are at lower, but significant, risk.

• advanced age

• prolonged use of some medications, such as excessive thyroid hormone; some antiseizure medications; and glucocorticoids (certain anti-inflammatory medications, such as prednisone, used to treat conditions such as asthma, arthritis and some cancers).

Risk factors may not tell the whole story. You may have none of these factors and still have osteoporosis. Or you may have many of them and not develop the condition. It's best to discuss your specific situation with your doctor.

—*C.J.S.*

very much to get most of the benefits of exercise," Recker says. He suggests 30 minutes of brisk walking five days a week. Add a little weightlifting, and that's even better. It's always smart to ask your doctor before starting a new exercise program, especially if you already have osteoporosis or other health problems.

Brighter Horizons

"A number of new things seem to be in the offing, eventually to come to us, and we're looking forward to getting some additional treatments for osteoporosis," says Troendle.

Uses of existing drugs may be broadened. Early drug trials are often conducted with patients who have severe disease, often after a fracture has oc-

curred or bone loss is quite serious. Some studies under way are testing to see if certain drugs are effective in less severe cases, if they can be started sooner, or used in combination.

The search for bone-building drugs continues. Some naturally occurring bone-specific growth factors have been identified and their use as drugs is being investigated. "The way I visualize the ideal future is that we'll be able to give Drug X that builds up bone to where it's stronger and the risk of fracture is no longer present, then Drug Y maintains it by preventing breakdown," says Stern.

In the realm of devices, researchers are exploring the use of ultrasound to assess bone health. Such tests would eliminate radiation exposure and probably cost less. The study of risk factors

also continues. "We consider that to be the research that has the greatest public health significance," says Sherry Sherman, Ph.D., of the National Institute on Aging. Last fall, the institute launched the Study of Women's Health Across the Nation, a large-scale national examination of the health of women in their 40s and 50s. Researchers expect to learn a great deal about the factors affecting women's health during these transitional years and beyond. Studies of genetics, biochemical markers, and life habits are already turning up new insights.

Osteoporosis has been described as an adolescent disease with a geriatric onset, highlighting the importance of beginning to take steps—in exercise and diet—early in life to reduce its disabling impact in later years.

Is Butter *Really* Better for Me?

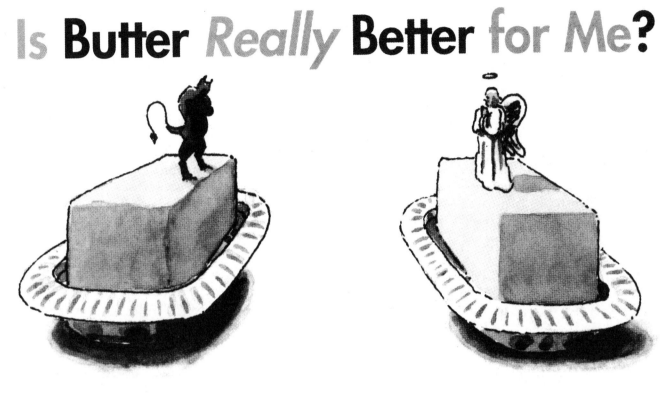

Kathleen Meister

ILLUSTRATION BY LARRY ANDERSON

KATHLEEN MEISTER, M.S., IS A FREELANCE MEDICAL WRITER AND FORMER ACSH RESEARCH ASSOCIATE.

IN THE DR. SEUSS STORY *The Butter Battle Book*, two nations go to war over the question of whether bread should be eaten butter-side-up or butter-side-down. In the United States in 1994, we are facing a different type of butter battle. We're fighting over the type of spread to use on our bread. Should it be butter or margarine?

Until very recently, the American public was firmly convinced that margarine was the healthier choice. And some people still believe that margarine has fewer calories than butter (it doesn't). However, the current controversy about margarine doesn't involve its calorie count. Instead, the principal concern is the possible effect of margarine

on the risk of heart disease. Traditionally, both scientists and the public believed that margarine was good for the heart because it is low in saturated fat. Now, however, people are concerned that margarine may actually be bad for the heart because it is made of partially hydrogenated oils that contain *trans* fatty acids.

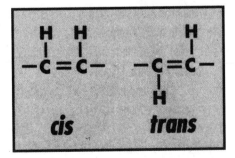

cis   *trans*

What Are *Trans* Fatty Acids Anyway?

The term *trans* refers to a seemingly trivial (but actually very important) aspect of the structure of an unsaturated

fatty acid. In a *trans* fatty acid, the hydrogen atoms surrounding a double bond are on *opposite* sides of the carbon chain. In ordinary unsaturated fatty acids (which chemists call *cis* fatty acids), the hydrogens are on the *same* side.

Why does this matter? It matters because the difference between *cis* and *trans* has a major impact on the shape of the fatty acid molecule. *Cis* fatty acids have bent chains, with a kink in the middle, while *trans* fatty acid chains are essentially straight. As a result of this difference in chain shape, *cis* and *trans* fatty acids have very different properties. For example, *trans* fatty acids have higher melting points and thus are semisolid at room temperature. *Cis* fatty acids are liquid at room temperature.

Practically all of the fatty acids in natural, unmodified vegetable oils are *cis*. However, when these oils are partially

Reprinted with permission from *Priorities*, Vol. 6, No. 4, 1994, pp. 9-11. © 1994 by the American Council on Science and Health, Inc., 1995 Broadway, 2nd Floor, New York, NY 10023-5860.

hydrogenated, substantial amounts of *trans* fatty acids are formed.

Not all *trans* fatty acids come from partially hydrogenated vegetable oils. Small amounts are present in fats derived from ruminant animals — beef, lamb, and dairy fats, including butter. However, the proportion of *trans* fatty acids in these animal fats is low. Butter contains 2-9% *trans* fatty acids, as compared to 25-30% in stick margarines and 13-20% in tub margarines.

Which Foods Contain *Trans* Fatty Acids?

Margarine is not the only food that contains *trans* fatty acids from partially hydrogenated vegetable oils. These oils are also found in vegetable shortenings; commercial deep-frying fats; baked goods such as cookies, cakes and crackers; and salted snacks such as potato and corn chips. In most of these food products, partially hydrogenated oils are used as a substitute for saturated fats such as lard, beef tallow and coconut oil.

Why don't food manufacturers use unmodified vegetable oils in these products? They can't use them because unmodified oils don't have the stability and texture needed for many food processing applications. Unmodified oils can't be used in deep-frying because they quickly turn rancid at high temperatures. They don't create the desired texture in many baked goods. Most obviously, American consumers, who are accustomed to using solid margarine or butter on bread and rolls, simply don't accept liquid oils as a substitute.

Health Concerns About *Trans* Fatty Acids

Trans fatty acids have aroused concern because they may raise blood cholesterol levels. Much attention has been devoted to this subject in recent months, both in scientific journals and in the popular press. Most notably, in a commentary in the *American Journal of Public Health,* two researchers from the Harvard School of Public Health shocked readers by claiming that *trans* fatty acids in partially hydrogenated vegetable oils may be responsible for more than 30,000 deaths per year. This estimate received widespread coverage by the news media. However, it has been seriously questioned by health experts.

The extent of the effect of *trans* fatty acids on blood cholesterol levels depends on the types of fat that you're comparing. If you compare a *trans*-rich fat such as margarine or vegetable shortening to an unmodified oil such as olive oil or corn oil, you will find that *trans* does indeed raise cholesterol levels. This fact is of little practical significance, however, since unmodified corn oil or olive oil cannot be substituted for partially hydrogenated vegetable oil in most food processing applications.

One major reason why many scientists doubt the "30,000 deaths" estimate is that it is based on a comparison between *trans* fatty acids and the type of *cis* unsaturated fatty acid that predominates in olive oil. But since olive oil and partially hydrogenated vegetable oil are not used for the same purposes, comparing them isn't very meaningful.

The more relevant comparison is between *trans*-rich fats and the saturated fats that can be be used in their place. Margarine, vegetable frying fats and shortening should be compared with other fats that can be used for the same purposes, such as butter, beef tallow and lard. Would people be better off if they chose these saturated fats, rather than

Choosing Salad and Cooking Oils

Today's supermarket shoppers face a bewildering array of choices in the salad and cooking oil aisle. From a nutritional standpoint, however, the variety is not as great as it may seem. The similarities among the various oils are actually more important than their differences.

All salad and cooking oils contain the same amount of fat — 14 grams per tablespoon. All provide the same number of calories — about 120 per tablespoon. All are low in saturated fat, and all are free from tropical oils. Some of the oils sold to restaurants and other food service establishments are hydrogenated, but the salad and cooking oil products sold directly to the public for household use are not.

The main difference among oils is that some (including olive, canola and peanut oils) are rich in monounsaturated fatty acids, while others (such as soybean, corn and sunflower oils) are rich in polyunsaturated fatty acids. Which type is better? Actually, there are benefits to each. Polyunsaturated oils may have a stronger cholesterol-lowering effect, but they tend to lower both the HDL (good) and LDL (bad) cholesterol fractions. Monounsaturated oils seem to lower just LDL (bad) cholesterol.

The bottom line: Since both monounsaturated and polyunsaturated oils have advantages, you can feel free to choose any oil that suits your taste. Remember, though, to use as little as possible of any oil, because all oils are very high in total fat and calories.

eating *trans*-rich fats? Unfortunately, no one knows for sure. Only a few studies in human volunteers have compared the effects of *trans*-rich fats with those of saturated fats, and the results of these studies have been inconsistent. More research is clearly needed.

Putting *Trans* Fat into Perspective

Until scientists learn more, the best advice is to be cautious about using *both* saturated fats and *trans*-rich fats. Many of the foods that contain these types of fats are high-calorie, low-nutrient foods that should be eaten in limited amounts anyway. Instead of making the choice of fats your top priority, it is better to concentrate on selecting nutritious foods that are not excessively high in any type of fat or in total calories. For example:

- Rather than worrying about whether your cookies and potato chips are made with coconut oil or partially hydrogenated vegetable oil, it makes sense to eat fewer cookies and potato chips and eat larger amounts of more nutritious snacks (such as fresh fruits and vegetables) instead.

- Rather than agonizing over whether your favorite fast-food chain cooks its foods in beef tallow or partially hydrogenated vegetable oil, it makes sense to eat *all* deep-fried foods less frequently and choose foods prepared in other ways more frequently. If you're grabbing fast food, grab salads, grilled chicken or charbroiled burgers rather than deep-fried chicken, fish or French fries.

Fatty Acid Composition of Popular Salad and Cooking Oils

- Rather than going to war over the choice between butter and margarine, it makes sense to use all table spreads in smaller amounts. Try using other, less fatty products to add flavor and moistness to foods (*e.g.*, syrup or honey on waffles and pancakes, jam or marmalade on toast, sliced tomatoes in sandwiches, salsa or lowfat yogurt on baked potatoes, herbs or lemon juice on vegetables.) Try serving some foods with no topping at all. Use oil instead of butter or margarine for cooking whenever possible (see "Choosing Salad and Cooking Oils"). Also, if you find the taste acceptable, you may want to select one of the newer margarine alternatives that contain less fat than either butter or traditional stick-type margarine (see "What Kind of Margarine Should You Choose?").

Finally, don't fight the butter battle so hard that you lose the health war. Choosing a table spread is only one of the many decisions you make that affect the overall quality of your diet, and diet is only one of the many aspects of your lifestyle that influence your risk of disease. You have more to gain from a comprehensive effort to improve the quality of your diet and from a broad-based program to reduce your risks of chronic diseases than from a narrow focus on any one dietary issue.

Which type of margarine is the best one to choose?

The kind that comes in a tub rather than a stick and calls itself a "spread" rather than "margarine."

Soft, tub-style products are better than hard, stick-type products because they contain smaller proportions of hydrogenated fats. Thus, they contain smaller amounts of saturated and *trans* fatty acids.

The products called "spreads" are better than true margarines because they are lower in total fat and calories. Unlike butter and margarine, which consist almost entirely of fat, spreads contain a substantial amount of non-fatty ingredients such as dairy whey. These ingredients contribute to the flavor of the products but not to their fat content.

An increasing proportion of the products in the "margarine" section of the supermarket are actually spreads rather than margarines. Check the label of your favorite brand. You may already be using a "spread" without even realizing it.

And remember: To cut back on fat and calories, use less of all these products!

Health Implications of Vegetarian Diets

By Ella Haddad, DrPH, RD • Associate Professor • Department of Nutrition • School of Public Health • Loma Linda University • Loma Linda, CA

As the number of individuals adopting vegetarian dietary practices increases, physicians and other healthcare professionals are called upon to provide guidance and advice. The benefits of largely plant-based diets of fruits, vegetables, cereal grains, beans and nuts are being promoted as the Mediterranean and Asian diet pyramids.[1]

Several populations in Mediterranean countries, and some areas in Asia where traditional diets consist largely of foods of plant origin, exhibit low rates of chronic diseases and long life expectancies. Strict vegetarians, or vegans, exclude all food of animal origin. Population studies have shown that vegetarians tend to have lower rates of obesity, heart disease, hypertension, adult-onset diabetes and some cancers. It is generally assumed that the benefits associated with vegetarian diets are due to the fact that these diets contain lower amounts of saturated fat and cholesterol and higher amounts of dietary fiber, antioxidants and phytochemicals.

Vegetarians vary with respect to dietary practices and beliefs. A vegetarian is someone who does not eat animal flesh (meat, poultry, or fish). Lacto-ovovegetarians usually include eggs and dairy products in their meals. Vegetarian diets have gained much respect in recent years and the practice is now generally accepted as a legitimate alternative eating style. The American Dietetic Association position paper states that vegetarian diets "are healthful and nutritionally adequate when appropriately planned."[2] In its latest edition, the Dietary Guidelines for Americans assures the public that vegetarian diets are consistent with the Guidelines and can meet the recommended dietary allowances for nutrients.[3]

Vegetarian Update

There is an increasing tendency among researchers to conclude that the reduced disease risk ob-

Vegetarian Diets: Nutrients and Diet

The adequacy of vegetarian diets depends on the range of foods consumed. Strictly plant-based diets are nearly devoid of vitamin B_{12}. Rauma and colleagues (*J Nutr* 25; 2511, 1995) studied the vitamin B_{12} status in long-term adherents of a strict uncooked vegan diet called the "living food diet" (LFD) in which most food items are fermented or sprouted. Serum vitamin B_{12} concentration and the dietary intakes of 21 long-term adherents of the LFD were compared with those of 21 omnivorous controls. In a longitudinal study, the LFD resulted in decreased serum vitamin B_{12} in six of nine subjects. The cross-sectional study revealed significantly lower serum vitamin B_{12} in the LFD adherents, compared to their matched omnivorous controls. Those consuming nori or chinerilla seaweeds had somewhat better B_{12} status than those who did not, but B_{12} levels fell over time in all but one subject.

Jannell and associates (*J Am Diet Assoc.*, 95:180; 1995) compared the nutrient intake of 23 vegetarian women to 22 nonvegetarian women in a six-month prospective study. Vegetarians were defined as those who excluded meat, fish and poultry from their diets. They were classified as vegans or lacto-vegetarians according to their intake of dairy products. Vegetarian women had significantly lower mean intakes of riboflavin, niacin, vitamin B_{12}, zinc and sodium. Vegans had lower intakes of riboflavin, calcium, and vitamin B_{12} than nonvegetarians; their mean intake of calcium, vitamin B_{12} and zinc were below the RDA for those nutrients. The authors expressed potential concern regarding B_{12} and possibly calcium intake among vegans.

Vegetarian Diet Low in Available Iron

Dietary assessment of iron intake and biochemical measurements were investigated in 55 vegetar-

From *Nutrition & the M.D.*, August 1996, pp. 1-7. © 1996 by Lippincott-Raven Publishers. Reprinted by permission.

served in vegetarians is not explained so much by their not eating meat, but by the fact that they eat more plant foods. There is consensus that dietary advice for those at risk for coronary artery disease should not just narrowly focus on the restriction of dietary saturated fat and cholesterol. Additional effort must be directed toward an increase in the intake of foods high in soluble fiber; vegetable protein; folic acid; antioxidants such as vitamin E, carotenoids, the isoflavonoids, and monounsaturated fat intake. These strategies translate into advice to significantly increase consumption of plant foods such as whole-grain cereals, vegetables, nuts, and legumes. In other words, a diet which is essentially vegetarian in its emphasis[4] is recommended.

That the vegetarian diet is helpful in the control of blood pressure continues to be supported. Melby CL, et al.,[5] found that among African-American Seventh-day Adventists (Seventh-day Adventists are vegetarians), a vegetarian diet (no consumption of animal flesh) is associated with lower blood pressure. In this population, a vegetarian diet was also associated with lower total cholesterol, low density lipoproteins (LDL), and triglycerides than in those consuming an omnivorous diet.

Because many young adult women adopt vegetarian diets, concern has been raised as to whether the practice is related to eating disorders such as anorexia. This does not appear to be the case. Janelle et al.[6] compared nutrient intake and eating behavior scores of vegetarian and nonvegetarian women between the ages of 20 to 40 years. Vegetarian women had lower dietary restraint scores. Dietary restraint is the perception of consciously limiting food intake to control weight. If weight loss were a major motivating factor for becoming vegetarian then it would be expected that vegetarians would have higher levels of dietary restraint.

Results of epidemiologic studies are traditionally expressed in terms of relative risk, a concept difficult for the public to grasp. In a recent re-examination of data from the Adventist Health Study[7], novel statistical calculations show how certain effects may delay or advance the first expression of disease. The Adventist Health Study is a cohort investigation of approximately 34,000 California non-Hispanic, white subjects living in Seventh-day Adventist households and followed for six years. Among its findings:

• Non-vegetarians develop coronary disease 1.77 years earlier than vegetarians.

• Among males, non-vegetarians have a remaining lifetime risk of developing coronary disease that is

ians and 59 nonvegetarians (*J Nutr*, 125; 212, 1995). In the vegetarian diet, soybean products replaced meat. Thus, the vegetarian diet rich in soybean products and restricted in animal foods, had limited bioavailable iron and did not maintain iron balance in men or women. There was a greater prevalence of low ferritin levels and anemia in the vegetarians, especially the women.

In a study by Alexander and associates (*Eur J Clin Nutr*; 48:538, 1994), similar calcium and zinc intakes were found in the vegetarians and omnivorous controls. Protein and vitamin D intake were significantly lower in vegetarians, particularly in vegans. Forty-five non-vegan vegetarians and five vegans were compared to 50 omnivorous controls in a prospective four-week study. Iron intakes were significantly higher in vegetarians than in omnivores. However, bioavailability of non-heme iron is known to be considerably lower and male vegetarians had lower ferritin levels compared to omnivores. All the vegans had B_{12} intakes below recommended levels and 35% of the long-term vegetarians and vegans had serum vitamin B_{12} concentrations below the reference range.

A vegetarian food guide has been developed for use by nutrition educators to assess vegetarian diets and to teach how to plan an adequate vegetarian diet. When all animal foods are avoided, consideration should be given to a source of vitamin D. Under certain conditions, sources of calcium may be needed in certain stages of life and additional sources of vitamin B_{12} are indicated for all vegans (*Am J Clin Nutr*; 59 [suppl]: 1248S, 1994).

11.9 percentage points higher (p < 0.05) than vegetarians.

• Non-vegetarian females have remaining lifetime risk of developing coronary disease that is 0.26 percentage points lower than female vegetarians.

• Those who rarely consume nuts develop coronary disease 2.64 years earlier and have an 11.9 percentage points greater remaining lifetime risk (p = 0.05) than persons who eat nuts at least five times each week.

The Physician and Vegetarian Patients

Physicians who may be called upon to evaluate their patients' diets must bear in mind that vegetarian dietary practices differ widely and individual assessment is needed to evaluate the nutritional quality of a given diet. To assist in such an evaluation, patients can keep a food diary or the physician can ask questions about intake and dietary habits.

1) Weight status

It is most important to evaluate the patient's weight status. Many plant foods are low in calories and meeting caloric needs may be a challenge for some vegetarians. This is especially true of children and adolescents, the elderly, vegans, and individuals who avoid all added fats and oils. Inadequate caloric consumption compromises protein and micronutrient intake. Adequate energy intake from a variety of foods to maintain desirable body weight is vital to nutrient sufficiency.

2) Vitamin B$_{12}$ (cobalamin)

Dietary deficiency of vitamin B$_{12}$ may result from a strict plant-based diet because the vitamin is absent from foods of plant origin. Analogs of the vitamin found in algae, spirulina, nori, or fermented soy products such as miso and tempeh, do not have vitamin activity for humans. Occasionally, lacto-ovo vegetarians may also have low serum B$_{12}$ if their intake of dairy products or eggs is low. Vegans and elderly vegetarians need to regularly consume a reliable source of the vitamin. This can be either cobalamin-fortified foods or vitamin preparations (a minimum of 50 µg per week).

Individuals with low serum B$_{12}$ may manifest paresthesia (numbness and tingling in the hands and legs), weakness, fatigue, loss of vibration and position sense, and a range of psychiatric disorders including disorientation, depression, and memory loss. The use of alcohol, tobacco and drugs such as antacids, neomycin, colchicine, and aminosalicylic acid may contribute to the problem by causing B$_{12}$ malabsorption in both omnivores and vegetarians. B$_{12}$ deficits may be fairly common in the elderly and may be associated with common neuropsychiatric disorders seen in the geriatric population. While oral B$_{12}$ supplements can restore serum levels of B$_{12}$ and eliminate macrocytic anemia, neurological disorders may persist for months after the initiation of treatment.

3) Vitamin D

In the U.S., milk is fortified with vitamin D. Vegans who avoid all animal foods and all dairy products need a supplementary source of vitamin D especially in northern climates and during the winter months.

4) Calcium

Studies on bone density, osteoporosis, and fracture rates have shown little differences between vegetarians and omnivores. In all such studies however, most of the subjects have been lactovegetarian. Vegans and those who avoid milk and dairy products must be encouraged to regularly consume calcium-rich vegetables (broccoli, Chinese cabbage, kale, mustard greens, turnip greens, and parsley) and food items such as calcium-containing tofu, calcium-fortified fruit juices and milk alternatives, or to take a calcium supplement.

5) Iron and zinc

Trace mineral intake is adequate in most vegetarians. Grains, legumes, nuts, green leafy vegetables contain substantial amounts of iron, zinc and other minerals. Some plant foods contain inhibitors of iron and zinc absorption (phytate in whole grains), but this does not seem to compromise status when the overall diet is varied and adequate. The absorption of iron is substantially enhanced by ascorbic acid. In Western countries, although ferritin levels are lower, iron deficiency anemia is not more prevalent among adult vegetarians than in omnivores.

Summary

Patients who show an interest in vegetarian diets as a dietary alternative should be encouraged by their physicians to do so. In general, patients must also be encouraged to have more meatless meals and consume more plant foods. A simple food guide (Table 1) provides the basic framework for daily intake.[8] A lactovegetarian diet, if properly selected, can meet all the nutritional needs of adults and children. There is, however, a clear case for supplementation of vitamin B$_{12}$ (and possibly vitamin D and calcium) for individuals following strictly vegan diets. Patients may be referred to Registered Dietitians for guidance or they may write to organizations which provide information.

References

1. Willett, W.C., et al. Mediterranean diet pyramid: a cultural model for healthy eating. *Am J Clin Nutr* 61:1402S; 1995.

2. Position of The American Dietetic Association: Vegetarian Diets. *J Am Diet Assoc* In comparison with vegetarians 93:1317; 1993.

3. Nutrition and Your Health: Dietary Guidelines for Americans. 4th ed. Washington, DC: U.S. Dept. of Agriculture and U.S. Dept. of Health and Human Services; 1995.

4. Roberts, W.C. Preventing and arresting coronary atherosclerosis. *Am Heart J* 130:580;1995.

5. Melby, C.L., et al. Blood pressure and blood lipids among vegetarian, semivegetarian, and non-

Table I. Food Guide for Vegetarians

Food Group	Servings	Serving Size
Breads, grains, cereals[1]	6 - 11	1 slice bread; 1/2 cup cooked cereal; 1 oz (3/4 - 1 cup) ready-to-eat cereal; 1 6-inch tortilla; small roll
Legumes, plant proteins	1 - 2	1/2 cup cooked dry beans, lentils, peas, limas. 1/2 cup soy products, meat analogs, tofu
Nuts, seeds	1 - 2	1/4 - 1/3 cup almonds, walnuts, sunflower seeds 2 tbsp peanut butter, almond butter, tahini
Vegetables, leafy greens[2]	3 - 5	1/2 cup cooked vegetable; 1 cup raw chopped vegetable or salad; 3/4 cup vegetable juice
Fruits	2 - 4	1 medium apple, orange, banana, etc.; 1/2 cup chopped, cooked, or canned fruit; 1/4 cup dried fruit; 3/4 cup fruit juice
Milk, yogurt, milk alternatives	2 - 3[3]	1 cup low-fat or nonfat milk or yogurt; 1-2 oz low fat cheese; 1 cup fortified soymilk (calcium, vitamin D, vitamin B_{12}); 1 cup tofu
Fats, oil	2 - 6	1 tsp oil, margarine, mayonnaise; 2 tsp salad dressing; 1/8 avocado; 5 olives
Sugar	0 - 9	1 tsp sugar, jam, jelly, honey, syrup, etc.

[1]*At least half of the servings from whole-grain breads and cereals*
[2]*Vegans must include at least 2 servings of green vegetables daily (broccoli, kale, collards, other green leafy)*
[3]*Three servings for women who are pregnant or breast-feeding, children, teenagers, young adults ≤24 years of age*

vegetarian African Americans. *Am J Clin Nutr* 59:103; 1995.

6. Janelle, K.C., Barr SI. Nutrient intakes and eating behavior scores of vegetarian and nonvegetarian women. *J Am Diet Assoc* 95:180; 1995.

7. Fraser, G.E., Lindsted, K.D., Beeson, W.L. Effect of risk factor values on lifetime risk of and age at first coronary event: The Adventist Health Study. *Am J of Epidemiol* 746; 1995.

8. Haddad, E.H. Development of a vegetarian food guide. *Am J Clin Nutr* 59 (suppl)1248S; 1994.

About the Author

Ella Haddad, DrPH, RD, is Associate Professor at the Department of Nutrition, School of Public Health, Loma Linda University. She has been a Registered Dietitian since 1957. Her main research interest is the nutrtional adequacy of vegetarian and/or vegan diets, especially with respect to zinc and calcium status.

For Further Reading

Eating for the Health of It, by Winston Craig, PhD, RD (Eau Claire, MI: Golden Harvest, 1993).

Simply Vegan, by Debra Wasserman and Reed Mangels, PhD, RD (Baltimore, MD: Vegetarian Resource Group, 1991).

The Dietitian's Guide to Vegetarian Diets: Issues and Applications, by Mark Messina, PhD and Virginia Messina, MPH, RD (Gaithersburg MD: Aspen Pub. Inc., 1996).

Sources of Information

Vegetarian Nutrition Dietetic Practice Group of the American Dietetic Association
216 West Jackson Boulevard
Chicago IL 60606-6995
(312) 899-0040

Seventh-day Adventist Dietetic Association
PO Box 75
Loma Linda CA 92354
(909) 793-8918

Vegetarian Resource Group
PO Box 1463
Baltimore MD 21203
(410) 366-8343

(continued)

What is a Vegetarian?

Vegan: Vegans eat only non-animal foods. They avoid all meats, fish, poultry, dairy products and milk. Some vegans also avoid honey.

Lacto-ovo vegetarian: These vegetarians include dairy products and eggs in their diet but avoid meats, poultry, and seafood.

Lacto-vegetarian: Lacto-vegetarians include dairy products in their diet, but avoid meats, fish, poultry, seafood and egg products.

Semi-vegetarians: These people usually avoid meat but occasionally eat some animal foods such as fish and poultry.

The Effects of Vegetarian Diets on Infants and Children

Vegetarianism has gained popularity in the West and has been practiced for centuries in Asia. Strict vegetarian or vegan diets may offer health advantages to adults who desire a low-saturated fat, high-fiber diet. However, the adequacy of these diets for infants and children may cause some concern. Risk of nutrient deficiency is greatest during periods of physiological stress and accelerated growth. Problems with dietary inadequacy are more likely to occur in children because their requirements relative to body weight are greater and they are less able to exert control over what they eat compared to adults. Severe malnutrition, as well as deficiencies of iron, vitamin B_{12}, calcium, and vitamin D, have been reported in infants and toddlers fed inappropriate vegetarian diets (*Am J Clin Nutr;* 59 [suppl]; 1176S, 1994).

Macrobiotic Diet

People who eat a macrobiotic diet advocate the use of locally grown whole foods such as grains, fresh vegetables, sea vegetables and beans. Sea salt and grain sweeteners such as rice syrup replace refined salt and sugar. Processed foods containing chemical additives are avoided, as are most concentrated fats. Animal foods (meat, poultry and dairy products) are not recommended except for small amounts of white fish (Source: *Becoming Vegetarian,* Melina, Davis and Harrison; Book Publishing Company, 1995; p.3).

Vegetarian diets that contain milk products and eggs are less likely to be inadequate than vegan diets. Meat and fish provide several nutrients that are scarce or absent from common foods of plant origin including iodine, taurine, vitamin B_{12}, vitamin D, and long-chain polyunsaturated fatty acids such as eicosapentaenoic and docosahexaenoic acid (DHA). Meat is also an important source of protein and iron in the diet, especially the heme iron that is well absorbed. Iron intakes of vegetarians are dependent on the iron content of the staple foods, wheat being superior to rice. Absorption of minerals such as iron, zinc, and calcium, are reduced in the presence of phytates common to plant sources and unrefined cereals favored by vegetarians.

Most vegan children are breast-fed into the second year of life. Problems of nutritional inadequacy may occur when infants are weaned onto an unsuitable breast-milk substitute. If fortified soya milk is used, most problems can be avoided. Iron-deficiency anemia in infancy is associated with late weaning practices and in macrobiotic vegetarians. Serum ferritin levels are low in vegetarian women of childbearing age. It has been reported that low ferritin levels ($<12\mu g/L$) in early pregnancy are associated with an increased risk of prematurity and low birth weight (ibid).

Severe malnutrition, as well as deficiencies of iron, vitamin B_{12}, calcium, and vitamin D, have been reported in infants and toddlers fed inappropriate vegetarian diets.

Factors known to influence the occurrence of rickets in vegetarians are the high phytate content of the macrobiotic diet, the dietary intake of vitamin D, exposure to sunlight, and the availability of dietary calcium. It has been proposed that high phytate diets increase vitamin D requirements. It is known that low availability of calcium from the diet increases parathyroid hormone production and increases the catabolism of vitamin D (ibid).

Differences in maternal diets result in infants born with different stores of essential fatty acids. Vegetarian, especially vegan diets, are rich in linoleic acid and have a high ratio of linoleic to linolenic acid. Some investigators believe this diet inhibits conversion of linolenic acid to DHA. It might be appropriate to suggest the use of soybean or canola oils for cooking, as they have lower such ratios.

Macrobiotic Diets

Bonny Specker summarized several studies regarding the calcium, vitamin D, and vitamin B_{12} status of lactating women consuming a vegetarian, mostly macrobiotic, diet. Vitamin D and calcium were not significant problems for the infants even though the intakes were low. A significant number of vegetarian women consuming a macrobiotic diet showed biochemical evidence of vitamin B_{12} deficiency. The prevalence of vitamin B_{12} deficiency did not appear higher in lactating women compared with non-lactating women. However, there was a relationship between maternal and infant vitamin B_{12} status with a large portion of infants showing vitamin B_{12} deficiency (*AJCN* 59[suppl]; 1182S, 1994).

Vitamin B_{12} deficiency usually presents with neurological signs and symptoms in infants. Many vegans are aware of the need to supplement their diets with vitamin B_{12}. J. Schneede, et al., studied omnivorous controls to determine the usefulness of metabolites in the diagnosis of dietary cobalamin deficiency. In the macrobiotic infants, both methylmalonic acid and total homocysteine were markedly increased (eight-fold and two-fold) over the controls. This represents a sensitive and specific test for the diagnosis and follow-up of functional cobalamin deficiency in infants (*Pediatric Research*, 36; 194, 1994).

Dagnelie and van Staveren conducted a population-based study on the nutritional status of children consuming macrobiotic diets in the Netherlands. They found that the macrobiotic diet consisting of whole-grain cereals (mainly unpolished rice), vegetables, and pulses, with small additions of seaweed, fermented foods, nuts, seeds and seasonal fruits caused ubiquitous deficiencies of energy, protein, vitamin B_{12}, calcium and riboflavin in macrobiotic infants. These deficiencies lead to retarded growth, fat and muscle wasting and slower psychomotor development. The breast milk of these mothers contained less vitamin B_{12}, calcium and magnesium (*AJCN*; 59[suppl]; 1187S, 1994).

Dagnelie and van Staveren suggest that certain modifications to the macrobiotic diet which are consistent with the macrobiotic philosophy could help to make the diet nutritionally adequate. These include:

1. The addition of dietary fat as a source of energy to >25-30% of energy intake in children e.g., from 4-5 tsp. of oil/day or twice this amount of nuts and seeds.

2. The inclusion of 3-5 oz per week of fatty fish to supply 2-3µg vitamin D/day.

3. Limited amounts of seaweed due to their content of vitamin B-12 analogues, which may block vitamin B-12 metabolism.

4. The inclusion of at least one serving per day of dairy products to provide a source of calcium, protein and riboflavin.

5. Reduction of fiber intake by children ≤2 years of age. This could be achieved by sieving the children's food and partly replacing whole cereal foods by lower-fiber food products (*AJCN*, 59 [suppl]; 1187S, 1994).

Fat and Weight Control

There have been times and places in history when being fat was considered beautiful. Harry Golden, writing in *Only in America* (Cleveland, Ohio: World Publishing Company, 1958), tells how it was on the Lower East Side of New York when he was a boy. For two cents and accompanied by lots of fanfare, the salesman would guess a person's weight and weigh him or her in public. It was a big social event on Saturday night in a society where women bragged about gaining five pounds and practiced ways to simulate double chins. Harry and his mother, however, had differing views:

> When I weigh myself I do not look at the results. I just listen to the gears grind and, when everything quiets down, I simply step off the scales and walk away. By this system I have won the battle, leaving the machine frustrated, if not useless. I was always a fat kid and once when I complained about it my mother said, "Nothing at all to worry about; in America the fat man is always the boss and the skinny man is always the bookkeeper."

Today's society, however, does not view fat pounds with pride. Thin is in. It is the willowy person who is seen as beautiful, socially acceptable, and appealing to the opposite sex. Those of us with bulges and bumps will knead and pound, use saunas, and starve ourselves—anything to lose a pound. Surveys indicate that as many as 40 percent of adult women and a quarter of adult men are dieting at any given time. Even more telling is the high number of grade school and adolescent girls who have reported weight loss attempts, often at the behest of their mothers.

In spite of these attitudes and values, and regardless of national goals to the contrary, America has gained weight. Following a steady trend, about one-third of the adult population has added an average of eight pounds in the last decade. Although whites of both genders have gained the most, weight increases cut across all ethnic, age, and gender groups. These findings are not unique to the United States; most of the industrialized world has seen a similar phenomenon since World War I. Still, the United States exceeds other countries in prevalence of overweight. This is not good news for the Healthy People 2000 goal, which calls for reducing overweight to no more than 20 percent of adults.

It is ironic that weight gain has occurred during the very time period when we have actually reduced fat consumption by about 3 percent of total calories. Perhaps there's a lesson to remember, one we'd like to forget and one that marketers of the hundreds of low- and no-fat foods would like us to ignore. Calories still count! Recipes can be changed to lower fat content, to be sure, but the fat is often replaced with high amounts of sugar. Some studies also suggest that we simply compensate for the reduced-fat foods at a later time. In addition, alcohol accounts for 6 percent of our caloric intake.

Questions about weight are still unanswered. Why do some of us gain too much with extraordinary ease when others try to gain and fail? How much *should* we weigh? Experts simply do not agree. The first two articles in this unit will discuss the uncertainties. We know a lot more than we did but still not enough to reach absolute conclusions. Yes, an obesity gene has been discovered, as have natural body chemicals that participate in the control of appetite. Any practical applications appear to be years away, however, although various news items indicate that companies will try to capitalize on this early information and public interest.

With the release of a major study from Cornell University, healthy weights are back in the news. Only recently we have, once again, been told to lower our view of appropriate weights and forget about increasing weight with age. But almost overnight higher weights are again in focus, as an intensive review of previous major longitudinal studies supports higher weights and shows health risks of moderate underweight equal to those of moderate overweight. That higher weights are especially protective for the elderly is borne out by a recent study from the National Institutes for Health and reported in "New Study Finds Higher Weight Protects Elderly."

One school of thought holds that, especially in the presence of other health risks, dieting must be attempted and can produce desired results. Others claim that it is far wiser to focus on lifestyle changes rather than on weight loss, and on health rather than on total weight. This philosophy espouses empowerment to increase self-awareness and effect gradual change, which is more likely to be permanent. If it works, it is a powerful argument, since most dieters regain their lost pounds within a few years.

One advantage of higher weights has stood over time, and that is protection against osteoporosis. This is a sig-

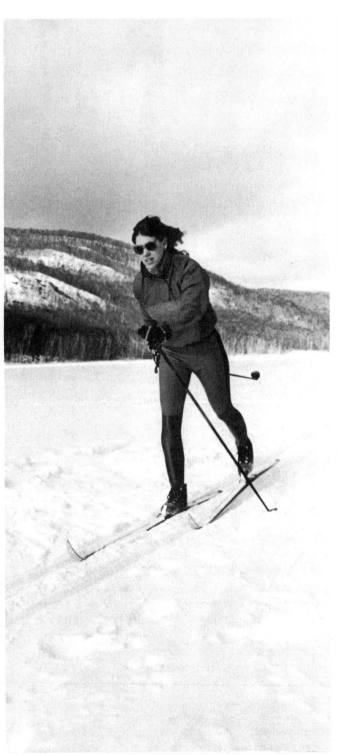

Weight Loss." Thus, in one's assessment of benefit and risk, the health advantages of weight loss must be counterbalanced by increased vulnerability to brittle bones.

If one does decide that losing weight is appropriate, doing so can become a major challenge. Health should be the focus, not societal pressure or fitting into a bathing suit. Most diets will work if adhered to, but weight loss alone is not cause for celebration. The trick is to keep it off, for only then is it effective. Just as important is losing it safely. Put together, this means loss that is slow and gradual, a permanent lifestyle change that includes exercise, and maintaining a diet that provides adequate nutrients and calories. This is not exciting, not dramatic, and not easy; in fact, it is just plain hard work. Even then, many Americans are not successful. Often, of course, people opt for weight-loss centers and achieve varying degrees of success. Periodically these centers become news items when they fail to disclose enough information about costs, success rates, and staff credentials. In the article "Losing Weight Safely" you will find guidelines for safe and effective weight loss. A more dramatic solution for the severely obese is described in "Surgery for Obesity." Where surgery is appropriate, gastric restriction may be viable.

Many experts see prevention of obesity as the most effective strategy for those still at healthy weights, and it is logical that childhood should be targeted as a time when future eating behaviors are established. The final article describes the responsibilities of both the parent and the child in the feeding process. Adhering to these roles is believed to enable the child to recognize internal regulatory cues and avoid overfeeding. However, even overweight children should grow up with emotionally healthy attitudes about themselves.

Given the intense interest among both health professionals and the public, other ways of controlling weight will no doubt be found in the future. Most people hope that any innovations or new strategies will permit appetite satisfaction and an occasional strawberry shortcake.

Looking Ahead: Challenge Questions

How does concern about your weight affect your life and that of your friends? Analyze your attitudes and behavior and describe what, if any, changes in these are appropriate.

What are the issues of benefit and risk that one should consider before deciding to go on a diet?

Find a description of a new trendy diet and evaluate it for effectiveness and safety.

Which of the many products with fat and sugar substitutes do you like? What was your purpose in using them? Did you reduce total calories by using these products?

Do you think weight reduction should be a national goal? Why or why not? What population groups would you target, and what strategies would you use?

nificant point, especially but not exclusively for the elderly, white female, as it accounts for most of the fractures of aging and millions of health care dollars annually. It is disconcerting to discover the negative effects of dieting on bone density, irrespective of the quality of one's diet or amount of exercise, that is described in "Dieting and

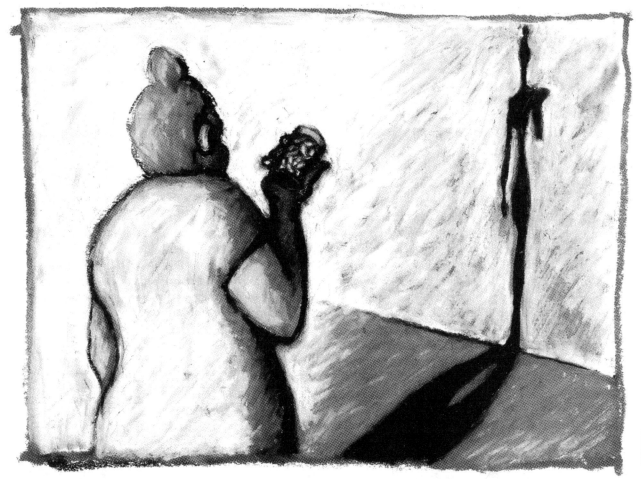

ILLUSTRATION: LARRY ANDERSON

OBESITY: NO MIRACLE CURE YET

KRISTINE NAPIER

People burdened with extra body fat know all too well that one size doesn't fit all—especially when it comes to weight loss. Many are hoping, though, that today's rapidly progressing research on the genetics of obesity will produce a one-size-fits-all approach to slimming down their bulging curves. But as exciting as this research is, the unfortunate reality is that most overweight people won't be able to squeeze a solution out of it.

Recently, U.S. health officials announced that the percentage of obese Americans—those packing 20 to 30 percent more than their ideal body weight—had grown from a decades-long level of a quarter of the population to a hefty third of the population. In everyday terms, that means that the average 5' 6" woman, who should weigh between 117 and 143 pounds (see box on page 119 to see how to figure your own healthy weight), is considered obese if her weight is above a range of 171 to 186 pounds.

Obesity. It's worse than a four-letter word. The condition ranks with the worst of physical afflictions. Obese people lug around enough extra weight to cause serious health problems. There is much evidence that obesity significantly increases a person's risk of developing high blood pressure, abnormal blood cholesterol levels, diabetes, gout and osteoarthritis. Indirectly, obesity is a major risk factor for dying too young. The collective impact of obesity on the nation's health—and on its health care costs—is enormous.

Americans express genuine concern about their excess weight. Of all their physical maladies, it's the one complaint that vast numbers of them focus on curing. But for all the talk there's very little action. Many Americans lose some weight with each dieting effort, but it's a paltry few that keep it off for more than a year. Repeated attempts at weight loss not only feed feelings of failure but also nurture tremendous frustration and negative self talk.

THE SKINNY ON ANTI-OBESITY DRUGS

People have long sought a "magic bullet" for obesity—a drink, injection or pill that would magically melt away those excess pounds. Cracking the obesity nut has also perplexed the scientists searching for an effective obesity cure. In the 50s and 60s many doctors prescribed amphetamines, also called "uppers." These drugs helped people lose weight by curbing their appetite, but they created more problems than they solved. Amphetamines were highly addictive; they also made users high or stimulated them to the point of euphoria and/or dangerous aggression.

Knowing that appetite could be controlled chemically, researchers began searching for a replacement for amphetamines—for a drug that could control appetite without producing amphetamines' harmful effects. Scientists today are still searching along three lines: They are investigating drugs that curb appetite, drugs that rev up the body's metabolic rate and burn fat faster and drugs that act like the body's own naturally occurring leptin (see main article).

The U.S. Food and Drug Administration (FDA) recently approved the first anti-obesity drug for long-term use. Dexfenfluramine, long available in Europe, will be sold in the U.S. later this year under the trade name Redux. This new drug is in the category of drugs that curb appetite.

Dexfenfluramine suppresses appetite—particularly carbohydrate cravings—by maintaining higher levels of serotonin, a so-called neurotransmitter, in the brain. Serotonin is a critical factor in mood control. Many antidepressant drugs work by controlling serotonin levels, and appetite control is linked to those mental processes that work to modulate mood and feelings of stress. High serotonin levels are desirable in people who need to lose weight because high serotonin levels help to reduce appetite. Dexfenfluramine works to keep serotonin levels high by preventing its breakdown and stimulating cells to produce even more.

There are concerns about using dexfenfluramine. Stopping it might cause a person to experience a sudden severe depression or might cause unpredictable, impulsive behavior. Rodent research has shown that serotonin levels can stay at abnormally low levels for months after the drug is discontinued—and normal serotonin levels are necessary for normal mood control. Another concern is whether it will be possible for a person to maintain weight loss without the drug. There is some speculation that indefinite, long-term use of dexfenfluramine may be necessary to prevent someone's regaining shed pounds.

Among the other drugs currently in use for weight loss are phentermine and fenfluramine. These two drugs are chemically related to amphetamines. Both phentermine and fenfluramine have been around for many years, but there has been a resurgence in their use as diet aids. Phentermine and fenfluramine are often prescribed together, and for a very good reason. "While fenfluramine can cause central nervous system depression, phentermine is more of a stimulant," says Mary Ann Stuhan, R.Ph., a clinical pharmacist at Cleveland's Mt. Sinai Medical Center.

Stuhan also points out that the FDA recommends that these two drugs be used for only a few weeks; among the reasons for this abbreviated use is that phentermine and fenfluramine are addictive. "Indeed, they are useful in appetite suppression short term, but the emphasis is on the short term. They should be used only in conjunction with education on how to change lifestyle. People have to remember that drugs alone will not cause any significant weight loss. Medications such as fenfluramine and phentermine should only be used in the first couple of weeks of weight loss effort when people are learning how to change their habits."

Some people have turned to what has been termed a natural weight loss aid—the mineral chromium. Its proponents claim that chromium, which is needed by the body in small amounts, can help overweight people shed excess pounds (this among other questionable health claims made for the mineral). But the studies conducted on chromium's weight-loss potential have themselves been questionable at best. In addition, preliminary research (and we stress *preliminary*) suggests that ingesting large quantities of chromium might cause chromosome damage. For now, experts say that chromium supplements simply cannot be recommended for weight loss or for any other condition.

What some people don't realize is that any weight-loss drug is only an aid. A drug must be accompanied by an intensive program of behavior modification—a program that helps define a healthier style of eating and exercising to be followed *forever*.

That's precisely why news of advances in understanding the genetic underpinnings of obesity sends ripples of excitement through the country. News of the obesity (ob) gene, of the newly discovered hormone leptin and of new weight-loss drugs has captured headlines for months. But what's the news all about?

Exciting Discoveries

The first wave of news came with the December 1994 discovery by researchers at New York's Rockefeller University that the portliness of a strain of overweight mice can be explained by their having a defective version of the ob gene.

In normal mice, a properly working version of the ob gene tells fat cells to make a special protein—a hormone called leptin—but to make it only when the body's fat cells have stored enough fat. The leptin travels through the bloodstream to the brain and tells the brain the body has stored a healthy amount of body fat. The mice then regulate their food intake and maintain normal body weight.

Mice with an absent or defective ob gene don't make leptin when they've eaten enough food and stored enough fat. No leptin, no message to the brain. The mice overeat and plump up.

Six months after the discovery of the ob gene, three teams of researchers, including the Rockefeller team, reported injecting the ob mice with leptin—with dramatic results. The once obese rodents ate less, slimmed down and even revved up their metabolism to burn calories at an increased rate. Even normal-weight mice injected with leptin lost body weight.

Obese people were ready to line up for leptin injections. Their hopes were quickly dashed by the next discoveries, however. Unlike their rotund rodent friends, obese humans do not have a mutated ob gene. What's more, obese humans aren't even lacking leptin. Surprisingly, tests revealed that obese people actually have leptin levels some 20 to 30 times higher than the levels found in lean people.

Researchers speculated that the obese human body wasn't "hearing" the leptin's message. Like other body hormones, leptin can't do its job of curbing the appetite unless the body heeds the hormone's call. In a fascinating and intricate system, the body "hears" a hormone's message via receptors. Receptors are basically antennae—the connections through which the messages carried by the hormones are transmitted to the brain. When the receptors are faulty, a message cannot be relayed to the brain. Unheard by the brain, the message—such as the one contained in leptin—cannot bring about any change.

A further advance will help researchers discover if the deaf-to-leptin theory is true. In December 1995 researchers from Millennium Pharmaceuticals in Cambridge, Massachusetts, and Hoffman-LaRoche in Nutley, New Jersey, reported finding the location of the leptin receptor in the human brain. The researchers are now probing to find out if the leptin receptors in the brains of obese people are faulty. The scientists' hunch is that only a very small percentage of obese people have defective leptin receptors.

> **Americans have developed very poor health habits. We drop off dry cleaning, library books and mail at drive-up windows, then drive through a fast-food line to order a fat-laden, thousand-calorie lunch.**

If any treatment is to result from this series of discoveries, it will probably come in the form of drugs devised to modulate or change the receptor to allow it to hook up with the leptin and receive its message. Scientists are engaged in promising research along these lines. Investigators in one line of research have discovered that when properly working leptin receptors in normal-weight mice are overstimulated, the mice eat less and become very thin. The investigators are hoping that overstimulating the properly functioning leptin receptors in obese humans will have the same effect—and will ultimately help those people to lose weight.

This solution would only work, however, if an obese person had enough properly working leptin receptors. Someone with severely abnormal leptin receptors or with very few normal receptors would need a far more complex type of therapy—therapy that could repair the severely defective gene responsible for making leptin receptors. This almost science-fiction solution is years away—probably even decades away. The first step is to identify leptin-receptor gene mutations in obese people—exactly what the researchers at Millennium are currently trying to do.

Other types of therapies would be necessary if an obese person's body produced normal amounts of leptin and had normal receptors—which might indeed be the case with some obese people. Such a person's brain cells might still be "deaf" to leptin's message. It's as if a television set had a normal antenna but a broken circuit board. This person would need a drug therapy that somehow could fix the broken circuit inside the cell to let leptin's message get through.

On still another front, investigators are conducting research they suspect will identify how leptin affects yet other genes to influence appetite and weight. One exciting research area involves a hormone called glucagon-like peptide-1 (GLP-1), a known appetite suppressant. It seems highly likely that leptin sends messages to genes that in turn signal cells to make more GLP-1.

It's Not All in the Genes

These discoveries have been reported well to a rapidly progressing scientific world. But a critical fact about these advances hasn't made it through the filter of the lay media to the consumer: These discoveries, however exciting, probably apply to only a small percentage of overweight Americans. Millennium researchers stress that very few obese Americans have a faulty leptin receptor or have cells deaf to leptin's message.

But how do scientists know this without having identified faulty leptin receptors yet? For one thing, they know that human genes haven't changed much for several generations—but the incidence of human obesity has. The researchers also know that we live in a world of caloric excess and activity deprivation. In short, Americans have developed very poor health habits. We drop off dry cleaning, library books and mail at drive-up windows, then drive through a fast-food line to order a fat-laden, thousand-calorie lunch. We replace too many home-cooked meals with higher fat frozen or carry-out versions. We snack in our easy chairs in front of the TV with remote in hand. A single convenience—an electric can opener or pencil sharpener, a garage-door opener, an extension phone in every room—doesn't make a huge difference in the number of calories burned, but taken together they turn us into sedentary blobs. Similarly, an occasional fast-food meal is perfectly fine; but the combination of a steady diet of fast food and convenience food with no regular exercise is deadly to the waistline.

Americans with 20 or 30 pounds to lose shouldn't wait for advancing obesity research to produce a magic pill. Instead, they should develop a lifestyle that focuses on fitness and health rather than on taste and convenience. They—and, indeed, most of us—need to eat less and exercise more. Even that small percentage of Americans whose obesity is due to genetic factors—and for whom new drugs may be developed one day—will have to eat less and exercise more. Some truths never change.

WHAT'S A HEALTHY WEIGHT?

Why does healthy weight vary so widely for people of the same height? Bone structure has a lot to do with it, as does the type of weight a person carries. Bigger boned people and people with dense muscle mass can safely carry around more weight than can people with large fat deposits.

The following is an easy, rule-of-thumb way to figure the range of normal body weight:

- For men: Figure 106 pounds for the first five feet of height and 6 additional pounds for each inch over five feet. Weights 10 percent over and 10 percent under this figure are within the normal range.

- For women: Figure 100 pounds for the first five feet and 5 additional pounds for each inch over five feet. Again, weights 10 percent over and 10 percent under this figure are normal

For example, for a woman 5' 6" tall (66 inches), the midpoint of healthy weight would be 130 pounds. That's 100 pounds plus the 6 additional inches times 5 pounds per inch, or 100 plus 30 pounds. This weight could be 10 percent lower (130 minus 13 pounds, or 117 pounds for a small-boned woman with low muscle) or 10 percent higher (130 plus 13 pounds, or 143 pounds for a large-boned woman who exercises and has a greater amount of muscle). A normal range of weight for a 5' 6" tall woman would thus be between 117 and 143 pounds.

KRISTINE NAPIER, M.P.H., R.D., IS A FREELANCE HEALTH AND SCIENCE WRITER AND EDITOR BASED IN CLEVELAND, OH. SHE CONTRIBUTES REGULARLY TO *PRIORITIES* AND OTHER ACSH PUBLICATIONS.

New study questions weight guidelines

Frances M. Berg, MS

The new U.S. guidelines for healthy weight were barely off the press when another study appeared which highlights the controversy surrounding the topic of healthy weight.

The impressive new Cornell University study suggests, first, that there is as much risk in being moderately underweight as overweight; second, that the recommended range of healthy weight may be set too low at both lower and upper limits; and third, that life insurance data on which weight recommendations have often been based does not accurately represent the U.S. population *(I J Obesity 1996;20:1:63-75).*

The optimal weight for men appears to be about 15 pounds heavier than most recommendations, or about the average weight of men in the United States, says Richard P. Troiano, PhD, RD, lead author in the Cornell study.

The evidence comes from an analysis of 22 longitudinal studies on weight as related to all-cause mortality. Some 1,000 citations were reviewed to find these studies, all that met the criteria and provided weight cut-off values and a comparison of at least three groups of healthy subjects.

Studies were combined through advanced analysis techniques to increase validity and obtain large sample sizes. Most of the analysis focused on the risks of white men, since there was limited information on white women and even less on minority men and women.

The white male sample consisted of 17 studies, 37 substudies and 235 weight groups which included 356,747 men, average age 50 years at entry. In this group there had been 38,032 deaths.

Lowest mortality

Analysis showed the lowest risk of death was between a body mass index of 23 and 29, with 27 as the point of lowest risk in 10-year follow-up

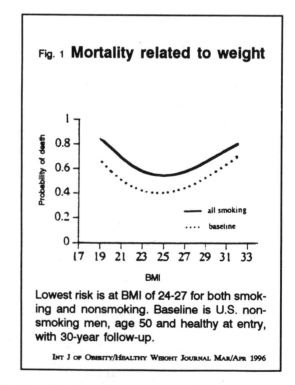

Fig. 1 **Mortality related to weight**

Lowest risk is at BMI of 24-27 for both smoking and nonsmoking. Baseline is U.S. nonsmoking men, age 50 and healthy at entry, with 30-year follow-up.

Int J of Obesity/Healthy Weight Journal Mar/Apr 1996

studies; this is for U.S. non-smokers, age 50 at entry, without evidence of disease at beginning of study.

For 30-year follow-up studies, the lowest risk of death was between a BMI of 24 and 27 with the lowest risk point as 24. Above and below this range, mortality was increased *(figure 1)*.

Current recommendations say a healthy weight range for a 5-foot 10-inch man is between 132 and 174 pounds. However, the Cornell study finds the optimal range between 167 and 188 pounds heavier at the lower level.

Troiano says, "Our analysis shows that for 50-year-old non-smoking white men of this height, mortality during 30 years of follow-up was higher only when these men weighed more than 195 lb or less than 160 lb."

Healthy weight ranges
Recommended and minimum mortality

Height	Dietary Guidelines (pounds)	Cornell study (pounds)
5'6"	118-155	148-167
5'8"	125-164	158-177
5'10"	132-174	167-188
6'	140-184	177-199
6'2"	148-195	186-210

The table "Healthy weight ranges" compares the recommended weight ranges from 1995 Dietary Guidelines (BMI 19-25) with ranges of minimum mortality risk for men age 50 found in the Cornell study (BMI 24-27):

Troiano says the optimal range found in the Cornell study is similar to the National Academy of Sciences weight recommendations for men age 45 to 54.

The relation of weight to mortality with 30 years follow-up is clearly U-shaped in this study. Body weights only slightly less than recommended values were associated with death rates comparable to that at the high end of BMI values. This does not appear to be due to smoking or existing disease.

For women, while information is limited, the study generally showed little relationship between weight and mortality for nonsmokers and for mixtures of smokers and nonsmokers, with 10 year follow-up.

Ironically, the new 1995 USDA/USDHHS Dietary Guidelines for healthy weight, just released, have dropped the higher weight allowances after age 35 which were used in the 1990 guidelines.

Smoking and preexisting illness

The higher death rates associated with underweight have often been discounted because of the belief they were due to smoking or pre-existing illness. The study investigated this and found no evidence of either.

With 30 years follow-up, smoking increased the death rate uniformly across all weight levels. Similarly, whether persons with disease were included or excluded made no difference with either short or long follow-up. The researchers conclude the same U-shape is observed even when studies stratify smoking or eliminate early deaths.

Results ignored

Troiano says the risks of underweight have been mistakenly dis-

---

'Optimal weight for men appears to be about 15 lbs heavier than most recommendations'

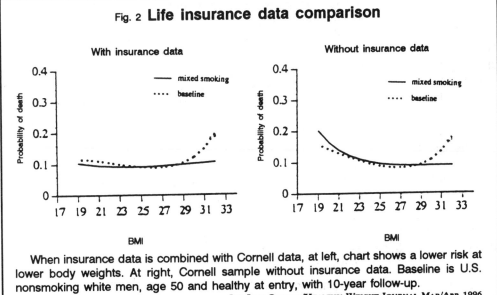

Fig. 2 **Life insurance data comparison**

When insurance data is combined with Cornell data, at left, chart shows a lower risk at lower body weights. At right, Cornell sample without insurance data. Baseline is U.S. nonsmoking white men, age 50 and healthy at entry, with 10-year follow-up.

INT J OF OBESITY/HEALTHY WEIGHT JOURNAL MAR/APR 1996

Healthy Weight Ranges for Men and Women

BMI 19—25

Height	Weight in pounds
4'10"	91-119
4'11"	94-124
5' 0"	97-128
5'1"	101-132
5'2"	104-137
5'3"	107-141
5'4"	111-146
5'5"	114-150
5'6"	118-155
5'7"	121-160
5'8"	125-164
5'9"	129-169
5'10"	132-174
5'11"	136-179
6'0"	140-189
6'1"	144-189
6'2"	148-195
6'3"	152-200
6'4"	156-205
6'5"	160-211
6'6"	164-216

1995 DIETARY GUIDELINES/HEALTHY WEIGHT JOURNAL MAR/APR 1996

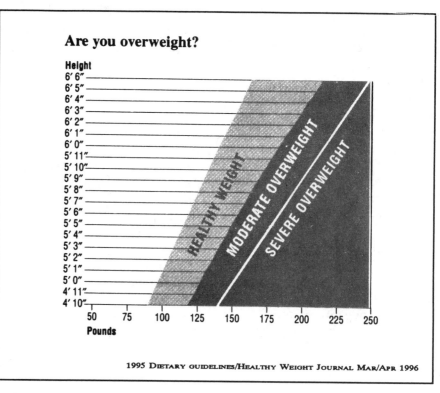

Are you overweight?

1995 DIETARY GUIDELINES/HEALTHY WEIGHT JOURNAL MAR/APR 1996

Guidelines for healthy weight
The 1995 Dietary Guidelines for Americans

"Balance the food you eat with physical activity — maintain or improve your weight."

This is the basic message of the healthy weight guidelines presented to the public in the new 1995 *Dietary Guidelines for Americans* published by the U.S. Department of Agriculture and the Department of Health and Human Services.

The guidelines offer a graphic with ranges of healthy weight, moderate overweight and severe overweight.

Healthy weight spans a body mass index range of 19 to 25. *Moderate overweight* includes BMIs of 26 and 27. *Severe overweight* begins at a BMI of 29.

The latest set of guidelines omit any upward weight shift with age.

After age 35, the 1990 guidelines had raised the healthy weight range from a BMI of 19-25 to 21-27, reporting that research showed "people can be a little heavier as they grow older without added risk to health."

This was dropped in the 1995 edition, and no increase was allowed.

The new guidelines warn against being too thin, and against excessive concern with weight.

They recommend adopting a more healthful lifestyle by starting a regular exercise program of accumulating 30 minutes or more of moderate physical activity on most — preferably all — days of the week, and by cutting fat intake to 30 percent or less of total calories. They recognize the difficulty of losing weight.

counted. He maintains that the scientific literature has emphasized the risks of overweight, while paying little attention to the risks of underweight.

The strong concern about overweight in the scientific and medical communities as well as the general public is shown "by the frequency of publications on overweight and weight control and the millions of dollars spent annually on weight loss efforts."

He quotes a report that states, "In affluent societies . . . survival is more likely in those as lean as possible," and cites the advice of one obesity specialist who claims the op-

timal weight for men is a BMI of 19.9 to 22.6.

"A major theme is that any excess body weight is hazardous, and lower

weight is always better . . . perhaps because thinness is considered attractive" and obesity stigmatized.

He suggests that researchers in

several studies have ignored their own data, even reporting a direct relationship between weight and mortality when their own data shows a curve or U-shape. Some have used selective emphasis to focus on the risks of overweight while downplaying the risks of low body weight that their own studies show.

Insurance data biased

Recommended weight ranges need no longer rely on life insurance data, Troiano contends, although using this kind of sample was justified in the past when others were unavailable.

The Cornell study for the first time investigates the often-criticized bias of insurance data. The researchers compared their baseline sample of white men with data from the Build studies of 1959 and 1979, which combine data from many insurance companies. The 10-year follow-up was used, since the Build studies had follow-ups of less than 10 years.

Using the insurance data shapes a very different curve of mortality than does the Cornell baseline sample. In particular it indicates lower risks at lower weights, as seen in *figure 2.*

The researchers conclude the general population has markedly higher mortality at low weights than life insurance policy holders, as well as higher overall mortality. Thus, the policy holders, who have higher socioeconomic status, are not representative of the population at large. Differences may be due to greater access to medical care, they suggest.

They conclude, "These results, combined with the poor success of maintaining weight loss and the potential risks of weight loss, suggest that it may be inappropriate to recommend that persons with BMIs in the range of 26 to 27 lose weight to increase longevity."

(Note: BMI tables are available in Healthy Weight Journal Sep/Oct 1993:93, and Health Risks of Obesity, page 112.)

New study finds higher weight protects elderly

Frances M. Berg, MS

Being slightly heavier than normal after age 70 protects against early death for both men and women, according to recent research at the NIH Obesity Research Center at St. Luke's-Roosevelt Hospital in New York. The study showed that being thinner than normal can be dangerous for elderly people.

If you graph the relationship between body mass index and mortality, the curve is clearly U-shaped. The base of the U-curve is fairly wide suggesting that a broad range of weights are well tolerated by older adults, said David Allison, PhD, lead researcher of the study, which was reported in October at the annual meeting of the North American Society for the Study of Obesity in in Baton Rouge, La.

The point of lowest risk of death for women was a body mass index of 30.2, and for men 28.4. The range of lowest risk was a BMI of about 28 to 32 for women, and 26 to 30 for men. For a 5-foot-5-inch woman this is 168 to 192 pounds; for a 5-foot-10 man, 181 to 207 pounds.

The findings are consistent with most other results, Allison says. "The BMIs associated with minimum mortality have generally been high in studies of older persons, typically ranging from approximately 25 to 32. This is in contrast to younger people, among whom optimal BMIs are generally thought to be in the range of about 20 to 25."

The study suggests higher weight may protect against diseases that primarily affect the aged. An example is the lower hip fracture risk in older women with higher BMIs.

Dieting after age 70

The findings are particularly important, say the researchers, because many elderly people believe they are overweight when they are not, and many moderately overweight elderly are trying to lose weight. They cite a Centers of Disease Control study that found 16 percent of men and 21.4 percent of women over age 70 years were trying to lose weight.

Subjects were 2,829 men and 4,568 women (total 7,397) in the Longitudinal Study of Aging, a nationally representative sample. They were interviewed in 1984 at age 70 or over, and followed through 1990.

The results were essentially the same whether analyses were weighted or unweighted, whether various disease states were controlled for or not, and when socioeconomic factors were considered. There was no evidence that weight affected the mortality of blacks any

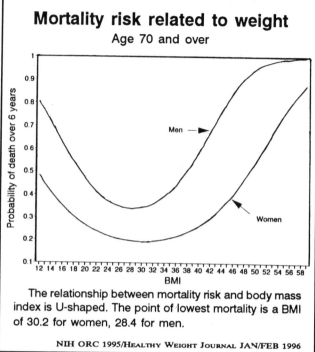

Mortality risk related to weight
Age 70 and over

The relationship between mortality risk and body mass index is U-shaped. The point of lowest mortality is a BMI of 30.2 for women, 28.4 for men.

NIH ORC 1995/HEALTHY WEIGHT JOURNAL JAN/FEB 1996

differently than it did for whites.

Although the overall predicted death rate was lower when the apparently unhealthy subjects (with markers for preexisting disease) were excluded, the shape of the U-curve and the BMI associated with minimum mortality were virtually unchanged.

Pre-existing health problems were all highly significant in relation to earlier mortality. But regardless of which disease states were considered, they did not appreciably affect the U-shape or the weight of lowest mortality. Researchers investigated the possible connection with subjects who'd had the following disease states for two years or more: cancer, Alzheimer's, osteoporosis, hip fracture, angina, hardening of arteries, hypertension, rheumatic fever, coronary heart disease, myocardial infarction, other heart attack, stroke, arthritis, diabetes, aneurism, blood clot and varicose veins.

The data set did not contain weight change history. This was identified as a research need, since weight changes may be important in old age. The study also did not provide smoking information, and Allison says it is plausible that at least some of the increased mortality with low BMIs could be related to smoking. However, he notes that numerous analyses of smoking data in other studies have failed to show much difference in total effect on the BMI mortality association.

The researchers conclude that until research shows otherwise, it appears unwise to encourage weight loss for all but the severely obese elderly.

Dieting and weight loss increase osteoporosis risk

Frances M. Berg, MS

Osteoporosis takes a huge toll in suffering and health care costs. Mainly affected are women after menopause and elderly men. Related hip fractures which can lead to death in the elderly are particularly severe.

Higher body weight is known as a protective factor against osteoporosis, fragile bones and related fractures.

Menopausal bone loss

Bone loss after menopause is less for obese women compared with nonobese women.

A French study of 155 healthy early postmenopausal women, followed over a 31-month period, showed that even moderate excess weight reduces postmenopausal bone loss.

The researchers found that within the first years after menopause, the annual rate of bone loss was much lower for women with a body mass index of 25 or above compared with women who had a BMI of less than 25. Moreover, urinary calcium excretion was lower, suggesting decreased bone resorption in this group.

This protective effect was independent of age and time since menopause, and may be related to increased conversion of estrogen due to higher body fat, the researchers suggest *(J Clin Endocrin & Metabol 1993;77:3:683-686).*

Women who were short, had low body weight, low calcium intake and were heavy smokers invariably had low radial bone mass in an Indiana study of 124 white women *(Annals of Intern Med 1990;112:96-101).*

Dieting lowers bone density

A lifetime body mass index of under 24 was associated with much lower bone density for both men and women in a study at the Dept. of Community and Family Medicine, University of California, San Diego *(Bone and Mineral 1993;20:141-149).*

A BMI of 26 or over was related to significantly higher age-adjusted bone mineral density than a BMI of less than 26. With increasing maximum weight, bone mineral density increased sharply and signifcantly at all sites tested (radial shaft, ultradistal

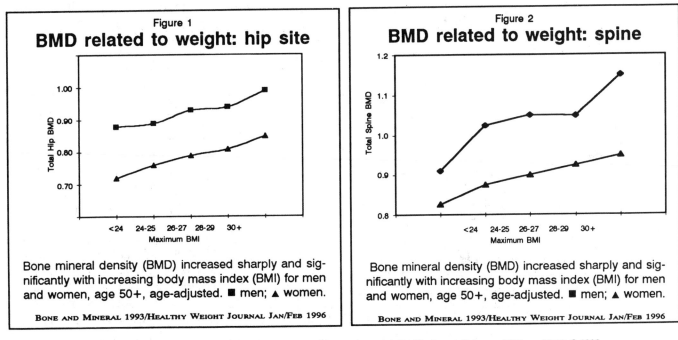

Figure 1
BMD related to weight: hip site

Bone mineral density (BMD) increased sharply and significantly with increasing body mass index (BMI) for men and women, age 50+, age-adjusted. ■ men; ▲ women.

BONE AND MINERAL 1993/HEALTHY WEIGHT JOURNAL JAN/FEB 1996

Figure 2
BMD related to weight: spine

Bone mineral density (BMD) increased sharply and significantly with increasing body mass index (BMI) for men and women, age 50+, age-adjusted. ■ men; ▲ women.

BONE AND MINERAL 1993/HEALTHY WEIGHT JOURNAL JAN/FEB 1996

wrist, total hip, lumbar spine) for both men and women *(figures 1, 2).*

Chronic dieting and weight loss were associated with markedly lower bone density, independent of weight.

In the study, weight gain of 10 pounds between ages 40 and 60, with or without subsequent loss, was related to higher bone density than weight loss and no weight change at all sites for both men and women.

Age-adjusted bone mineral density increased significantly with each increasing weight gain category for all sites, except for ultradistal wrist in women, even when controlled for current smoking, current weight, and weight at age 18 *(figure 3).* Weight fluctuation of 10 pounds or more had the same favorable effect. Weight gain after age 18 was associated with higher bone density at all sites.

Women who reported that they had to "stay on a diet" to maintain their weight had lower levels of bone density, and were thinner, than women who reported they could eat as they liked to maintain appropriate weight.

In the study, 427 white men and 616 white women were surveyed five times, measured at the first, fourth and fifth visits, between 1972-74 and 1988-1990. The mean age at the fifth visit was 76 years (range 57-97) for men, 75 years (57-94) for women. In addition, subjects gave recalled weight at age 18 and lifetime maximum weight. The study was adjusted for age and smoking.

Weight loss thins bones

Weight loss decreases mineral content in women's bones even with adequate nutrition and aerobic exercise, in research at the USDA Human Research Center in Grand Forks, N.D.

In a five-month residential weight loss program at the center, 14 women lost an average of 8.1 kg (18 pounds). Their changing bone status during weight loss was measured with dual energy x-ray absorptiometry. Both bone mineral density and bone mineral content decreased significantly: 36 g and .01 g/cm2, respectively.

Potentially some bone mineral may be regained with weight regain, said the Grand Forks researchers, but it is unknown whether bone quality is as good as before, or how essential trace elements are affected.

Similar results were found at the Osteoporosis Research Centre in Copenhagen, Denmark, where 51 obese patients averaged a 5.9 percent loss of total body bone mineral during 15 weeks of weight loss. Postmenopausal women who were not on estrogen replacement had higher bone loss *(Abstract Am Soc Clin Nutr 1992; J Bone Mineral Res 1994;9:4:459-463; HWJ Sep/Oct 1994;8:5:85-86).*

Amenorrhea

Bone density is decreased in young amenorrhoeic women. Osteoporosis in women with anorexia nervosa is a serious problem that is not rapidly reversed by weight regain, say Allan Kaplan and Paul Garfinkel in *Medical Issues and the Eating Disorders (1993, Brunner/Mazel, NY).*

They cite research that shows patients with anorexia nervosa and former anorectics with current bulimia nervosa have significantly lower bone mineral density than do normal weight bulimics and controls. This increased the risk of pathological bone fractures up to seven fold in one study. They suggest this is related to low levels of estrogen and calcium.

They also cite research that found, while there was improvement in bone density for adolescents with anorexia nervosa who regained weight, even after one year it remained significantly below that of healthy girls.

Causes of bone loss

Why weight has such an impact on bone mass is being investigated in the elderly by the Framingham osteoporosis study.

Is it because heavier persons subject their weight-bearing bones to more load than do thin persons, thus strengthening them? Or because, through the conversion of androstenedione to the metabolically active estrogen, estrone, the extra fat tissue in obese postmenopausal women provides them with higher estrogen levels than nonobese women?

Or is it that bone mineral density reaches a higher peak in early adulthood for obese persons, and thus remains higher after bone loss than for thinner adults?

A recent report on this study by David Felson, MD, and colleagues

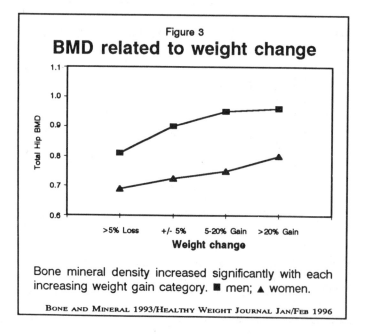

Figure 3
BMD related to weight change

Bone mineral density increased significantly with each increasing weight gain category. ■ men; ▲ women.

<small>BONE AND MINERAL 1993/HEALTHY WEIGHT JOURNAL JAN/FEB 1996</small>

provides strong evidence that weight affects bone density differently at different sites and in each sex, providing evidence that both weight-bearing and estrogen effects may be important *(J Bone and Mineral Res 1993;8:5:567-573).*

The 693 women and 439 men in the study, average age 76 years, were assessed according to numerous factors related to bone status in 1988-1989, after having been weighed and measured every two years for over 40 years. Information was available on the level of physical activity, and for women the age at menopause (average 48 years) and estrogen use.

Weight change during 40 years was the strongest factor to explain bone mineral density among women at all sites. But weight change did not affect radius bone mineral density in men. The effect of weight and weight change on bone mineral density was in general much less in men than in women.

The results suggest that the strong effect of weight on bone mineral density is due to load on weight-bearing bones in both sexes. The sex difference is unexplained but may be due to adipose tissue production of estrogen in women after menopause.

The predominant source of estrogen in women who had never used estrogen replacement was adipose tissue. These women had a stronger link between weight and bone mass than women who used estrogen.

No relationship was found between central obesity and bone mass in either sex.

The osteoporosis study looked at both men and women, so the effect of sex-based variables such as estrogen could be observed. It assessed both weight-bearing and non-weight-bearing sites, such as the spine versus the wrist, indicating the effect of weight on bone mass. The subjects were weighed repeatedly for 40 years, so weight changes since early adulthood could be studied.

If weight loss is deemed desirable to improve the health status of female patients, this practice should include adequate nutrient intake and physical activity to help maintain bone health in the process. A history of dieting in a woman suggests the need for careful evaluation of osteoporosis risk at menopause.

Losing Weight Safely

Marilynn Larkin
Marilynn Larkin is a writer in New York City.

Americans trying to lose weight have plenty of company. According to a 1995 report from the Institute of Medicine (IOM), tens of millions of Americans are dieting at any given time, spending more than $33 billion yearly on weight-reduction products, such as diet foods and drinks.

Yet studies over the last two decades by the National Center for Health Statistics show that obesity in the United States is actually on the rise. Today, approximately 35 percent of women and 31 percent of men age 20 and older are considered obese, up from approximately 30 percent and 25 percent, respectively, in 1980.

The words obesity and overweight are generally used interchangeably. However, according to the IOM report, their technical meanings are not identical. Overweight refers to an excess of body weight that includes all tissues, such as fat, bone and muscle. Obesity refers specifically to an excess of body fat. It is possible to be overweight without being obese, as in the case of a body builder who has a substantial amount of muscle mass. It is possible to be obese without being overweight, as in the case of a very sedentary person who is within the desirable weight range but who nevertheless has an excess of body fat. However, most overweight people are also obese and vice versa. Men with more than 25 percent and women with more than 30 percent body fat are considered obese.

Many people who diet fail to lose weight—or, if they do lose, fail to maintain the lower weight over the long term. As the IOM report, "Weighing The Options: Criteria for Evaluating Weight-Management Programs," points out, obesity is "a complex, multifactorial disease of appetite regulation and energy metabolism."

Because many factors affect how much or how little food a person eats and how that food is metabolized, or processed, by the body, losing weight is not simple. For example, recent studies suggest a role for genetic makeup in obesity. This area is still controversial, and more studies will be needed before scientists can say with certainty that a person's genes may set limits on how much weight can be lost and maintained.

Yet many people persist in seeking simple cures to this complex health problem. Lured by fad diets or pills that promise a quick and easy path to thinness, they end up disappointed when they regain lost weight.

"When it comes to weight loss, if something sounds too good—or too easy, or too delicious—to be true, it probably is," says Victor Herbert, M.D., J.D., professor of medicine and director of the Nutrition Center at the Mount Sinai School of Medicine and Bronx VA Medical Centers in New York City, and member of the board of directors of the National Council Against Health Fraud. "If a weight loss claim is sensational, it is not true; if it is true, it is not sensational."

No Shortcuts

"There are no shortcuts—no magic pills," adds Lori Love of the Food and Drug Administration's Center for Food Safety and Applied Nutrition. Losing weight sensibly and safely requires a

The first step in losing weight safely is to determine a realistic weight goal.

From *FDA Consumer*, January/February 1996, pp. 16-21. Reprinted by permission of *FDA Consumer*, the magazine of the U.S. Food and Drug Administration.

To help consumers plan a healthful diet, FDA

and USDA have revamped food labels.

multifaceted approach that includes setting reasonable weight-loss goals, changing eating habits, and getting adequate exercise. Appetite suppressants (diet pills) or other products may help some people over the short term, but they are not a substitute for adopting healthful eating habits over the long term.

The first step in losing weight safely is to determine a realistic weight goal. Two types of tables are commonly used as guidelines. One is the weight-for-height table developed in 1990 by the U.S. Department of Agriculture and the Department of Health and Human Services. This table offers a range of suggested weights for adults based on height and age.

Another table uses body mass index (BMI), a mathematical formula that correlates weight with body fat. In 1993, the National Institute of Diabetes and Digestive and Kidney Diseases developed a table that correlates height, weight and BMI.

A physician or other health provider can help you set a reasonable goal with these tables. To reach the goal safely, plan to lose 1 to 2 pounds weekly by consuming approximately 300 to 500 fewer calories daily than usual (women and inactive men generally need to consume approximately 2,000 calories to maintain weight; men and very active women may consume up to 2,500 calories daily).

Moderation, Variety and Balance

After determining a reasonable goal weight, devise an eating plan based on the cornerstones of healthful eating—moderation, variety and balance, suggests Herbert.

"Moderation means not eating too much or too little of any particular food or nutrient; variety means eating as wide a variety as possible from each, and within each, of the five basic food

Obesity a Disease

Obesity is now considered a disease—not a moral failing. According to a new report from the Institute of Medicine, "obesity is a heterogeneous disease in which genetic, environmental, psychological, and other factors are involved. It occurs when energy intake exceeds the amount of energy expended over time. Only in a small minority of cases is obesity caused by such illnesses as hypothyroidism or the result of taking medications, such as steroids, that can cause weight gain."

Public health concerns about this disease relate to its link to numerous other diseases that can lead to premature illness or death. The report notes that overweight individuals who lose even relatively small amounts of weight are likely to:

- lower their blood pressure (and thereby the risk of heart attack and stroke)

- reduce abnormally high levels of blood glucose (associated with diabetes)

- bring blood levels of cholesterol and triglycerides (associated with cardiovascular disease) down to more desirable levels

- reduce sleep apnea, or irregular breathing during sleep

- decrease the risk of osteoarthritis of the weight-bearing joints

- decrease depression

- increase self-esteem.

Of course, losing excess weight is also likely to improve appearance, which is a strong motivation for many people.

To order a copy of the IOM report, call (1-800) 624-6242 (in Washington, D.C., call 202-334-3313). The cost is $30 plus $4 shipping and handling.

—M.L.

groups; and balance refers to the balance achieved by following moderation and variety, as well as the balance of calories consumed versus calories expended," he explains. To lose weight, fewer calories should be consumed than expended; to maintain weight loss, the number of calories consumed and expended should be about the same.

The five basic food groups and the recommended number of servings from each are incorporated into the Food Guide Pyramid developed by USDA and HHS. These groups are (1) bread, cereal, pasta, and rice; (2) vegetables; (3) fruits; (4) milk, yogurt and cheese; and (5) meat, poultry, fish, dry beans, eggs, and nuts. A sixth group (fats, oils and sweets) consists mainly of items that are pleasing to the palate but high in fat and/or calories; these should be eaten in moderation.

Using the Food Label

To help consumers plan a healthful diet, FDA and USDA have revamped food labels. By law, most food labels now must display a Nutrition Facts panel containing information about how the food can fit into an overall daily diet. Nutrition Facts state how much saturated fat, cholesterol, fiber, and certain nutrients are contained in each serving. Serving sizes must now be based on standards set for similar kinds of food, so the nutritional value of similar products may be compared.

On the food label, %Daily Value shows what percentage of a given nutrient is provided in one portion for daily diets of 2,000 and 2,500 calories.

Whether or not a given food fits into a weight-loss diet depends on what other foods you eat that day. For most people, the goal is to select a variety of foods that together add up to approximately 100 percent of the Daily Value for total carbohydrate, dietary fiber, vitamins, and minerals; total fat, cholesterol and

sodium each may add up to less than 100 percent.

This system permits a good deal of flexibility. No food is inherently "bad"; it is the total diet for the day that counts. You may compensate for an occasional rich dessert or serving of fried food by eating foods that are low in fat, oil or sugar for the rest of the day. However, high-fat foods should be limited, because they can quickly use up a day's supply of calories without providing high percentages of vital nutrients.

Simple modifications in food selection and preparation allow you to include traditional favorites and snacks within the context of a healthful weight-loss diet; for example, select 1 percent or skim milk products instead of those made with whole milk, lean cuts of meat and poultry, and nonfat frozen yogurt instead of ice cream. Low-fat plain yogurt may be substituted for sour cream in dips, dressings or spreads; reduced-fat cheeses may be used instead of those made from whole milk. Broil, roast or steam foods instead of frying.

Look on the nutrition label for words such as "low," "light" or "reduced" to describe the calorie and fat content per serving. These foods must have significantly fewer calories or significantly less fat than similar products that do not make these claims. Foods that are advertised as "low in cholesterol" also must be low in saturated fat.

Foods that claim to contain fewer calories or less fat than similar servings of similar products must show the difference on the label. For example, on a container of low-fat cottage cheese, the label would show that a serving of the low-fat product contains 80 calories and 1.5 grams of fat while regular cottage cheese contains 120 calories and 5 grams of fat per serving.

Include small portions of desserts or high-fat snacks rather than attempting to cut them out altogether. Eliminating fa-

vorite foods may result in cravings that can lead to binge eating and weight gain.

Avoid low-calorie fad diets that exclude whole categories of food such as carbohydrates (bread and pasta) or proteins (meat and poultry). These diets may be harmful because they generally do not include all nutrients necessary for good health. "Every fad diet that demands an unusual eating pattern, such as emphasizing only a few types of foods, deviates from one or more of the guidelines of moderation, variety and balance," says Herbert. "The greater the deviation, the more harmful the diet is likely to be."

Exercise

Regular exercise is important for overall health as well as for losing and maintaining weight. There is evidence to suggest that body fat distribution affects health risks. For example, excess fat in the abdominal area (as opposed to hips and thighs) is associated with greater risk for high blood pressure, diabetes, early heart disease, and certain types of cancer. Vigorous exercise can reduce abdominal fat and thus lower the risk of these diseases.

A half hour of brisk walking or other aerobic activity three times weekly can help the body use up calories consumed daily as well as excess calories stored as fat. Weight-bearing exercises also help tone muscles and may reduce the risk of osteoporosis.

Diet Pills

The 1991/1992 Weight Loss Practices Survey, sponsored by FDA and the National Heart, Lung, and Blood Institute, found that 5 percent of women and 2 percent of men trying to lose weight use diet pills. Products considered by FDA to be over-the-counter weight control drugs are primarily those containing the active ingredient phenylpropanolamine (PPA), such as Dexatrim and Acutrim. PPA is available OTC for weight control in a 75-mg controlled-release dosage form, when combined with a restricted diet and exercise.

Using diet pills containing PPA will not make a big difference in the rate of weight loss, says Robert Sherman of FDA's Office of OTC Drug Evaluation.

Eliminating favorite foods may result in cravings

that can lead to binge eating and weight gain.

Regular exercise is important to overall health, as well as for losing and maintaining weight.

"Even the best studies show only about a half pound greater weight loss per week using PPA combined with diet and exercise," he adds. Sherman cautions that the recommended dosage of these pills should not be exceeded because of the risk of possible adverse effects, such as elevated blood pressure and heart palpitations.

Since PPA is also used as a nasal decongestant in over-the-counter cough and cold products, consumers should read the labels of OTC decongestants to see if they contain PPA. They should not take PPA in two products labeled for different uses.

Sherman notes that FDA has received a small number of reports indicating that PPA use might be associated with an increased risk of stroke. A large-scale safety study was begun in September 1994 to explore the possibility. Based on available data, the agency does not believe that an increased risk of stroke is a concern when PPA is used at recommended dosages.

Weight-Loss Programs

Many people turn to weight-loss programs for help in planning a daily diet and changing lifestyle habits. The IOM report provides guidelines for evaluating the potential effectiveness of such programs.

"To improve their chances for success, consumers should choose programs that focus on long-term weight management; provide instruction in healthful eating, increasing activity, and improving self-esteem; and explain thoroughly the potential health risks from weight loss," according to the report. Consumers should also demand evidence of success. If it is absent or consists primarily of testimonials or other anecdotal evidence, "the program should be viewed with suspicion."

IOM recommends that potential clients be given a truthful, unambiguous, non-misleading statement about the program's approaches and goals, and a full disclosure of costs. The cost breakdown should include initial and ongoing costs, as well as the cost of extra products.

The basic tenet of weight loss—to eat fewer calories than you burn and to stay active—is easy to say but, like most lifestyle changes, not so easy to do. With realistic goals, and a commitment to losing weight slowly, safely and sensibly, the chances of long-term success improve dramatically.

Surgery for Obesity

THE STORY

An under-used operation that closes off much of the stomach not only helps seriously obese people lose weight and keep it off, but also helps control their diabetes, among other benefits.

The procedure, called gastric bypass, essentially blocks off most of the stomach, reducing its functional size from a little more than a quart to about two ounces, or about five tablespoons of food. The new, tiny stomach fills up quickly, so one feels full after eating only a small amount. This limits the amount of food that can be eaten and, thus, the calories the body can absorb. Weight losses of 100 pounds or more after a gastric bypass are not uncommon.

Equally important, the operation appears to resolve a variety of serious weight-related health problems. Diabetes, which is very common in overweight people and which can lead to blindness, nerve degeneration, and death, is often cured by a gastric bypass. In the September *Annals of*

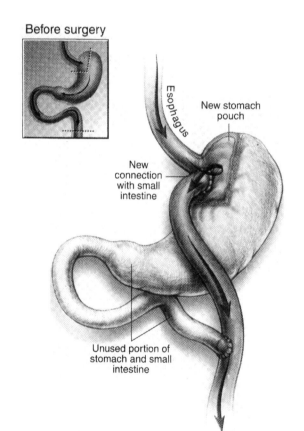

Before surgery

Esophagus

New stomach pouch

New connection with small intestine

Unused portion of stomach and small intestine

Surgery, researchers from East Carolina University report that 83 percent of their obese diabetic patients no longer needed daily insulin shots after the surgery. And 98 percent of those with sugar-control problems but not full-blown diabetes regained normal blood-sugar levels.

A paper in the September *Neurology* shows that gastric bypass can also stop idiopathic intracranial hypertension (IIH), or high pressure in the fluid surrounding the brain and spinal cord, a potentially fatal problem that may be related to obesity. Cerebrospinal fluid pressure dropped 50 percent in eight women with

IIH who had the operation at the Medical College of Virginia. The surgery relieved symptoms of IIH such as headaches and ringing in the ears, and improved obesity-related urinary incontinence.

Gastric bypass should not be confused with the intestinal bypass operations that were the rage in the 1970s. These procedures "re-plumbed" the digestive tract so food passed through the stomach and then bypassed the first few feet of the small intestine, making it difficult for the body to absorb nutrients. While people lost weight after this operation, a large number suffered serious vitamin and mineral deficiencies and constant diarrhea. Some experienced kidney or liver failure, and a number of deaths were attributed to intestinal bypass.

— *The Editors*

THE PHYSICIAN'S PERSPECTIVE

George Blackburn, MD, PhD

It is unfortunate that the widely publicized failure of intestinal bypass continues to overshadow other surgical treatments for obesity. Since the first gastric restriction was performed 30 years ago at the University of Iowa, a growing body of evidence suggests that this procedure should be used more widely.

Two consensus conferences sponsored by the National Institutes of Health, one in 1980 and another in 1991, endorsed gastric restriction for the treatment of severe obesity, not only because it can reduce excess body weight but also because it can correct some of the serious health problems that accompany it. The reports described above are but two examples of how gastric restriction can correct deadly obesity-related diseases.

In addition, medical insurance companies in almost every state approve of the operation and cover its costs, which range from $10,000 to $15,000.

So why is gastric restriction a well-kept secret, with only 15,000 operations performed each year in the United States? In large measure because of the widespread prejudice against obese people. Many people, physicians included, wrongly believe that obese people merely need to stop eating so much and they will lose weight. In reality, severe obesity is a potentially deadly disease that sometimes requires a treatment as dramatic as surgery.

The principle behind gastric restriction is quite simple — reduce the size of the stomach so less food fits into it. This can be accomplished by either stapling off part of the stomach (a gastroplasty) or

STAGES OF OBESITY			
STAGE	BODY-MASS INDEX*	% IDEAL WEIGHT	ADULT CHANGE IN BODY WEIGHT
I	25-27	100-120%	10-20 lbs
II	27-30	120-140%	20-40 lbs
III	30-40	140-180%	40-100 lbs
IV	>40	>180%	>100 lbs

*(Weight in kilograms) / (Height in meters)^2

creating a small pouch in the top of the stomach and connecting the intestines to it (a gastric bypass). The rest of the digestive system remains in place, so normal digestion and nutrient absorption occur, thus avoiding the pitfalls of the old intestinal bypass operations.

We have had the opportunity over the course of many years to follow thousands of men and women who have had gastric bypass surgery. The results are very encouraging. The majority of people see their weight drop by 50 percent within a year, and many manage to keep much of this weight off over the long term. In addition to diabetes, high blood pressure, high cholesterol levels, sleep apnea (failing to breathe for periods of time while asleep), incontinence, and joint pains, all consequences of excess weight, are often controlled or eliminated. Just as important is the improved quality of life. I often hear people talk about the happiness and confidence that shedding so much weight has given them.

This operation is certainly not for every overweight person. **I only recommend a gastric restriction for someone in stage IV obesity (see table). These are people who have gained a large amount of weight during adulthood – generally in excess of 100 pounds – or who are gaining weight at an alarming pace and are developing one or more of the weight-related health problems mentioned earlier.** And then I advise it only if their weight does not respond to exercise, a very-low-calorie diet, or appetite-suppressing medication. The procedure requires major surgery, something that obese people do not tolerate as well as thinner people do. Serious complications can follow the operation, and people can die because of it. In the study from East Carolina University, nine of 608 patients (1.5 percent) died as a result of gastric bypass surgery.

While that number sounds high, let's put it into perspective. The risk of dying from gastric bypass surgery is far less than that of dying from obesity — an estimated 300,000 Americans die as a direct result of obesity each year. In the ongoing Swedish Obesity Study, 2,000 obese men and women were randomly assigned to either gastric restriction surgery or drug therapy. While the total number of deaths won't be disclosed until the end of the experiment, only three deaths

occurred as a result of surgery during the first six years, or one-fifth the rate of deaths from surgery in the East Carolina study. Among the nonsurgery group, 27 people died during the first two years from diabetes, heart attacks, or strokes that were brought on by obesity.

Although gastric restriction may sound like a "quick fix," it isn't. In fact, the operation won't work without postoperative attention and support. For long-term weight control, a patient must learn to develop healthy eating habits and increase physical activity. This can take as long as five years, which is apparently the time required to re-engineer adult habits involving food and exercise. Ongoing participation in a support group is critical.

Obviously the first approach to excess weight is controlling diet and increasing the amount of daily activity. In some people, however, these strategies just don't work very well. For them, gastric bypass represents an effective way to reduce weight and control other serious weight-related problems.

Dr. Blackburn is director of the nutrition support service at the Deaconess Hospital in Boston and the vice president-elect of the North American Society for the Study of Obesity.

FOR MORE INFORMATION

▼ *American Society for Bariatric Surgery, San Francisco, 415-753-6029; Massachusetts Medical Society's Committee on Nutrition, Waltham MA, 617-893-4610*

The new paradigm of trust

Ellyn Satter, MS, RD

We are in the midst of a paradigm shift in our attitudes about obesity and the treatment of obesity. The current paradigm assumes that all obesity is harmful and must be treated. Primary prevention is identifying individuals at risk and preventing them from becoming obese. This current paradigm is a control paradigm.

In contrast, the emerging paradigm assumption about fatness is that it may be normal for some people. Growing out of acceptance of size variation, primary prevention in the emerging paradigm becomes building positive feeding interactions and life style patterns that allow children to develop bodies that reflect their genetic endowment.

The emerging paradigm is a trust paradigm, based on observations that children have tendencies for a particular body build, including the food regulation processes and inclinations for movement that support those ten-

---

> 6 *Children can get too fat when parents feed in a restrained fashion, hesitating to gratify children's appetites for fear they will get fat.* 9

---

dencies (*Pediatrics 1968*: 41:18–29). The task for the growing child is not to remain slim, but to maintain energy balance in response to variations in caloric density of the diet, activity level and growth.

The emerging paradigm of prevention is based on the hypothesis that children who are more grounded in their internal regulatory processes are less likely to make errors of energy balance, and thus more likely to sustain appropriate body weight regulation throughout life.

Parents' trust is prevention key

Within the trusting model of primary prevention, parents are supported in feeding and nurturing well. Fat (or potentially fat) children can be fed like other children when parents observe a division of responsibility in feed-

ing. Parents take responsibility for providing wholesome and appealing food at predictable and pleasant times, then trust children to manage their own eating and decide how much to eat of what parents have made available. Primary prevention can also be helping parents to raise an emotionally healthy fat child.

Fat children grow up to think less of themselves primarily if their parents think less of them. Fat children and their parents need particular help in learning to deal with the prejudice and social and emotional challenges obesity presents.

If a child gains too much weight, feeding dynamics, parenting, food selection and activity should be examined to detect what is interfering with the child's ability to regulate growth. The key question is, "What changed at the point that the child began gaining too much weight?" However, it is important to be wary of assuming causation.

Research illustrates what happens when internal regulation is undermined. Children whose parents controlled their food intake were less able to adjust how much they ate in response to changes in energy density of food (*Pediatrics 1994;94:653-661*). Children followed longitudinally were fatter when they had feeding problems early on, and when their parents were preoccupied with keeping them from being fat (*HWJ/Obesity & Health May/Jun 1991;3:40–41*).

Abnormal fatness

The emerging paradigm definition of obesity is not fatness, per se, but fatness that is abnormal or unnecessary for the individual. Fatness can be normal for children who grow at the 95th percentile weight for height, or above, if they show a consistent and predictable pattern of growth, and any growth adjustments are gradual and occur over an extended time. If fatness is the result of unstable body weight with abrupt or acute weight gain, it is likely to be abnormal.

Children can get too fat when a parent or primary care provider systematically overfeeds them. Ordinarily, if a parent errs and overfeeds a child or the child errs and eats too much, the child compensates by eating less the next feeding or next day.

Children can get too fat when parents feed in a restrained fashion, hesitating to totally gratify children's appetites for fear they will get fat. And children can get too fat when they don't feel safe. Stress in the family or the environment may interfere with parents' ability to provide for their children. Stress is passed along to the children who may gain weight. Among typical responses to stress, children may overdemand food as a way of attracting the parents' attention or become underactive because they are despondent.

In all cases, rather than attempting to shift calorie balance with diet and exercise, it is essential to identify and resolve underlying causes in order to restore the child's normal regulatory and growth patterns. That outcome goal is achievement of the child's weight, not some externally defined (even modest) standard of weight. Striving for a particular body weight creates distortions with eating and feeding and interferes markedly with nurturing the child.

Does the new paradigm work?

Whether or not the emerging paradigm "works" depends on the outcome goal.

If the goal is to help children grow in a stable and consistent fashion and to achieve the adult body that is right for them, then, yes, the emerging paradigm works. What results from such humanistic and realistic strategies is normal growth. And normal growth works.

If the goal of preventive intervention with children's

> *"The emerging definition of obesity is fatness that is abnormal or unnecessary for the individual."*

weight is the current one of keeping children from growing up fat, probably not. But the current paradigm proponents haven't kept children thin, either, even when they try harder. In fact, trying to externally control food intake and activity can undermine children's ability to maintain energy balance and make them fatter than they otherwise would be.

Children have their own considerable capability with eating, activity and growth and the best approach is to support that capability rather than trying to outwit it. Working with rather than against these natural regulatory abilities enhances the likelihood of maintaining stable body weight throughout life *(Healthy Weight Journal Nov/Dec 1995;9:6:107-108).*

Ellyn Satter, MS, MSSW, RD, is a registered dietitian and family therapist in Clinical Social Work specializing in the treatment of eating disorders. She is the author of How to Get Your Kid to Eat . . . But Not Too Much, *and* Child of Mine: Feeding with Love and Good Sense.

Current and emerging paradigms of obesity

Issues for children

Issue	Current "Control" Paradigm	Emerging "Trust" Paradigm
Body weight	Primarily optional	Primarily a genetic given
Assumption about fatness	Fatness is always bad and should be treated Everyone should be slim	Fatness is normal for some people It is OK for some people to be fat
Definition of obesity	Weight or BMI outside a particular range Children: Above certain %tile weight/height	Fatness that is excessive *for the individual* Unstable growth with excessive weight gain
Cause of obesity	Overeating and underexercise	We don't know. Likely genetic predisposition plus multiple environmental distortions.
Solution to obesity	Undereat and over exercise	Establish consistent and positive eating and exercise Identify and resolve disrupting factors
Outcome	Achieve a defined body weight or BMI Children: Keep them slim	Behavioral: Positive eating and activity Let weight evolve Let children grow up to reflect their genes
Recommendation to patient	Manipulate eating and exercise to restrict weight Keep on manipulating	Develop the weight that is right for them For children, provide well for them and keep on providing

SOURCE: ELLYN SATTER, 1995/HEALTHY WEIGHT JOURNAL NOV/DEC 1995

Food Safety

The dichotomization of risk distorts the reality that nothing is absolutely safe or absolutely dangerous.
—Peter Sandman, in "Determining Risk,"
FDA Consumer, June 1990.

In 1906, with the passage of the first Food and Drug Act, the federal government began to assume some responsibility for food safety. Increased governmental involvement has been an inevitable trend ever since. With the 1950s came a fear that chemicals in the food supply, especially additives, might be carcinogenic. Congress responded with tighter control on the use and testing of additives. In 1958, the Delaney Clause prevented the use of any additive found to induce cancer in man or experimental animals, and the GRAS (Generally Recognized as

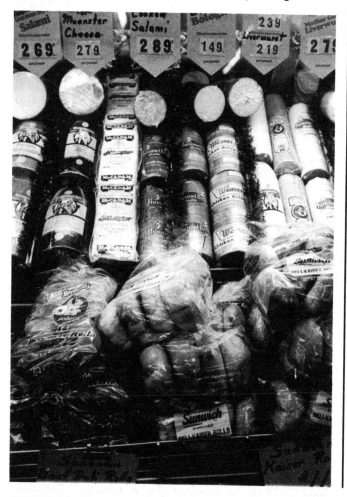

Safe) list identified those believed by scientists to be safe for human consumption. This list is periodically revised, and the testing and retesting of additives continues. The Food and Drug Administration (FDA) governs all of these procedures, and books of regulations cover all aspects of food production and service.

The concept in the quote at the top of this page is not new. A sixteenth-century physician, Paracelsus, said, "All things are poison. Nothing is without poison." Thus, it is appropriate for critics to question the continued usefulness of the Delaney Clause. When this law was passed, they argue, only about 50 carcinogens were known. Today thousands are known, and advances in analytical methods enable the detection of amounts with no biological or toxicological significance, causing useful products to be banned needlessly. Some prominent scientific groups believe that the FDA should not be allowed to "concern itself with trifles." This is known as a "de minimis" policy. Recent removal of some pesticide regulations is a step in this direction.

But today's consumers frequently fail to assess risk and benefit rationally. With little knowledge to draw upon, they do not understand that even an essential nutrient can be both life-giving and life-threatening. Sodium, for example, is absolutely necessary for life, but if put into an infant's formula instead of sugar, it can (and has) resulted in death. Likewise, arctic explorers have become very ill from eating a small portion of polar bear liver due to its excessive vitamin A content. Nor do consumers always understand that the word "natural" is not a guarantee of safety. This can be illustrated easily by pointing out the risks associated with snake venom or amanita mushrooms growing on the lawn or in the woods.

Given the complexity of biological interactions, the uniqueness of each human organism, and the multitude of chemicals that could potentially interact, few knowledgeable people would contend that the absolute safety of anything can be ensured. Yet activist groups demand just that and have become experts at escalating a minor or nonexistent issue into a major catastrophe. It has been argued that if it takes programs like *60 Minutes,* or a partisan political group such as the National Resources Defense Council, or a self-appointed watchdog group such as Food and Water, Inc., to create a public issue, then it probably isn't a safety issue at all. Alar—a growth regulator used in apple orchards—is a good example. The scare in 1989 over Alar's safety appears to have been nothing more than media hype, but it seriously hurt the apple industry and shook parents' confidence in apple juice for their children. The Food Marketing Institute finds that, although the consumer's confidence in the food supply has risen (see the first article in this book), food safety is still a key consumer issue. In this unit you will find articles on additives, naturally occurring toxins, and irradiation. A related article on genetic engineering is also in the first unit.

Food-borne illnesses continue to be a major threat to health. On a yearly basis, total costs of these illnesses come to nearly $10 billion, deaths reach at least eight thousand, and total cases are estimated at between several and tens of millions. Some of the most prevalent illness-producing organisms today were not public health issues twenty years ago, a sign that conditions and lifestyles have changed. One of these is *E. coli* 0157:H7, which became infamous for causing a 1991 outbreak of food poisoning in Washington State from undercooked hamburger. A number of fatalities and several outbreaks later (including one of immense proportions recently in Japan), it is clear that this is truly serious. Many people blame the packing industry or the government's food inspection procedures for the presence of illness-producing organisms, but most outbreaks could easily be prevented with proper food-handling procedures.

All of us must learn about safe food handling. While many people assume that food-borne illness is contracted primarily in restaurants, it is revealing to discover that each of us is his or her own worst enemy. Food properly handled in home kitchens could reduce the incidence of disease significantly. This always includes conformance with rules governing bacterial growth, time, and temperature. A case in point is undercooked ground meat and the *E. coli* organism. Equally likely is the very common bacterium, salmonella, which is found in a high percentage of raw poultry and may be in raw eggs as well. Sometime in the future, eggs pasteurized in the shell will be available. In the meantime, handle all foods carefully. Look for safe food-handling instructions on labels and leaflets at your meat counters. The first three articles in this unit discuss the food-borne illnesses that should be of concern to the consumer.

An article follows on mad cow disease primarily because of the amount of press it has received. Almost certainly this is like the Alar scare and is much ado about nothing, but conjecture over a linkage to Creutzfeldt-Jakob Disease, a chronic degenerative disease of the central nervous system in humans, has escalated fears. Several cases in England caused speculation that beef was infected through the consumption of supplements made from infected sheep. The European community subsequently refused to import British beef, which created a major political issue abroad. The United States has not imported British beef for years.

Consumer groups periodically force a focus on pesticide usage on crops and residues in food. In "How Much Are Pesticides Hurting Your Health?" the mythology sur-

rounding the values and dangers of pesticides is discussed. Users of organic foods should realize that it is impossible to grow food completely free of pesticides. The National Academy of Sciences (NAS), in response to public concern over a possible connection between pesticides and cancer, points out that the incidence of lung cancer alone is rising. A major NAS report on pesticides in the diets of infants and children finds no current cause for concern and certainly no reason to reduce the consumption of fresh produce.

Another issue that sometimes concerns the public is the additive monosodium glutamate (MSG). Still another review of the safety of MSG has found no linkage between amounts normally consumed and negative reactions in either adults or children. Food irradiation, as discussed by Alan Morton in "After the Glow," is both a food safety issue and a political issue. Some activist groups, such as Food and Water, Inc., have used very aggressive scare tactics to persuade the public to boycott irradiated products. Fortunately, although Food and Water, Inc., delayed its use in the United States, irradiation has been approved for a number of products. It does not produce radioactive food, but it will destroy bacteria that cause food-borne diseases. Irradiation also helps to maintain high-quality produce over a prolonged shelf life, both of which are advantages to the consumer.

Finally, there is the issue of toxins, including carcinogens, that occur naturally in food. While their presence may be a surprise to some of us, under most circumstances there is no reason for alarm bells. Once again the dose makes the poison, and few of us live on a single food item such as cabbage. Scientists will continue their search for new knowledge of these chemicals.

All would agree that it is appropriate to raise questions about the safety of our food supply. Sometimes there is disagreement on the extent of the problem and on how to solve it. As consumers, we must accept personal responsibility for safe food handling. We must also continue to expect our regulatory agencies to do their best. Problems arising over the safety of food supplies can be documented throughout history. Clearly, solutions are not easy.

Looking Ahead: Challenge Questions

If you were to consume only those foods for which complete safety could be proven, what would you eat?

Rank order three issues of food safety that you think are the most important, and justify your selection.

What measures would you suggest to counteract misinformation about food safety and the tactics used by activist organizations?

Observe yourself when you handle food. In what ways might you be the vector of food-borne illness?

Choose your favorite meal and determine which natural ingredients are known to be toxic in some way. Why is this not a problem?

FOODBORNE ILLNESS: ROLE OF HOME FOOD HANDLING PRACTICES

The Principal author of this Scientific Status Summary was S. J. Knable, Ph.D., The Pennsylvania State University

Outbreaks of foodborne illness, such as the highly publicized outbreaks of *Escherichia coli* O157:H7 in the western United States in early 1993 that led to the tragic deaths of four children (CDC, 1993), remind us that under certain circumstances, familiar foods can lead to serious consequences, even death. Despite progress in improving the overall quality and safety of foods produced in the U.S., significant foodborne illness and death due to microbial pathogens still occur. . . .

FACTORS CONTRIBUTING TO NEW MICROBIOLOGICAL CHALLENGES

Several interrelated factors contribute to new microbiological challenges and risks throughout the food system.

Demographics and lifestyles. Demography and lifestyle of U.S. consumers have changed dramatically during the past two decades. The U.S. population has increased and family size has decreased. There are more families with both parents working outside the home and more single-parent households than previously. More children are shopping for and preparing their own food because no parent is home during the day (Goldman, 1990). In addition, the proportion of elderly individuals in the population has also increased and the number of people at increased risk for foodborne illness has grown.

Preference for quick methods of food preparation, convenience foods, fresh and "fresh-like" foods," minimally processed foods, and foods that meet specific health/dietary needs has increased. To meet these preferences and the needs of a growing population, new processing, preservation, and packaging techniques have been incorporated into the manufacturing of food products. Distribution networks have become large, centralized, and complex. Changes such as these affect the epidemiology of foodborne illnesses and present new microbiological risks.

Minimally processed foods, for example, are designed for convenience, "fresh-like" state, and extended shelf life. Minimally processed foods present concerns to food manufacturers in maintaining product safety. These foods may receive a lower heat treatment than required for commercial sterility. They may be vacuum packaged or packaged in atmospheres modified by the addition of nitrogen and/or carbon dioxide. Such processing and packaging conditions alter the microbial ecology of foods. The heat treatment may destroy some microorganisms but not others, e.g., bacterial spores. The modified atmospheres may inhibit the growth of some microorganisms surviving the heat treatment, but may enhance the growth of others, even at refrigeration temperatures. The extension of shelf life may allow time for growth of undesirable, harmful microorganisms. This is of particular concern in ready-to-eat products not requiring cooking before consumption. . . .

Several microorganisms that were not previously recognized as important foodborne pathogens have emerged during the past two decades, adding to our microbiological challenges. These pathogens include Norwalk virus, *Campylobacter jejuni*, *E. coli* O157:H7, *Listeria monocytogenes*, *Vibrio vulnificus*, *Vibrio cholera*, and *Yersinia enterocolitica* (IOM, 1992; Doyle, 1991; Doyle, 1985). Some of these microorganisms, *Campylobacter*, for example, may have come to our attention through investigative surveillance and ability of laboratories to identify them (Hedberg et al., 1994). *E. coli* O157:H7 appears to be a new pathogen that acquired genetic determinants for new virulence factors (Whittam et al., 1993; Griffin and Tauxe, 1991). *E. coli* O157:H7 was first recognized as a foodborne pathogen in 1982 and is now known as an important cause of the diarrheal form of hemorrhagic colitis (painful bloody diarrhea) and renal failure in humans (Padhye and Doyle, 1992; Griffin and Tauxe, 1991; Doyle, 1985). In its report on a small outbreak in California, the CDC noted that many unrecognized sporadic cases and small outbreaks of *E. coli* O157:H7 due to

Table 1—Common Foodborne Diseases Caused by Bacteria. *From Cliver (1993)*

Disease (causative agent)	Latency Period (duration)	Principal Symptoms	Typical Foods	Mode of Contamination	Prevention of Disease
(*Bacillus cereus*) food poisoning, diarrheal	8–16 hr (12–24 hr)	Diarrhea, cramps, occasional vomiting	Meat products, soups sauces, vegetables	From soil or dust	Thorough heating and rapid cooling of foods
(*Bacillus cereus*) food poisoning, emetic	1–5 hr (6–24 hr)	Nausea, vomiting, sometimes diarrhea and cramps	Cooked rice and pasta	From soil or dust	Thorough heating and rapid cooling of foods
Botulism; food poisoning (heat-labile toxin of *Clostridium botulinum*)	12–36 hr (months)	Fatigue, weakness, double vision, slurred speech, respiratory failure, sometimes death	Types A&B: vegetables; fruits; meat, fish, and poultry products; condiments; Type E: fish and fish products	Types A&B: from soil or dust; Type E: water and sediments	Thorough heating and rapid cooling of foods
Botulism; food poisoning infant infection	Unknown	Constipation, weakness, respiratory failure, sometimes death	Honey, soil	Ingested spores from soil or dust or honey colonize intestine	Do not feed honey to infants —will not prevent all
Campylobacteriosis (*Camplyobacter jejuni*)	3–5 days (2–10 days)	Diarrhea, abdominal pain, fever, nausea, vomiting	Infected food-source animals	Chicken, raw milk	Cook chicken thoroughly; avoid cross-contamination; irradiate chickens; pasteurize milk
Cholera (*Vibrio cholerae*)	2–3 days hours to days	Profuse, watery stools; sometimes vomiting, dehydration; often fatal if untreated	Raw or undercooked seafood	Human feces in marine environment	Cook seafood thoroughly; general sanitation
(*Clostridium perfringens*) food poisoning	8–22 hr (12–24 hr)	Diarrhea, cramps, rarely nausea and vomiting	Cooked meat and poultry	Soil, raw foods	Thorough heating and rapid cooling of foods
(*Escherichia coli*) foodborne infections enterohemorrhagic	12–60 hr (2–9 days)	Watery, bloody diarrhea	Raw or undercooked beef, raw milk	Infected cattle	Cook beef thoroughly pasteurize milk
(*Escherichia coli*) foodborne infections entroinvasive	at least 18 hr (uncertain)	Cramps, diarrhea, fever, dysentery	Raw foods	Human fecal contamination, direct or via water	Cook foods thoroughly; general sanitation
(*Escherichia coli*) foodborne infection enterotoxigenic	10–72 hr (3–5 days)	Profuse watery diarrhea; sometimes cramps, vomiting	Raw foods	Human fecal contamination, direct or via water	Cook foods thoroughly; general sanitation
Listeriosis (*Listeria monocytogenes*)	3–70 days	Meningoencephalitis; stillbirths; septicemia or meningitis in newborns	Raw milk, cheese and vegetables	Soil or infected animals, directly or via manure	Pasteurization of milk; cooking
Salmonellosis (*Salmonella* species)	5–72 hr (1–4 days)	Diarrhea, abdominal pain, chills, fever, vomiting, dehydration	Raw, undercooked eggs; raw milk, meat and poultry	Infected food-source animals; human feces	Cook eggs, meat and poultry thoroughly; pasteurize milk; irradiate chickens
Shigellosis (*Shigella* species)	12–96 hr (4–7 days)	Diarrhea, fever, nausea; sometimes vomiting, cramps	Raw foods	Human fecal contamination, direct or via water	General sanitation; cook foods thoroughly
Staphylococcal food poisoning (heat-stable enterotoxin of *Staphylococcus aureus*)	1–6 hr (6–24 hr)	Nausea, vomiting, diarrhea, cramps	Ham, meat, poultry products, cream-filled pastries, whipped butter, cheese	Handlers with colds, sore throats or infected cuts, food slicers	Thorough heating and rapid cooling of foods
Streptococcal foodborne infection (*Streptococcus pyogenes*)	1–3 days (varies)	Various, including sore throat, erysipelas, scarlet fever	Raw milk, deviled eggs	Handlers with sore throats, other "strep" infections	General sanitation, pasteurize milk
Vibrio parahaemolyticus foodborne infection	12–24 hr (4–7 days)	Diarrhea, cramps; sometimes nausea, vomiting, fever, headache	Fish and seafoods	Marine coastal environment	Cook fish and seafoods thoroughly
Vibrio vulnificus foodborne infection	In persons with high serum iron: 1 day	Chills, fever, prostration, often death	Raw oysters and clams	Marine coastal environment	Cook shellfish thoroughly
Yersiniosis (*Yersinia enterocolitica*)	3–7 days (2–3 weeks)	Diarrhea, pains mimicking appendicitis, fever vomiting, etc.	Raw or undercooked pork and beef; tofu packed in spring water	Infected animals especially swine; contaminated water	Cook meats thoroughly, chlorinate water

Reprinted with permission from the American Council on Science and Health (ACSH), New York, NY

undercooking of hamburger in the home probably occur throughout the U.S. (CDC, 1994a).

Listeria monocytogenes has been recognized as a human pathogen for several decades but the importance of food as a vehicle for transmission has only recently been identified (Doyle, 1985). *L. monocytogenes* is widely distributed in the environment and carried in the intestinal tracts of a variety of animals and humans (Doyle, 1985). Of significance to food safety, the microorganism can grow, although slowly, at refrigeration temperatures. *Listeria monocytogenes* causes illness primarily in individuals at increased risk for foodborne illness. Infection with *L. monocytogenes* may result in meningitis, miscarriage, and perinatal septicemia (Doyle, 1985). *S. enteriditis* can contaminate whole shell eggs when infected hens transmit the pathogen to the egg when it is produced. The global incidence of this serotype increased dramatically from 5% of all isolates in the U.S. in the 1970s to 20% of isolates in 1989 (St. Louis et al., 1988).

Emergence of these microbial health threats (diseases and their causative agents) may be due to several factors. These include: emergence of new microorganisms, recognition of existing diseases previously undetected, and changes in the environment that provide an epidemiologic "bridge" (IOM, 1992). The potential for foods to be involved in the emergence or reemergence of microbial threats to humans is great, largely because there are many points in the food system at which food safety can be compromised (IOM, 1992). . . .

FACTORS CONTRIBUTING TO FOODBORNE ILLNESS IN THE HOME

The extent of the hazards associated with pathogenic microorganisms and the risk of acquiring foodborne illness depend on several factors. These include type of pathogen, number of microorganisms ingested, and the consumers' susceptibility to the pathogen.

Pathogens. Pathogenic bacteria, viruses, fungi, parasitic protozoa, other parasites, and marine phytoplankton may cause foodborne illness. One way foodborne illness may arise is from infection by microorganisms and parasites. Infection occurs when pathogens, such as *Campylobacter* or *Salmonella*, in the ingested food, grow in the host's intestine. The infection may involve subsequent growth in other tissues or the production of toxin, in which case the illness is classified as a toxicoinfection. Foodborne illness may also stem from intoxication. Intoxication occurs when pathogens, such as *S. aureus*, produce toxin in a food or when a toxic chemical occurs in food before consumption. Common foodborne diseases caused by pathogenic microorganisms or their toxins are described in Tables 1–4. Depending on host susceptibility, foodborne illness may be mild to severe or lead to serious chronic complications such as arthritis, carditis, Guillain-Barre' syndrome, and hemolytic anemia (CAST, 1994; Smith, 1994; Archer and Young, 1988; Mossel, 1988; Archer 1985) or death. The complications that may be associated with certain foodborne illnesses are listed in Table 5.

Among outbreaks of known etiology reported to the Centers for Disease Control and Prevention (CDC) between 1973 and 1987, bacterial pathogens were responsible for most of the outbreaks (66%) and cases (92%; Bean et al., 1990). . . .

About 60% of the foodborne illnesses reported to CDC from 1973–1987 were of unknown etiology. The inability to determine the etiologic agent in reported outbreaks may be attributable to late or incomplete laboratory investigations, lack of recognition of the pathogen as a disease agent, or inability to identify the pathogen with available laboratory techniques (Bean and Griffin, 1990; Bean et al., 1990). . . .

The ability of several bacterial pathogens to multiply rapidly to dangerous levels in foods allowed to warm up or to remain warm for an extended period is responsible for their frequent implication in foodborne illness. Some pathogens, however, such as *L. monocytogenes*

"The potential for foods to be involved in the emergence or reemergence of microbial threats to humans is great ... (IOM, 1992)."

Table 2—Common Foodborne Diseases Caused by Viruses. *From Cliver (1993)*

Disease (causative agent)	Onset (duration)	Principal Symptoms	Typical Foods	Mode of Contamination	Prevention of Disease
Hepatitis A (Hepatitis A virus)	15–20 days (weeks to months)	Fever, weakness, nausea discomfort; often jaundice	Raw or undercooked shellfish; sandwiches, salads, etc.	Human fecal contamination, via water or direct	Cook shellfish thoroughly; general sanitation
Viral gastroenteritis (Norwalk-like viruses)	1–2 days (1–2 days)	Nausea, vomiting, diarrhea, pains, headache, mild fever	Raw or undercooked shellfish; sandwiches, salads, etc.	Human fecal contamination, via water or direct	Cook shellfish thoroughly, general sanitation
Viral gastroenteritis (rotaviruses)	1–3 days (4–6 days)	Diarrhea, especially in infants and young children	Raw or mishandled foods	Probably human fecal contamination	General sanitation

and *Y. enterocolitica*, can grow at refrigeration temperatures and others, such as *E. coli* O157:H7, and viruses, can cause illness at very low levels in foods.

Certain pathogens may be a greater problem in the home than in foodservice establishments or in commercially prepared foods. Approximately 92% of the 231 outbreaks of botulism from 1973–1987 were associated with food prepared in the home, especially home-canned foods (Bean and Griffin, 1990). . . .

Foods. A variety of foods are associated with foodborne illnesses, including foods of animal origin, such as fish and shellfish, red meats, poultry, fruits and vegetables, eggs, and dairy products (CAST, 1994; Bean and Griffin, 1990; Bryan, 1988a). In recent years, foodborne illnesses have been associated with novel substrates, such as potatoes, sauteed onions, garlic-in-oil mixtures, cooked rice, and sliced fruits. Vegetables grown in the ground or close to it are likely to be contaminated by the spore-forming bacteria *C. botulinum*, *C. perfringens*, and *B. cereus* (Bryan 1988a). Outbreaks of botulism have been associated with foil-wrapped baked potatoes left at room temperature, sauteed onions, and garlic-in-oil mixtures. Outbreaks of *B. cereus* food poisoning have been associated with cooked rice held at room temperature.

Mishandling Factors. From 1973–1987, 7,458 outbreaks and 237,545 cases of foodborne illness were reported to the CDC. Among the 7,219 outbreaks in which it was reported, the site of preparation of the implicated food was a commercial or institutional establishment in 79% of outbreaks and the home in 21%, with variations for different illness etiologies (Bean and Griffin, 1990). Sporadic cases and small outbreaks in homes, however, are considered far more common than cases constituting recognized outbreaks and comprise most of the foodborne illness cases in the U.S. (Schuchat et al. 1992; Tauxe, 1992, 1991; Bean and

Table 3—Common Foodborne Diseases Caused by Protozoa and Parasites. *From Cliver (1993)*

Disease (causative agent)	Onset (duration)	Principal Symptoms	Typical Foods	Mode of Contamination	Prevention of Disease
(PROTOZOA) Amebic dysentery (*Entamoeba histolytica*	2–4 weeks (varies)	Dysentery, fever, chills; sometimes liver abscess	Raw or mishandled foods	Cysts in human feces	General sanitation; thorough cooking
Cryptosporidiosis (*Cryptosporidium parvum*)	1–12 days (1–30 days)	Diarrhea; sometimes fever, nausea, and vomiting	Mishandled foods	Oocysts in human feces	General sanitation; thorough cooking
Giardiasis (*Giardia lamblia*)	5–25 days (varies)	Diarrhea with greasy stools, cramps, bloat	Mishandled foods	Cysts in human and animal feces, directly or via water	General sanitation; thorough cooking
Toxoplasmosis (*Toxoplasma gondii*)	10–23 days (varies)	Resembles mononucleosis fetal abnormality or death	Raw or undercooked meats; raw milk; mishandled foods	Cysts in pork or mutton, rarely beef; oocysts in cat feces	Cook meat thoroughly; pasteurize milk; general sanitation
(ROUNDWORMS, Nematodes) Anisakiasis (*Anisakis simplex, Pseudoterranova decipiens*)	Hours to weeks (varies)	Abdominal cramps, nausea, vomiting	Raw or undercooked marine fish, squid or octopus	Larvae occur naturally in edible parts of seafoods	Cook fish thoroughly or freeze at -4° F for 30 days
Ascariasis (*Ascaris lumbricoides*)	10 days –8 weeks (1–2 years)	Sometimes pneumonitis, bowel obstructions	Raw fruits or vegetables that grow in or near soil	Eggs in soil from human feces	Sanitary disposal of feces; cooking food
Trichinosis (*Trichinella spiralis*)	8–15 days (weeks, months)	Muscle pain, swollen eyelids, fever; sometimes death	Raw or undercooked pork or meat of carnivorous animals (e.g., bears)	Larvae encysted in animal's muscles	Thorough cooking of meat; freezing pork at 5° F for 30 days; irradiation
(TAPEWORMS, Cestodes) Beef tapeworm (*Taenia saginata*)	10–14 weeks (20–30 years)	Worm segments in stool; sometimes digestive disturbances	Raw or undercooked beef	"Cysticerci" in beef muscle	Cook beef thoroughly or freeze below 23°F
Fish tapeworm (*Diphyllobothrium latum*)	3–6 weeks (years)	Limited: sometimes vitamin B-12 deficiency	Raw or undercooked fresh-water fish	"Plerocercoids" in fish muscle	Heat fish 5 minutes at 133°F or freeze 24 hours at 0°F
Pork tapeworm (*Taenia solium*)	8 weeks–10 years (20–30 years)	Worm segments in stool; sometimes "cysticercosis" of muscles, organs, heart, or brain	Raw or undercooked pork; any food mishandled by a *T. solium* carrier	"Cysticerci" in pork muscle; any food —human feces with *T. solium* eggs	Cook pork thoroughly or freeze below 23°F; general sanitiation

Table 4—Common Foodborne Diseases Caused by Toxins in Seafood. *Adapted from Cliver (1993)*

Disease (causative agent)	Onset (duration)	Principal Symptoms	Typical Foods	Mode of Contamination	Prevention of Disease
(TOXINS IN FINFISH) Ciguatera poisoning (ciguatoxin, etc.)	3–4 hr (rapid)	Diarrhea, nausea, vomiting, abdominal pain	"Reef and island" fish: grouper, surgeon fish, barracuda, pompano, snapper, etc.	(Sporadic); food chain, from algae	Eat only small fish
	12–18 hr (days–months)	Numbness & tingling of face; taste & vision aberrations, sometimes convulsions, respiratory arrest, and death (1–24 hrs)			
Fugu or pufferfish poisoning (tetrodotoxin, etc.)	10–45 min to ≥ 3 hr	Nausea, vomiting, tingling lips and tongue, ataxia, dizziness, respiratory distress/arrest, sometimes death	Pufferfish, "fugu" (many species)	Toxin collects in gonads, viscera	Avoid pufferfish (or their gonads)
Scombroid or histamine poisoning (histamine, etc.)	minutes to few hours (few hours)	Nausea, vomiting, diarrhea, cramps, flushing, headache, burning in mouth	"Scombroid" fish (tuna, mackerel, etc.); mahimahi, others	Bacterial action	Refrigerate fish immediately when caught
(TOXINS IN SHELLFISH) Amnesic shellfish poisoning (domoic acid)		Vomiting, abdominal cramps, diarrhea, disorientation, memory loss; sometimes death	Mussels, clams	From algae	Heed surveillance warnings
Paralytic shellfish poisoning (saxitoxin, etc.)	≤ 1 hr (≤ 24 hr)	Vomiting, diarrhea, paresthesias of face, sensory and motor disorders; respiratory paralysis, death	Mussels, clams, scallops, oysters	From "red tide" algae	Heed surveillance warnings

Reprinted with permission from the American Council on Science and Health, New York, NY

Table 5–Medical Complications Associated with Certain Foodborne Infections. *From CAST (1994)*

Bacterial Infections Transmitted by Foods	Complications/sequelae
Aeromonas hydrophila enteritis[a]	Bronchopneumonia, cholecystitis
Brucellosis	Aortitis, epididymo-orchitis, meningitis, pericarditis, spondylitis
Campylobacteriosis	Arthritis, carditis, cholecystitis, colitis, endocarditis, erythema nodosum, Guillain-Barre' syndrome, hemolytic-uremic syndrome, meningitis, pancreatitis, septicemia
Escherichia coli (EHEC-types) enteritis	Erythema nodosum, hemolytic uremic syndrome, seronegative arthropathy, thrombotic thrombocytopenic purpura
Q-fever	Endocarditis, granulomatous hepatitis
Salmonellosis	Aortitis, cholecystitis, colitis, endocarditis, epididymoorchitis, meningitis, myocarditis, osteomyelitis, pancreatitis, Reiter's disease, rheumatoid syndromes, septicemia, splenic abscesses, thyroiditis, septic arthritis (sickle-cell anemic persons)
Shigellosis	Erythema nodosum, hemolytic-uremic syndrome, peripheral neuropathy, pneumonia, Reiter's disease, septicemia, splenic abscesses, synovitis
Vibrio parahaemolyticus enteritis	Septicemia
Yersiniosis	Arthritis, cholangitis, erythema nodosum, liver and splenic abscesses, lymphadenitis, pneumonia, pyomyositis, Reiter's disease, septicemia, spondylitis, Still's disease
Parasitic Infections Transmitted by Foods	**Complications/sequelae**
Cryptosporidiosis[b]	Severe diarrhea, prolonged and sometimes fatal
Giardiasis[b]	Cholangitis, dystrophy, joint symptoms, lymphoidal hyperplasia
Taeniasis	Arthritis, cysticercosis (*T. solium*)
Toxoplasmosis	Encephalitis and other central nervous system diseases, pancarditis, polymyositis
Trichinosis	Cardiac dysfunction, neurologic sequelae

[a]Suspected to be foodborne or waterborne.
[b]Waterborne.

Griffin, 1990; Schwartz et al., 1988). Foodborne illness in the home is reported much less frequently than institutional outbreaks because fewer people are typically involved. Additionally, sporadic cases of mild illnesses are less likely than more serious illnesses to result in medical attention, reporting, and investigation.

Bryan (1988b) reviewed the handling errors leading to foodborne illness outbreaks in the U.S. reported to CDC between 1961 and 1982. The top 12 factors contributing to 345 outbreaks resulting from mishandling/mistreatment of foods in the home are listed in Table 6. Use of contaminated foods or raw ingredients, inadequate cooking/canning/heat processing, and obtaining food from an unsafe source were the three leading factors contributing to foodborne illness in the home. Raw animal products may contain low levels of pathogenic microorganisms and cause illness if not properly cooked. For example, poultry may contain various species of *Salmonella* and *Campylobacter*; shell eggs may contain species of *Salmonella,* especially *S. enteritidis;* and ground beef may contain various pathogens, including *E. coli* O157:H7. Shellfish from sewage-polluted waters, raw milk, and wild mushrooms are foods obtained from unsafe sources. Microorganisms associated with these foods may be spread during preparation and may survive inadequate heating. Bacterial spores may be present on soil-grown cereals, vegetables, and fruits and may survive heating that is less severe than heating in a pressure cooker.

The fourth and fifth factors, improper cooling and lapse of time between preparation and eating, are time and temperature violations. The sixth factor is contamination of food by food handlers. People who carry foodborne pathogens in their intestinal tracts or touch fecally contaminated surfaces and fail to completely remove traces of fecal contamination by proper hand washing may contaminate any food they touch.

Bean and Griffin (1990) listed the mishandling factors thought to contribute to 1,678 foodborne illness outbreaks occurring during 1973–1987 with corresponding etiologies. Improper storage or holding temperature was the factor most often reported in *B. cereus* (94%), *C. perfringens* (97%), *Salmonella* (84%), *S. aureus* (98%), and group A *Streptococcus* (100%) outbreaks. Inadequate cooking was the factor most often reported in outbreaks due to *C. botulinum* (91%), *V. parahaemolyticus* (92%), and *Trichinella spiralis* (100%). Food from an unsafe source was the factor most often cited for outbreaks due to *Brucella* (100%), *Campylobacter* (67%), ciguatoxin (83%), mushroom poisoning (98%), and paralytic shellfish poisoning (100%). Personal hygiene was most frequently reported in *Shigella* (91%), Hepatitis A (96%), Norwalk virus

(78%), and *Giardia* (100%) outbreaks. For each year from 1983–1987, Bean et al. (1990) reported that the most common practice that contributed to foodborne disease was improper

Table 6–Top Twelve Factors Contributing to 345 Outbreaks of Foodborne Disease Caused by Mishandling and/or Mistreatment of Foods in Homes in the U.S., 1973-1982. From Bryan (1988b)

Rank	Contributing Factor	Percent[a]
1.	Contaminated raw food/ingredient	42.0
2.	Inadequate cooking/canning/heat processing	31.3
3.	Obtained food from unsafe source	28.7
4.	Improper cooling	22.3
5.	Lapse of 12 or more hours between preparing and eating	12.8
6.	Colonized person handling implicated food	9.9
7.	Mistaken for food	7.0
8.	Improper fermentations	4.6
9.	Inadequate reheating	3.5
10.	Toxic containers	3.5
11.	Improper hot holding	3.2
12.	Cross-contamination	3.2

[a]Percentage exceeds 100 because multiple factors contribute to single outbreaks.

storage or holding temperature, followed by poor personal hygiene of the food handler.

Usually several sequential factors result in foodborne illness (Bryan, 1988b). These are: (1) a pathogen must reach the food, (2) it must survive there until ingested, (3) in some cases, it must multiply to reach infectious levels or produce toxins, and (4) the person ingesting the food must be susceptible to the levels ingested. For example, in staphylococcal food poisoning, *S. aureus* typically reaches cooked food during handling. With sufficient time at room temperature or during inadequate cooling in too large a container in the refrigerator, the pathogen produces enterotoxin. The first six of the top 12 factors contributing to foodborne illness outbreaks (listed in Table 6) are either contamination and/or time and temperature-related errors. These errors account for the vast majority of foodborne illnesses in the home.

PREVENTING FOODBORNE ILLNESS IN THE HOME

Everyone in the food system, from those

"Everyone in the food system, from those who produce food to those who prepare it, has a role in food safety."

who produce food to those who prepare it, has a role in food safety. People in each segment of the food system need to understand the compelling reasons for proactive control of food safety. These reasons include: (1) microorganisms are ubiquitous in the environment and are found on raw agricultural products, (2) pathogens may survive minimal preservation treatments, (3) humans may introduce pathogens into food products during production, processing, distribution and/or preparation just before consumption, (4) depending on individual susceptibility, foodborne illness can range from mild to severe and life-threatening, with chronic complications.

People need to be aware of the control they have in their own kitchen for foodborne illness. They also need to understand how important food handling practices—acquisition, storage, preparation, serving, and dealing with leftovers—affect food safety. The top four mishandling factors cited in Table 6 are the most critical food handling practices to stress in food safety programs (Bryan, 1988b). Messages to the public about handling practices important in maintaining the safety of new unfamiliar food products may also be useful.

Messages and Educational Strategies. The most effective and practical strategy for controlling hazards and assuring food safety throughout the food system is the Hazard Analysis and Critical Control Points (HACCP) concept (Bauman, 1990). Successful application of the HACCP concept requires monitoring the points, processes, or practices that are critical for food safety and then actively controlling them to prevent problems from occurring. The food processing industry has effectively applied HACCP to the control of foodborne pathogens since the 1970s (Bauman, 1990). HACCP is relevant to all stages of the food system, from production to consumption. Education and training of people in each segment of the food system—from producers, retailers, foodservice operators, to preparers—should be an integral part of HACCP. Educational efforts, varying appropriately for different target audiences, should be proactive and messages should be HACCP-based, clear, consistent, and persuasive.

The U.S. Dept. of Agriculture (USDA, 1989) applied the HACCP concept in developing educational material for consumers. The agency identified five "educational critical control points" defined as the points most important in preventing foodborne illness but least understood by consumers. The points identified were: acquisition, storage, preparation, service, and handling leftovers. For example, in "A Quick Consumer Guide to Safe Food Handling" the agency provides the following advice based on the five critical control points:

- When you shop, buy cold food last, get it home fast.
- When you store food, keep it safe, refrigerate.
- When you prepare food, keep everything clean, thaw in refrigerator.
- When you're cooking, cook thoroughly.
- When you serve food, never leave it out over two hours.
- When you handle leftovers, use small, shallow containers for quick cooling.
- When in doubt, throw it out.

Similarly, the agency's safe food handling labels, shown in Fig. 1, required in July 1994 on packages of raw and partially cooked meat and poultry products, provide advice based on critical control points.

Some foodborne pathogens present few risks to most individuals but life-threatening risks to others, e.g., those with immunosuppression due to illness or medications, infants, pregnant women, and elderly individuals. Special educational emphasis should be given to these "at risk" groups. These individuals need to understand that they are more susceptible to foodborne illness even if they consume very low levels of foodborne pathogens, and therefore, must vigilantly use proper food handling practices. They must understand the need to avoid eating raw or undercooked animal foods, such as unpasteurized milk, avoid eating raw or undercooked seafood, particularly molluscan shellfish, and prevent cross-contamination between raw and cooked foods during preparation and storage. Individuals in these "at risk" groups and those who serve them need to understand that they should thoroughly cook raw animal foods to at least 160°F to kill any pathogens that may be present, promptly refrigerate leftovers in small shallow containers, and reheat leftovers to 165°F before consumption. Because outbreaks involving many deaths have occurred in nursing homes as a result of consumption of undercooked eggs or products made from raw eggs, the CDC recommends use of pasteurized eggs for institutions such as nursing homes and hospitals (CDC, 1990). The CDC recommends that, to avoid listeriosis, people at high risk use proper food handling practices and thoroughly wash raw vegetables before eating, avoid eating soft cheeses (e.g., Mexican-style and feta) and reheat ready-to-eat foods (e.g., hot dogs) thoroughly to at least 165°F. The CDC also said that these individuals may choose to avoid foods from delicatessen counters and to thoroughly reheat cold cuts to at least 165°F before eating (CDC, 1992; Schuchat et al., 1992).

Caregivers of infants younger than age one must understand the need for close attention to their use of sanitary containers, potable water (safe drinking water), good personal hygiene

"Education and training of people in each segment of the food system—from producers, retailers, foodservice operators, to preparers—should be an integral part of HACCP."

(hand washing), and sanitary practices in the preparation of infant formula. If possible, individuals who change diapers in institutional day care centers should refrain from preparing foods for infants. Because microorganisms may be introduced into the formula from the infant during feeding, leftover infant formula should be discarded after each feeding and a new container should be prepared immediately before the next feeding.

The CDC (1994b) suggested that because messages about behaviors that prevent or foster emerging infections are often most effective before unsafe behaviors develop, educational efforts targeting children and adolescents should be emphasized. Similarly, the National Advisory Committee on Microbiological Criteria for Foods (NACMCF), formed in 1988 by agencies of the U.S. Depts. of Agriculture, Health and Human Services, Commerce, and Defense, recommended the development of a basic food safety curriculum and specific lesson plans with accompanying audiovisual materials for public and private school systems (Rhodes, 1991). The NACMCF also advised that training be provided for teachers of children, initially, in grades 4–6. Further, the committee said that public service announcements were needed to foster the awareness of food safety principles (Rhodes, 1991). Additional strategies for reaching consumers include providing information in leaflets at retail markets, in recipes, in computer programs, and on computer networks. Safe food handling educational programs for national television audiences similar to those targeted at preventing AIDS and automobile injuries would be helpful.

As new innovative foods, such as minimally processed foods, are developed, clear, HACCP-based information about the importance of refrigeration and other handling practices would be useful. The NACMCF recommended the development of a mandatory, uniform logo, to read "*Important* Must Be Kept Refrigerated," for perishable refrigerated items for which temperature is the key element of safety (Rhodes, 1991). Because temperature maintenance can be extremely important, the committee also recommended that manufacturers use time/temperature indicators where possible to show product mishandling. Sherlock et al. (1992) suggested that consumer education may be necessary to ensure the success of time/temperature indicators. Incorporation of food handling information into product labels may be useful to actively and continuously educate consumers about new food products and the necessary safe food handling practices.

Resources for Consumers and Educators. A variety of information about food safety, including food handling tips, is available for

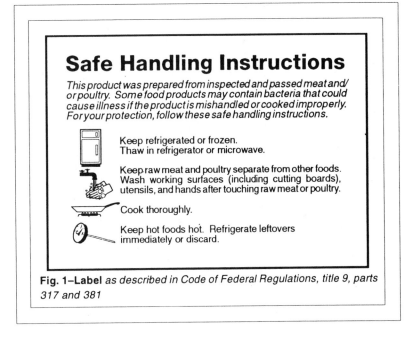

Fig. 1—Label as described in Code of Federal Regulations, title 9, parts 317 and 381

consumers and educators from several sources including: federal agencies (Food and Drug Administration, USDA, CDC), food industry trade organizations, scientific societies, food science and nutrition departments at land grant colleges and universities, and other organizations. Information formats include printed materials and videos for educators, other professionals, and the public. Much of the material is free or available for a nominal cost. Some material is written specifically for certain groups of people, such as people at high risk for foodborne disease. Information published by federal agencies may also be available from the local offices of these agencies.

As part of a national campaign to reduce the risk of foodborne illness and to increase knowledge of food-related risks from food production through consumption, the FDA and USDA established in 1994 the Foodborne Illness Education Information Center (Beltsville, MD). The Center is developing an educational database that will be made available to educators, trainers, and organizations producing educational and training materials for food workers and consumers. The database is accessible through a variety of electronic networks such as Internet, the National Agriculture Library electronic bulletin board, and PENpages' International Food and Nutrition Database.

The USDA's Food Safety and Inspection Service also operates a Meat and Poultry Hotline (1-800-535-4555) to answer questions about safe handling of meat and poultry. The number of consumer calls to the Hotline has grown steadily since 1985. Journalists, cookbook authors, and extension agents also use the Hotline for the latest information about food safety (USDA, 1994, 1991a,b). Similarly, the FDA operates a Seafood Hotline (1-800-FDA-4010) to answer questions about seafood safety.

Conclusion

Because microorganisms are ubiquitous in the environment they naturally occur on plants and animals. A small percentage of these microorganisms are pathogenic and, therefore, require control measures. Humans may also introduce pathogens into foods during production, processing, distribution, and/or preparation. Everyone in the food system, from people who produce food to those who prepare it, has a significant role in food safety, including activities broadly defined as food handling.

Surveys have found that some people consider homes the least likely place for food safety problems to occur. In contrast, epidemiologic studies indicate that sporadic cases and small outbreaks in homes comprise most of the foodborne illness cases in the U.S. Botulism, campylobacteriosis, and listeriosis are often caused by mishandling of foods in the home. Additional epidemiologic studies on sporadic cases of *Salmonella* and *E. coli* O157:H7 are urgently needed to help determine the magnitude of problems associated with these pathogens and to determine common causes and sites of preparation of implicated foods.

Several changes in society contribute to microbiological challenges. People have expressed concern about food safety, but some appear to be unaware of the home food handling practices that can affect their risk of acquiring a foodborne illness. Education, with specific programs targeted at individuals at high risk, is the key means for increasing public awareness of foodborne disease risks and preventing foodborne illness. To enable the public to make informed food safety decisions affecting their health, educational efforts must provide compelling reasons for the need for vigilance in proper food handling practices. Information about the means for preventing, controlling, or eliminating microbial hazards must be clear, consistent, and science-based.

References

Archer, D.L. 1985. Enteric microorganisms in rheumatoid diseases: Causative agents and possible mechanisms. J. Food Protect. 48: 538-545.

Archer, D.L. and Kvenberg, J.E. 1985. Incidence and cost of foodborne diarrheal disease in the United States. J. Food Protect. 48: 887-894.

Archer, D.L. and Young, F.E. 1988. Contemporary issues: Diseases with a food vector. Clin. Microbiol. Rev. 1: 377-398.

Bauman, H. 1990. HACCP: Concept, development, and application. Food Technol. 44(5): 156-158.

Bean, N.H. and Griffin, P.M. 1990. Foodborne disease outbreaks in the United States, 1973-1987: Pathogens, vehicles, and trends. J. Food Protect. 53: 804-817.

Bean, N.H., Griffin, P.M., Goulding, J.S., and Ivey, C.B. 1990. Foodborne disease outbreaks, 5-year summary, 1983-1987. J. Food Protect. 53(8): 711-728.

Bennett, J.V., Holmberg, S.D., Rogers, M.F., and Solomon, S.L. 1987. Infectious and parasitic diseases. In "Closing the Gap: The Burden of Unnecessary Illness," Oxford University Press, New York.

Bryan, F.L. 1988a. Risks associated with vehicles of foodborne pathogens and toxins. J. Food Protect. 51: 498-508.

Bryan, F.L. 1988b. Risks of practices, procedures and processes that lead to outbreaks of foodborne diseases. J. Food Protect. 51: 663-673.

Buchanan, R.L. and Deroever, C.M. 1993. Limits in assessing microbiological food safety. J. Food Protect. 56(8): 725-729.

CAST. 1994. Foodborne Pathogens: Risks and Consequences. A report of a Task Force of the Council for Agricultural Science and Technology, Ames, Iowa.

CDC. 1990. Update: *Salmonella enteritidis* infections and shell eggs-United States, 1990. Morbid. Mortal. Wkly. Rept. 39: 909-912, Centers for Disease Control and Prevention, Atlanta, Georgia.

CDC. 1992. Update: Foodborne listeriosis—United States, 1988-1990. Morbid. Mortal. Wkly. Rept. 41(15): 251-258, Centers for Disease Control and Prevention, Atlanta, Georgia.

CDC. 1993. Update: Multistate outbreak of *Escherichia coli* O157:H7 infections from hamburgers-Western United States, 1992-1993. Morbid. Mortal. Wkly. Rept. 42: 258-263, Centers for Disease Control and Prevention, Atlanta, Georgia.

CDC. 1994a. *Escherichia coli* O157:H7 outbreak linked to home-cooked hamburger—California, July 1993. Morbid. Mortal. Wkly. Rept. 43: 213-215, Centers for Disease Control and Prevention, Atlanta, Georgia.

CDC. 1994b. Addressing Emerging Health Threats: A Prevention Strategy for the United States. Centers for Disease Control and Prevention, Atlanta, Georgia.

Cliver, D.O. 1990. Organizing a safe food supply system. IV. Consumer's role in food safety. In "Foodborne Diseases," ed. D.O. Cliver, pp. 361-367. Academic Press, New York.

Cliver, D.O. 1993. "Eating Safely: Avoiding Foodborne Illness," ed. A. Golaine, American Council on Science and Health, New York.

Cousin, M.A., Jay, J.M., and Vasavada, P.C. 1992. Psychrotrophic microorganisms. In "Compendium of Methods for the Microbiological Examination of Foods," ed. C. Vanderzant and D.F. Splittstoesser, 3rd ed., pp. 153-168. American Public Health Association, Washington, D.C.

Doyle, M.P. 1985. Food-borne pathogens of recent concern. Ann. Rev. Nutr. 5: 25-41.

Doyle, M.P. 1991. A new generation of foodborne pathogens. Contemp. Nutr. 16(6), General Mills Nutrition Department, General Mills, Stacy, Minn.

FMI. 1994. Trends in the U.S.: Consumer Attitudes and the Supermarket 1994. Food Marketing Inst. Washington, D.C.

Goldman, D. 1990. The new consumer, superbrands 1990. Adv. Weekly Suppl., Sept. 17, pp. 25-32.

Griffin, P.M. and Tauxe, R.V. 1991. The epidemiology of infections caused by *Escherichia coli* O157:H7, other enterohemorrhagic *E. coli*, and the associated hemolytic uremic syndrome. Epidemiol. Rev. 13: 60-98.

Hauschild, A.H.W. and Bryan, F.L. 1980. Estimate of cases of food- and waterborne illness in Canada and the United States. J. Food Protect. 43: 435-440.

Hedberg, C.W., MacDonald, K.L., and Osterholm, M.T. 1994. Changing epidemiology of food-borne disease: A Minnesota perspective. Clin. Infect. Dis. 18: 671-682.

IOM. 1992. "Emerging Infections: Microbial Threats to Health in the United States," ed. J. Lederberg, R.E. Shope, and S.C. Oaks, Jr., Institute of Medicine, National Academy Press, Washington, D.C.

Jay, J.M. 1992a. Microbiological food safety. Crit. Rev. Food Sci. Nutr. 31(3): 177-190.

Jay., J.M. 1992b. "Modern Food Microbiology," 4th ed. Van Nostrand Reinhold, New York.

Jones, J.M. 1992. "Food Safety." Eagan Press, St. Paul, Minn.

Lechowich, R.V. 1988. Microbiological challenges of refrigerated foods. Food Technol. 42(12): 84-89.

Lee, L.A., Gerber, A.R., Lonsway, D.R., Smith, J.D.,

Carter, G.P., Puhr, N.D., Parrish, C.M., Sikes, R.K., Finton, R.J., and Tauxe, R.V. 1990. *Yersinia enterocolitica* O:3 infections in infants and children, associated with the household preparation of chitterlings. N. Engl. J. Med. 14: 984-987.

Ollinger-Snyder, P. and Matthews, E. 1994. Food safety issues: Press reports heighten consumer awareness of microbiological safety. Dairy, Food, Environ. Sanita. 14(10): 580-589.

Mossel, D.A.A. 1988. Impact of foodborne pathogens on today's world, and prospects for management. An. Hum. Health. 1: 13-23.

Padhye, N.V. and Doyle, M.P. 1992. *Escherichia coli* O157:H7: Epidemiology, pathogenesis, and methods for detection in food. J. Food Protect. 55: 555-565.

Penner, K., Kramer, C., and Frantz, G. 1985. Consumer food safety perceptions. MF774. Kansas State Univ. Ext. Service, Manhattan, Kansas.

Potter, J.E. 1994. The role of epidemiology and risk assessment: A CDC perspective. Dairy, Food, Environ. Sanita. 14(12): 738-741.

Rhodes, M.E. 1991. Educating professionals and consumers about extended-shelf-life refrigerated foods. Food Technol. 45(4): 162-164.

Roberts, T. 1993. Cost of foodborne illness and prevention interventions. In "Proceedings of the 1993 Public Health Conference on Records and Statistics. Toward the year 2000 - Refining the Measures," pp. 514-518. U.S. Dept. of Health and Human Services, Washington, D.C.

Schuchat, A., Deaver, K.A., Wenger, J.D., Plikaytis, B.D., Mascola, L., Piner, R.W., Reingold, A.L., and Broome, C.V. 1992. Role of foods in sporadic listeriosis: I. Case-control study of dietary risk factors. J. Am. Med. Assn. 267(15): 2041-2045.

Schwartz, B., Broome C.V., Brown, G.R., Hightower, A.W., Ciesielski, C.A., Gaventa, S., Gellin, B.G., and Mascola, L. 1988. Association of sporadic listeriosis with consumption of uncooked hot dogs and undercooked chicken. Lancet 2: 779-782.

Sherlock, M., Fu. G., Taoukis, P.S., and Labuza, T.P. 1992. Consumer perceptions of consumer type time-temperature indicators for use on refrigerated dairy foods. Dairy, Food, Environ. Sanita. 12: 559-565.

Smith, J.L. 1994. Arthritis and foodborne bacteria. J. Food Protect. 57(10): 935-941.

St. Louis, M.E., Morse, D.L., Potter, M.E., DeMelfi, T.M., Guzewich, J.J., Tauxe, R.V., and Blake, P.A. 1988. The emergence of grade A eggs as a major source of *S. enteritidis* infections: New implications for the control of salmonellosis. J. Am. Med. Assn. 259: 2103-2107.

Tauxe, R.V. 1991. Salmonella: A postmodern pathogen. J. Food Protect. 54: 563-568.

Tauxe, R.V. 1992. Epidemiology of *Campylobacter jejuni* infections in the United States and other industrialized nations. In "*Campylobacter jejuni*—Current Status and Future Trends," eds. I. Nachamkim, M.J. Blaser, L.S. Tompkins, p. 9-19. American Society for Microbiology, Washington, D.C.

Tauxe, R.V. 1995. Personal communication. Centers for Disease Control and Prevention, Atlanta, Georgia.

Todd, E.C.D. 1989. Preliminary estimates of the cost of foodborne disease in the United States. J. Food Protect. 52: 595-601.

USDA. 1989. A margin of safety: The HACCP approach to food safety education. Project Report. U.S. Dept. of Agriculture, U.S. Government Printing Office, Washington, D.C.

USDA. 199la. The Meat and Poultry Hotline. A retrospective, 1985-1990. U.S. Dept. of Agriculture, U.S. Government Printing Office, Washington, D.C.

USDA. 1991b. USDA's Meat and Poultry Hotline links scientists and consumers. Food News for Consumers 7(4): 4-5. U.S. Dept. of Agriculture, Food Safety and Inspection Service, Washington, D.C.

USDA. 1994. Making the connection: An update - USDA's Meat and Poultry Hotline, 1993. U.S. Dept. of Agriculture, U.S. Government Printing Office, Washington, D.C.

USDA/FDA. 1991. Results of the Food and Drug Administration's 1988 health and diet survey—Food handling practices and food safety knowledge for consumers, U.S. Dept. of Agriculture and Food and Drug Administration, Washington, D.C.

Whittam, T.S., Wolfe, M.L., Wachsmuth, K., Orskov, F., Orskov, I., and Wilson, R.A. 1993. Clonal relationships among *Escherichia coli* strains that cause hemorrhagic colitis and infantile diarrhea. Infect. Immunol. 61(5): 1619-1629.

Williamson, D.M. 1991. Home Food Preparation Practice: Results of a National Consumer Survey. M.S. thesis. Cornell University, Ithaca, New York.

Williamson, D.M., Gravani, R.B., and Lawless, H.T. 1992. Correlating food safety knowledge with home food-preparation practices. Food Technol. 46(5): 94-100.

New risks in ground beef revealed

It looked as though the government acted effectively. Less than a year after undercooked, bacteria-laden hamburgers led to hundreds of illnesses and four deaths in the infamous Jack-in-the-Box incident of 1993, the U.S. Department of Agriculture declared the offending strain of bacteria—*E. coli* 0157:H7—an "adulterant." The legal implication: meat containing the bug is not considered fit for sale and is subject to federal seizure.

Nevertheless, illness-producing bacteria have become the leading cause of acute kidney failure among children in the United States, causing some 40,000 illnesses and 250 to 500 deaths each year. According to a team of Tufts University researchers, the government may be missing the forest for the trees by focusing primarily on *E. coli* 0157:H7. Judging by a new report from the group, as much as 25 percent of ground meat sold in supermarkets may contain other types of bacteria that are just as capable of causing kidney failure and related complications.

For a closer look at the state of the meat supply and some answers on how you can protect yourself and your loved ones, we spoke with the lead researcher of the new study, David W. Acheson, MD, of the Division of Geographic Medicine and Infectious Diseases at the Tufts New England Medical Center.

Q: *Ever since the Jack-in-the-Box story hit the media, fingers have been pointed at* E. coli *0157:H7 as the emerging culprit in food-borne illness. Why are you saying it's not the only one that's so lethal?*

Dr. Acheson: To answer that, let me roll back a bit. Bacteriologists discovered *E. coli* 0157:H7 back in 1982. It caused two very unusual outbreaks of grossly bloody diarrhea—one in Oregon and the other in Michigan. That was really when it got on the scientific map. By the mid to late '80s, it was determined that *E. coli* 0157 was making a toxin that was essentially identical to a toxin that had been discovered about a hundred years ago, called Shiga toxin.

Over the past ten years it has become very clear that Shiga toxin, not the bacteria themselves, is causing the problems associated with *E. coli* 0157:H7. It has also become clear that many other strains of bacteria are capable of producing Shiga toxin. What's happened is that the toxin genes have been moving around the world. Particles called bacteriophages are able to jump from one strain of bacteria and land in another. The bacteriophages then give the bacteria the genes that enable them to produce Shiga toxin.

Q: *So shouldn't the government be looking for Shiga toxin rather than* E. coli *0157:H7?*

Dr. Acheson: Yes, that's where the logic is. Look for the toxins, or look for *all* the toxin-producing bacteria and get away from the dogma of just checking for 0157. That's what has led us down this track here at Tufts.

Q: *How many types of bacteria can make Shiga toxin?*

Dr. Acheson: So far in North America more than 50

different types of *E. coli* have been linked to illness caused by Shiga toxin. The same numbers are coming out of Europe, South America, and Australia. In fact, in Australia there's almost no 0157:H7. But in January of last year there was a really nasty outbreak of illness due to an 0111 strain of *E. coli* in sausage. About two dozen people ended up with serious kidney complications, and one child died.

We've been trying to get Australians to realize that they need to move away from 0157. They test for it, even though they don't have it, and what they don't routinely test for is 0111.

Ironically, the United States imports a lot of beef from Australia, and according to my colleagues in Australia, the USDA makes the Australian meat companies test their beef for 0157 before they export it. There's evidence that 0111 is killing people in Australia, and it's in Australian cattle. But do we look for it in our imported Australian meat? No—we test for the bug they *don't* have in Australia. It's like a head-in-the-sand mentality.

Q: *It sounds like* E. coli *is the big problem, and we should try to get rid of all strains of it.*

Dr. Acheson: Actually, most strains of *E. coli* are "good" bacteria. We've all got millions of them in our guts, and we'd be a mess without them. It's just the toxin-producing strains that are a problem.

In the last couple of years it has also come out that Shiga toxin genes seem to be able to jump into bacteria other than *E. coli*. There was an outbreak in Europe in 1994 linked to a bacterium called *Citrobacter freundii*. It's part of the same general family as *E. coli*, but it's somewhat different. The outbreak occurred among a group of kids who had eaten something known in Germany as green butter, which is regular butter mixed with parsley. It turned out the parsley had been grown with cow manure or hadn't been washed properly. When these kids got sick, the illness was traced to Shiga toxin genes in the *Citrobacter*.

A similar thing was reported in Australia this year. A 5-month-old girl got sick from a strain of bacteria called *Enterobacter cloacae*, which had Shiga toxin genes in it.

Q: *Is there a test on the market that labs can use to check for Shiga toxin rather than just 0157?*

Dr. Acheson: Yes, we've been working on the Shiga toxin for years, and one of the things we developed was a rapid, accurate test that detects its presence. Following the Jack-in-the-Box outbreak, we decided we should try to do something to get the test out there where it could be useful. So Meridian Diagnostics in Cincinnati took it and made it suitable for use in hospital clinics. This way when a patient presents with diarrhea or bloody diarrhea, you're not just looking

for 0157. You can also use a variation of the test to check for toxins in, say, ground beef.

Q: *Are many people using the test?*

Dr. Acheson: No, not routinely. Many labs don't even check for 0157 in the stools of potentially affected patients. The Centers for Disease Control and Prevention published a survey this year showing that only about 50 percent of labs are looking for 0157. It's really quite scary how little attention is being paid to this.

Q: *What about the meat industry? Why isn't it testing for Shiga toxin or for bacteria other than 0157?*

Dr. Acheson: According to our research, 25 percent of ground beef is contaminated. If the results of our study are borne out with larger studies, I can see why the meat industry doesn't want to test for the toxin. It's going to cost them to do the test, and it's going to cost them to deal with the meat that comes up positive for Shiga toxin.

Still, it's only fair that consumers know that it's not just 0157 that's a problem, and the meat they're buying off their supermarket shelves is potentially as deadly as the half-cooked meat served in Jack in the Box in 1993.

Q: *What led you to conclude that 25 percent of ground beef may be contaminated with Shiga toxin?*

Dr. Acheson: We wanted to see whether the test we had developed to check for Shiga toxin in human stool was able to identify it in ground beef. So we bought ground beef and spiked it with different strains of toxin-producing bacteria. But we found that some of our "controls," non-spiked beef samples used for comparison, were kicking over positive for the toxin.

Of course, that set us all wondering what was going on here. So we mounted a very small scale study in which various members of the lab just went to supermarkets and bought ground beef, both here in Boston and in Cincinnati. We used several different tests and found that 25 percent of the samples contained toxin-producing bacteria. And none of it was *E. coli* 0157:H7.

Q: *It's enough to make a person never want to eat another hamburger. Is it safe to eat ground beef?*

Dr. Acheson: Yes, so long as it's thoroughly cooked and properly handled. [See box on next page.] You know, I think people have learned to be very careful with chicken because of *Salmonella* bacteria. They've woken up to the fact that if they prepare chicken on the countertop, they get out the bleach and make sure that everything is washed. But they may not do the same with ground beef. And it's fun to play with. The kids will come in and say, "Oh, let's make hamburgers." But in reality beef with toxin-producing bacteria is potentially as deadly, if not more so, than chicken with *Salmonella*.

Q: *Why are Shiga toxin-producing bacteria so harmful?*

Dr. Acheson: One of the things is that the infectious dosage seems to be really small. From studying the Jack-in-the-Box incident, scientists reckon that some of the hamburgers they rescued from the distributors contained only 100 or 200 toxin-producing bacteria per quarter-pound burger. That's much different than *Salmonella* food poisoning, in which it might take a million bacteria to get sick. This probably explains why person-to-person transmission is such a big deal. In fact, about 20 percent of U.S. outbreaks of 0157:H7 occurred in daycare settings and nursing homes and were caused by relatively few bacteria spread, for example, by not washing hands after changing diapers.

Another reason Shiga-producing bacteria are so harmful is that they are likely to make you much sicker than you would be with *Salmonella*. Roughly 5 to 10 percent of people who get sick enough to seek the attention of a physician end up with hemolytic uremic syndrome (HUS), a serious illness that often leads to kidney failure. Of those who get HUS, about 5 percent die during the acute stages of the disease, and 5 percent suffer major medical complications such as stroke or permanent kidney damage requiring transplant or dialysis. Of the remainder, 2 or 3 years later, probably half of them will still have significant kidney damage. So although it's not a frightfully common problem, it's not just like your regular food poisoning where you spend a couple of days in the bathroom and it's all over.

Q: *Most of the media coverage of hemolytic uremic syndrome seems to focus on children as the victims. Can, say, a middle-aged person suffer serious illness from Shiga toxin?*

Dr. Acheson: It can hit at any age, but it seems that children and the elderly are the most vulnerable. If you want to put numbers on it, I'd say that consumers under 10 and over 75 are the two populations that are hardest hit. We don't know exactly why, but it's probably related to the immune system. In young children, immunity hasn't fully kicked in yet, and in the elderly it's waning.

Q: *How can a parent tell if a child is sick with Shiga toxin?*

Bacteria busters: Tips for keeping food safe

To prevent illness from *E. coli* 0157:H7 and other Shiga toxin-producing bacteria, heed the following advice.

- At the supermarket, make sure meat and poultry are bagged separately from fruits and vegetables or that the meat is wrapped in a small plastic bag. Produce bagged along with meat can become contaminated with bacteria if the meat's juices seep out of the package and onto the fruits and vegetables. And since fruits and many vegetables are not cooked, any toxin-producing bacteria that reach them will not be destroyed.

- Rinse fruits and vegetables thoroughly with cold water before serving. Toxin-producing bacteria reside in animal feces rather than produce. But some outbreaks of illness due to *E. coli* 0157:H7 have been linked to lettuce and other produce that apparently had been exposed to fecal matter during growing or transport to the supermarket. Even cantaloupe and other melons with inedible skins should be rinsed carefully. The knife used to cut the fruit can carry bacteria lurking on the exterior into the fleshy inside of the fruit.

- During cooking, flip steaks with tongs or a spatula rather than a fork. Unlike ground beef, in which bacteria are mixed throughout the meat during the grinding process, steak harbors bacteria only on the surface. Sticking a fork into the meat, however, injects the interior with bacteria from the outside.

- Cook all meat and poultry to 160 degrees Fahrenheit. The meat should not look pink, and the juices should run yellow, with no trace of pink or red.

- Wash with hot soapy water hands, utensils, cutting boards, and countertops that have come into contact with raw meat or poultry. Also wash sponges and dishcloths used to wipe surfaces exposed to raw meat.

- When dining out, order hamburgers and other ground beef items well-done.

- Buy pasteurized apple cider or heat fresh cider to 160 degrees Fahrenheit. In 1991, about two dozen people were infected with *E. coli* 0157:H7 after drinking fresh cider at a mill in Massachusetts. Public health officials suspect that the contaminated cider was made with unwashed apples that had fallen off the tree and come into contact with animal feces on the ground.

- Do not drink raw milk.

- Wash hands thoroughly after changing diapers. If your child is in a daycare setting, make sure the staff does the same.

Dr. Acheson: That's one of the big problems, because its initial presentation is like any other illness a kid gets. Symptoms usually start 1 or 2 days after exposure. There isn't much of a fever, and about half the kids have vomiting and generalized abdominal pain, and they just feel bad. Often, they will have non-bloody diarrhea, which may or may not progress to bloody diarrhea.

Then, typically, the gut part of the disease—the abdominal pain, vomiting, and diarrhea—begins to get better. But as the gut part is improving or is even gone altogether, the child re-presents with a stroke, seizure, or kidney failure. One thing we're working on in our lab is figuring out how the toxin gets from the inside of the gut, where the bacteria produce it, across the gut wall and to the brain and kidneys. We don't know whether it is actually getting into the bloodstream or whether something else is going on.

Of course, the important thing for parents is that you're not going to want to run and have a checkup done every time your child gets diarrhea. But if the child has *bloody* diarrhea, unquestionably ask for a Shiga toxin test.

Q: *If parents start talking Shiga toxin, won't some pediatricians think they're crazy? Are physicians even aware of this problem?*

Dr. Acheson: Probably not as aware as they should be. We've got a real education job to do. There have been multiple cases in the literature of kids going to a doctor with these kinds of symptoms and then having their appendixes taken out or, in adults, having surgery to check for intestinal disease. In the meantime, somebody sends a stool sample off for a test, and then 3 days after the surgery they find toxin-producing bacteria. Some poor kid has gone through an operation and general anesthesia just because people don't think of Shiga toxin.

But consumers can go into the physician's office with an article like this and say, "Look, it may be Shiga toxin."

Q: *Once someone is diagnosed with Shiga toxin, what kind of treatment is available?*

Dr. Acheson: There is a drug called Synsorb-Pk being tested in Canada that mops up Shiga toxin in the gut. It looks moderately promising, but it's not a panacea. Unfortunately, there isn't a wonder drug.

But for me both as a physician and a parent, I'd want to know if my child had Shiga toxin. I mentioned the two phases: the diarrhea, vomiting, and fever that seem to get better; and the second stage where a child presents with a seizure or stroke. If you know that a child is infected with toxin-producing bacteria, you can at least watch for signs of kidney failure and for the other things we know happen. And you can be in there with supportive therapy. Being aware, watching fluid balance and other vital signs, can help avoid dialysis and may prevent strokes.

BOTULINUM TOXIN

A Poison That Can Heal

Luba Vangelova

Botulinum toxin can heal as well as harm. The bacterial toxin that can paralyze and kill if consumed in contaminated food is now safely used, in a purified form, as a medicine to control certain conditions marked by involuntary muscle contractions.

The history and lethality of botulism would seem to make it an unlikely source for a curative substance. Although death rates from botulism poisoning are just a fraction of what they were 30 years ago, botulism continues to strike dozens of people every year—most of them infants, according to statistics from the national Centers for Disease Control and Prevention in Atlanta.

"Botulism is still lurking, and if our guard is not up, it will create a problem," says Richard C. Swanson, director of the Food and Drug Administration's division of emergency and investigational operations and one of the agency's representatives to the Interagency Botulism Research Coordinating Committee.

> **T**here are three types of botulism poisoning: foodborne, wound and infant.

Botulism-causing *Clostridium botulinum* bacteria and their spores are everywhere. Prevalent in soil and marine sediments worldwide, their spores are often found on the surfaces of fruits and vegetables, and in seafood. The bacteria and spores themselves are harmless; the dangerous substance is the toxin produced by the bacteria when they grow. There are seven varieties of botulinum toxin, designated by the letters A through G.

Botulinum toxin is "the most poisonous substance known," says Stephen S. Arnon, M.D., head of the Infant Botulism Prevention Program at the California Department of Health Services. For this reason, anyone with symptoms of botulism should receive emergency treatment, and public health officials should be notified to locate the source of the contamination and prevent other cases.

Once in the body, the toxin binds to nerve endings at the point where the nerves join muscles. This prevents the nerves from signaling the muscles to contract. The result is weakness and paralysis that descends from the cranium down, affecting, among other things, the muscles that regulate breathing.

Before the development of mechanical ventilators, the respiratory paralysis caused by botulism claimed many more victims than it does today. Between 1910 and 1919, for example, the death rate from botulism was 70 percent. By the 1980s the rate had dropped to 9 percent, and in 1993 it was less than 2 percent. But recovery is still slow; assuming the patient receives proper care to ensure continued breathing, recovery occurs only when the affected nerves grow new endings, a process that can take several months, although the length of time varies greatly from case to case.

If botulism is caught in the early stages, injection of an antitoxin made from horse serum can lessen the severity of disease by neutralizing the toxin that has not yet bound to nerve endings. But because of the risk of serious side effects such as anaphylaxis, a life-threatening allergic reaction, and serum sickness (an unpredictable allergic reaction to the horse serum, which can lead to anaphylaxis), the equine antitoxin cannot always be used, and it is never given to infants.

The condition in which *C. botulinum* spores germinate and toxin is produced—absence of oxygen, low acidity levels, and temperatures between 40 and 120 degrees Fahrenheit (4.5 to 49 degrees Celsius)—can easily develop in improperly stored home-cooked or commercial foods, as well as in canned foods that have not been prepared with proper canning procedures. Infant intestinal tracts, which haven't yet developed the full range of beneficial bacteria, can also present an environment inviting to *C. botulinum* toxin production, as can some deep wounds.

Three Types

There are three types of botulism poisoning, distinguished by the manner in which they are contracted: food-borne, wound and infant. In infant botulism the toxin is produced when *C. botulinum* spores germinate in the intestine. (Rarely, adults can acquire the disease this way.) In wound botulism, which is very rare, the toxin is produced by *C. botulinum* bacteria in an infected wound. In the food-borne form of the disease, the person ingests the toxin itself by eating food contaminated with it. Statistically, infant botulism, which was recognized in the mid-'70s, is the most common form of the disease. But the public still generally associates botulism with food poisoning in adults and children. The food-borne disease is the most avoidable form of botulism.

Symptoms usually develop within a day of eating the food, although they can take up to 10 days to manifest. Apart from weakness and paralysis, common complaints include fatigue, dry mouth, and difficulty swallowing. Unfortunately, doctors sometimes misdiagnose the symptoms as Guillain-Barré syndrome, stroke, intoxication, or a handful of other conditions. For this reason, federal health officials suspect that botulism poisoning is underdiagnosed.

Home Canning

One of the most common culprits in food-borne botulism is home-canned food, especially vegetables such as asparagus, green beans, and peppers. More than 90 percent of food-borne botulism outbreaks between 1976 and 1985 were due to home-processed foods.

"If you home-can products, make sure you use proper equipment, proper containers to can in, and use the up-to-date process," Swanson advises. U.S. Department of Agriculture home canning guidelines are available from county extension offices. One basic recommendation is to cook food to be canned in pressure cookers because they can maintain temperatures high enough (above 212 F, or 100 C) for 10 minutes to kill the spores, which are remarkably heat-resistant.

One of the most common culprits in food-borne botulism is home-canned food.

Foods cooked at home should not be left at temperatures between 40 F and 140 F (4.5 C to 60 C) for more than four hours. Toxin that may have formed can readily be destroyed by boiling the food for 10 minutes.

Commercial foods have also been involved in botulism outbreaks. Some outbreaks have been attributed to improperly handled food, such as potato salad, served in restaurants. But many commercial food outbreaks are due to consumer mishandling, such as disregarding labels that indicate the food should be refrigerated. Some food companies acidify their products or lower their moisture content as an extra precautionary measure in case the refrigeration warning is not heeded. Consumers can best protect themselves by reading the labels and following the storage instructions, Swanson says, and by discarding rusty, swollen or otherwise damaged cans.

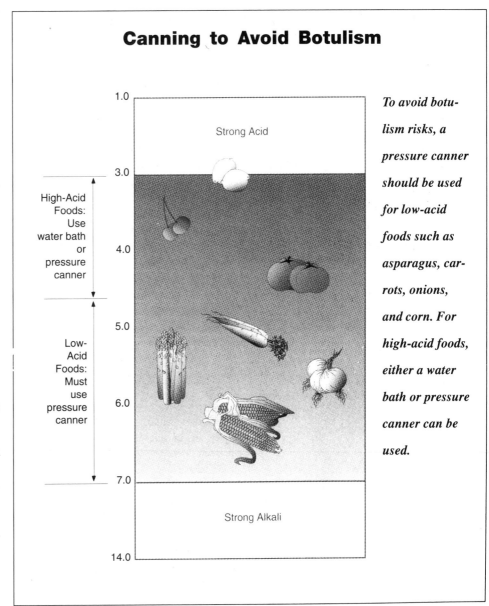

Canning to Avoid Botulism

1.0

Strong Acid

3.0

High-Acid Foods: Use water bath or pressure canner

4.0

5.0

Low-Acid Foods: Must use pressure canner

6.0

7.0

Strong Alkali

14.0

To avoid botulism risks, a pressure canner should be used for low-acid foods such as asparagus, carrots, onions, and corn. For high-acid foods, either a water bath or pressure canner can be used.

Infant botulism is serious, but rare and not usually fatal.

Infant Botulism

Infant botulism differs from food-borne botulism in that the toxin itself is not ingested. Instead, *C. botulinum* spores swallowed by the infant germinate and produce the toxin in the favorable environment of the baby's large intestine.

Because the spores are nearly everywhere in the environment, children and adults regularly ingest them, yet very rarely suffer ill effects. In a few cases, adults who have had intestinal surgery or whose intestinal tracts have otherwise been altered have contracted the disease the way infants do. This has led researchers to conclude that infants' as-yet "incompletely-developed intestinal flora," may be to blame, says Arnon, one of the co-discoverers of infant botulism in 1976.

Infant botulism is serious, but rare and not usually fatal. From 1976 through the end of 1993, 1,206 infant botulism cases were confirmed in the United States. About 75 to 100 cases are reported annually, about half of them in California (presumed to be due to the prevalence of *C. botulinum* spores in the state, its high number of births, and the pediatric community's familiarity with the disease, which results in more correct botulism diagnoses). All of the infant cases involve babies less than 1 year old; the disease is most common in the second month of life.

Infants' immature intestinal tracts offer a "window of vulnerability, and if a baby has the bad luck to swallow a botulism spore during that period, the spore has an opportunity to germinate," Arnon says. The spores travel with microscopic dust particles, so the researchers have concluded that most affected infants have simply inhaled the spores. "They mix with saliva, they're swallowed, and that's how they reach the intestine," Arnon says. Unfortunately, there is no way to prevent the disease in such cases.

But parents and other caregivers can prevent babies acquiring infant botulism from one source—honey. California researchers have isolated *C. botulinum* spores from about 10 percent of store-bought honey samples, and although less than 5 percent of infant botulism patients contract the disease from honey, health officials and pediatricians agree that honey should not be fed to infants under 1 year of age (it is perfectly safe for older children and adults).

The first sign that an infant has botulism is usually constipation, although this isn't always apparent to parents. Often the baby isn't brought to a doctor until parents notice other symptoms, such as lethargy and poor feeding as the paralysis begins to affect the baby's gag reflex and swallowing ability.

Because breathing is affected in the most severe stage of botulism-induced paralysis, researchers suspect a link between infant botulism and sudden infant death syndrome (SIDS), also known as crib death. One study done 15 years ago showed that about 5 percent of children in California whose deaths were attributed to SIDS actually had died from infant botulism. Because of the difficulty of conducting such studies, the link between SIDS and infant botulism remains poorly understood.

The infant botulism fatality rate is less than 2 percent, and recovery is usually complete. Often, however, infants have to spend weeks or months on a ventilator. Horse-derived antitoxin is not given to infants because of the risk of side effects such as anaphylaxis and serum sickness. But in February 1992, the California Department of Health Services began a new clinical trial that may provide a way of lessening the effects of the disease.

With funds from the FDA's Orphan Products Grants Program, the trial is evaluating a human-derived antitoxin obtained from laboratory workers who for occupational safety reasons have been immunized with botulinum toxoid, which is toxin whose poisoning potential has been removed.

The California investigators will assess whether infants given the antitoxin will have shorter hospital stays, fewer complications, and a halt to the progression of disease. Infant botulism represents the only opportunity to evaluate the safety and efficacy of human-derived botulism antitoxin (known formally as Botulism Immune Globulin) because of the sporadic and even less frequent occurrence of food-borne and wound botulism.

Use as Medicine

Meanwhile, purified botulism toxin is the first bacterial toxin to be used as a medicine. FDA licensed botulinum toxin as Oculinum in December 1989 for treating two eye conditions—blepharospasm and strabismus—characterized by excessive muscle contractions. It is now marketed under the trade name Botox.

Small doses of the toxin are injected into the affected muscles. As happens with botulism, the toxin binds to the nerve endings, blocking the release of the chemical acetylcholine, which would otherwise signal the muscle to contract. The toxin thus paralyzes or weakens the injected muscle but leaves the other muscles unaffected. The injections "block extra contraction [of the muscle] but leave enough strength for normal use," says Barbara Karp, M.D., deputy clinical director of the National Institutes of Health's National Institute of Neurological Disorders and Stroke.

Although the two eye conditions are the only indications for which it is licensed, botulinum toxin has been used investigationally for a variety of other conditions. "The main disease [group] the toxin is being used for is dystonias—neurologic diseases involving abnormal muscle posture and tension," Karp says. Examples include spasmodic torticollis (contractions of the neck and shoulder muscles), oral mandibular dystonia (clenching of the jaw muscles), and writers' and musicians' cramps.

Other investigational uses include: spasmodic dysphonia (which results in speech that is difficult to understand), urinary bladder muscle relaxation (such as in cases where muscle contraction is severe enough to require catheterized urination), esophageal sphincter muscle

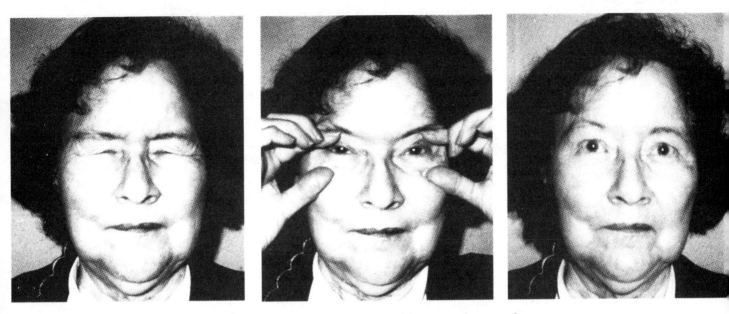

At left, a patient with blepharospasm before injection with Botox is unable to open her eyes due to abnormal muscle contractions. At center, still pre-injection, she uses her fingers to keep her eyes open. At right, after injection, her eyes stay open without difficulty.
(Photos courtesy Joseph Jankovic, M.D., professor of neurology, Baylor College of Medicine, Houston, Texas)

relaxation, and the management of tics.

Experience shows that "it works better for some things than others," NIH's Karp says. For example, "it works better for disorders that involve small muscles than large muscles," she says. But for about 2 to 5 percent of patients, the injections simply don't work at all, she adds.

Injections usually have to be repeated, as the effects usually only last about three to four months, although sometimes they can last over a year. Because of this, up to 10 percent of patients eventually develop antibodies to the toxin; this is more likely in patients who receive higher doses at more frequent intervals. Therefore, the makers of the biologic recommend that its dosage be kept as low as possible.

There are seven different types of

Not for Wrinkles

Botulinum toxin type A has been promoted for use as a wrinkle remedy. Apparently, some practitioners have been injecting the substance to ease wrinkles by weakening face muscles. In a Nov. 18, 1994, *Federal Register* notice, FDA denounced the promotion of such unapproved use as "an egregious example of promoting a potentially toxic biologic for cosmetic purposes."

botulinum toxin, and the currently marketed therapeutic toxin is type A. NIH is studying whether patients who have become immune to injections of type A toxin can successfully be treated by toxins of other types. So far, the research indicates that using type F to treat people with antibodies to type A seems to work, Karp says.

Botulinum toxin has "an amazing safety record," says Bill Habig, Ph.D., the recently retired deputy director of FDA's division of bacterial products in the Center for Biologics Evaluation and Research. "Considering it's one of the most toxic materials known and there was a lot of concern about it, it's turned out to be very safe," he says.

Luba Vangelova is a writer in Takoma Park, Md.

Mad Cow Madness

Julie Corliss

When the British government announced in March that 10 Britons with a rare, incurable brain affliction may have been infected with "mad cow disease," a stampede of mad cow stories hit the news. Countries around the world banned imports of British beef, amid fears that eating steaks and burgers from mad cows might cause Creutzfeldt-Jakob disease, or CJD. Like mad cow disease, CJD is a deadly, degenerative malady that leaves victims' brains riddled with tiny holes, leading to neurological problems such as muscle twitching and dementia.

There is, however, no direct evidence that eating beef from cows with the illness (known as bovine spongiform encephalopathy, or BSE) can cause brain disease in humans. But scientists have been hard pressed to come up with another explanation for the 10 recent cases of CJD, all of which share some unusual features that differ from the textbook description of the disease.

Suspicions of a possible link between the human and cow diseases actually began a decade ago, when BSE was first identified in British cattle herds. The disease is thought to have been transmitted to cows through feed that con-

tained the remains of sheep infected with another related brain disease, called scrapie.

Between 1986, when mad cow disease was first identified, and 1989, when Britain banned the use of sheep and cattle remains in cattle feed and began destroying any cows that showed disease symptoms, some cows with BSE were presumably turned into chops, roasts, and burgers. Control measures to curb the disease apparently worked — cases of BSE dropped to 7,000 in 1995, after peaking at nearly 37,000 in 1992. But because the disease has an average incubation period of five years, meat from diseased cows that weren't yet showing symptoms could have ended up on the dinner table after 1989.

That fact — combined with the handful of odd CJD cases occurring at the same place and time — triggered the recent panic. In the April 6 *Lancet,* members of Britain's National CJD Surveillance Unit describe the new cases, deeming them "cause for great concern."

Part of the concern arises from the many unknowns that still surround these mysterious diseases. *HealthNews* consulted experts around the country to clarify what *is* known and to explain why it's hard to determine how serious a threat BSE

poses to humans. Despite the uncertainty, most agree that any potential danger from eating mad cow meat pales in comparison to known hazards like smoking or driving a car.

How are scrapie, BSE, and CJD similar?

According to Fred Cohen, MD, professor of medicine and pharmacology at the University of California, San Francisco, the three are similar diseases in different animals. All are fatal, neurodegenerative diseases thought to be caused by prions — tiny, infectious particles made entirely of protein that are distinctly different from bacteria or viruses. Prions are remarkably stable and can survive freezing and heating to normal cooking temperatures. The hallmark of prion diseases is sponge-like holes in the brain, which can cause a host of bizarre behaviors. Sheep try to scrape the wool off their bodies (hence the name), cattle acquire a strange, high-stepping gait, while humans exhibit a loss of coordination and dementia.

How do people get CJD or other prion diseases?

CJD is exceedingly rare, striking on average only one in a million people each year world-

wide. About 15 percent of cases are caused by a genetic disorder. The rest are known as sporadic CJD, arising from unknown — possibly environmental — factors. However, a high percentage of people with sporadic CJD also have a genetic variation that makes them more vulnerable to the disease.

Prion diseases have been transmitted experimentally by injecting infectious material (which includes brain, spinal cord, spleen, and possibly other organs) directly into the brains of animals, including mice, hamsters, cows, and monkeys. Eating the infectious material is a much less effective means of getting the disease, but it does happen. In Papua New Guinea, natives who ate the brains of dead relatives as part of funeral rites contracted a CJD-like affliction known as kuru, a disease that largely disappeared when the cannibalism stopped. Monkeys, mink, cats, and other animals have acquired spongiform-type diseases after being fed infectious material. But it's never been proven how cattle get BSE. Six years ago, researchers at the US Department of Agriculture fed tissue from sheep with scrapie to cattle, but none of the cows have come down with BSE so far, says Randall Cutlip, DVM, PhD, research leader of the government's Respiratory and Neurologic Disease Research Unit in Ames, Iowa.

Other than through eating infected animal parts, the disease doesn't appear to be transmitted from animal to animal. Studies to see if the disease is passed from cow to calf are currently under way.

Should anyone who ate British beef in the past decade worry about getting CJD?

Experts agree that the risk of contracting BSE from beef is probably very, very small. Even though less than two percent of Britain's cows were known to be infected with BSE, meat from hundreds of thousands of diseased cows might have ended up in butcher shops. In theory, all British beef-eaters over the age of seven — which includes close to 50 million people — could have eaten mad cow meat. But as Kenneth Tyler, MD, a neurology professor and CJD expert at the University of Colorado Health Sciences Center, points out, only 10 cases of the unusual form of CJD have been reported to date.

As to how the unlucky 10 might have gotten the new CJD variant, scientists can only guess. Eight of the victims had the genetic susceptibility to sporadic CJD, but none had any other known risk factors. They had all eaten beef in the past decade, but the animal products that people typically eat — meat and milk — have never been shown to transmit disease, leading some scientists to speculate that the infection was more likely to have been passed on by accidentally eating some infectious material. "Maybe they encountered a chunk of brain or spleen in their steak and kidney pie," says Richard Marsh, DVM, PhD, a virologist at the University of Wisconsin who has studied prion diseases for over three decades. Others say that a concurrent infection, or taking certain drugs or alcohol, might have made the victims more susceptible to the disease.

What's special about the new CJD cases in Britain?

According to the recent *Lancet* report, the average age of the 10 patients — eight of whom have died — is 27, compared to an average age of about 65 in typical CJD cases. Their symp-

toms started with anxiety, depression, and behavioral problems and progressed more slowly than is typical with CJD. Autopsy reports also showed much larger clumps of prion protein in their brains. Researchers are currently testing to see if the prion is the same type as that seen in cattle — a painstaking process that may take up to two years.

Is there any risk in the US?

The risk of a mad cow disease epidemic similar to the one in Britain is negligible. Although several hundred British cattle were imported to this country in the 1980s before that practice was halted in 1989, it's unlikely those cattle pose any threat. The US Department of Agriculture reports that no cases of BSE have been detected since it began monitoring herds 10 years ago, and officials recently stepped up surveillance efforts. A voluntary ban on the use of cattle and sheep carcasses in animal feed has been in place for 11 years, and a mandatory ban from the US Food and Drug Administration is currently in the works.

According to the US Centers for Disease Control and Preven-

tion, the number of cases of CJD in the US has remained stable since 1979. The age distribution of these cases has not changed significantly, in contrast to those recently described in Britain.

Is there any chance that CJD could become an epidemic?

"We just don't know the dimensions of the problem in Britain yet, but based on our current understanding of pathogenic diseases, I would say it's probably not a massive public health threat," says Dr. Tyler, the Colorado CJD expert.

HealthNews associate editor and infectious disease specialist Abigail Zuger, MD, agrees, noting that diseases like CJD bear little resemblance to AIDS or influenza. "Prion diseases simply do not behave like bacterial and viral infections in human beings. Their patterns of infectivity are quite different, and, most importantly, they are not transmitted from person to person by casual or even sexual contact. Thus, even if the British cases of CJD do prove to be related to BSE, a spiraling epidemic is highly unlikely to occur."HN

How much are pesticides hurting your health?

Pesticides. Just the word conjures up images of ruined cropland and diseased wildlife. For many consumers, even scarier than those images are the things they can't see: potentially cancer-causing chemical residues tainting otherwise healthful-looking fruits and vegetables.

It's a catch-22. At the same time that health experts keep pushing for more consumption of fruits and vegetables to lessen cancer risk, alarming headlines and news stories warning of the risks of dietary pesticide residues constantly leach into the public stream of consciousness.

Are pesticides the cancer threat many are afraid of? Should you spend the extra money on organically grown produce? What about children? Should they be given anything but pesticide-free food? Following is a look at some of the common beliefs about pesticides in the food supply—and the realities behind them.

Myth: Pesticides and other chemicals rank as the most significant diet-related cancer threat.

Reality: In the United States, diets too rich in calories, fat, and alcohol pose a far greater cancer threat than pesticides and other chemical residues, according to a 400-plus page report just released by the National Research Council, which scrutinized the data on more than 200 known carcinogens in food. What's more, a wealth of research indicates that a diet rich in fruits and vegetables protects against cancer. Thus, the risks incurred by avoiding fruits and vegetables for fear of ingesting pesticide residues far outweigh any risks that come from eating a produce-rich diet.

Myth: The only cancer-causing compounds found in produce and grains are synthetic chemicals added during farming and processing.

Reality: The number of naturally occurring chemicals found in the food supply probably exceeds a million, and some of these are known to be potent carcino-gens. For example, a class of substances called myco-toxins, which are produced by fungal growth on food crops either in the field or during harvesting, are highly toxic and play a role in liver cancer. Many countries, including the United States, impose strict limits on the levels of mycotoxins allowed in foods.

Myth: To determine the amount of pesticide residues allowed in foods, the Environmental Protection Agency finds out what dose of the chemical is toxic and then sets the legal limit slightly below that level.

Reality: To come up with limits, the EPA looks at animal studies that help project the maximum amount of a pesticide residue that a person could consume daily during a 70-year life span without suffering any harm. Once they determine this level, they set the legal limit at just a small fraction of that amount—generally 100 times lower—just to be on the safe side.

Myth: Pesticides are more toxic to children than to adults.

Reality: While most people assume that children's small size leaves them much more vulnerable than adults to the effects of pesticides and other chemicals, that's not necessarily the case. The ability of a child's rapidly developing body to metabolize, detoxify, and excrete chemicals is profoundly different from that of adults and plays a major role in their vulnerability to pesticides. Children's metabolic rates are much higher than adults', which may allow youngsters to excrete certain pesticides and other chemicals much more quickly.

That's not to say pesticides do not pose a problem for youngsters. Infants and children eat a far less varied diet than adults and so consume much more of certain foods for their body weight, which could boost their exposure to certain pesticide residues. This difference and others are not considered thoroughly when the government determines what levels of pesticides will be allowed in the food supply, according to a major report from the National Research Council issued in 1993.

Still, the report concluded that when it comes to pesticide exposure and physiologic responses, differences between children and adults are usually less than 10-fold. Given that the EPA typically factors in a 100-fold margin of safety, the problem certainly doesn't warrant keeping fruits and vegetables out of a child's diet.

Myth: All fruits and vegetables should be washed in detergent and peeled carefully to eliminate all traces of pesticide residues.

Reality: All fresh fruits and vegetables should be

To find out everything from how to dispose of an insect repellent used in your garden to whether the chemicals your exterminator is using are safe, call the National Pesticide Telecommunications Network's toll-free hotline at 1-800-858-7378. Operators are available from 9:30 a.m. to 7:30 p.m. Eastern time, Monday through Friday.

rinsed thoroughly with water to remove any dirt, bacteria, and surface chemicals that may have come into contact with the food. Fruits and vegetables with edible peels should also be scrubbed thoroughly with a brush, and the outer leaves of lettuce, cabbage, and other greens should be removed. Most experts advise against cleaning produce with detergents, however, because soapy products may leave behind traces of other chemicals not intended for consumption.

As for peeling, it does help rid produce of pesticides, since some chemicals tend to remain on or just under the skin of fruits and vegetables. That's particularly true of waxed products, like cucumbers; the wax that gives the fruit or vegetable its shiny appearance sometimes contains fungicides. On the other hand, you might not want to make a habit of peeling every vegetable and fruit you eat; much of the fiber and cancer-fighting nutrients in produce concentrate in or just beneath the skin.

Myth: Media reports that caution consumers about pesticide residues in certain foods should be taken as warnings to avoid those foods.

Reality: Headlines and news bites alarming consumers about pesticide residues should be viewed with a skeptic's eye. Scientists have developed sophisticated techniques that enable them to detect residues of pesticides so minute as to be virtually meaningless in many cases. In other words, the mere presence of a pesticide doesn't mean it's concentrated in a large enough dose to do any harm. The real question to ask is whether the pesticide level exceeds federal limits.

Keep in mind that residues are expressed in parts per million (ppm), parts per billion (ppb), and parts per trillion (ppt). Just what does that mean in practical terms?

1 ppm = 1 cent in $10,000, *or*
　　　　1 pancake in a stack four miles high

1 ppb = 1 second in 32 years, *or*
　　　　1 inch in 16,000 miles

1 ppt = 1 second in 32,000 years, *or*
　　　　1 square foot of tile in a floor the size
　　　　of Indiana

Myth: Once the government determines that a pesticide is unsafe for the public in any amount, its production in the United States is prohibited.

Reality: Unfortunately, between 1991 and 1994 alone, U.S. companies exported some 58 million pounds of pesticides banned for use in this country to other nations with more lax pesticide laws. This practice creates what has been dubbed "the circle of poison." Pesticides prohibited in the United States can travel the globe, boomeranging back to us through wind, rain, waterways, even imported food products. The scenario raises numerous ethical questions and highlights the necessity of considering the global, rather than just the national, impact of pesticides and other environmental contaminants.

Myth: Foods labeled organic must meet strict federal standards.

Reality: The federal government has yet to set a legal definition of "organic." Granted, 11 states currently have their own organic certification programs in place, as do 33 private organizations. Nevertheless, these programs vary in their definition of "organic" as well as in the degree to which the standards are enforced. As a result, consumers have no assurance what an organic label means.

The major roadblock to an all-encompassing federal definition has been financial. While the 1990 Farm Bill called for establishment of a national "organic" standard, funding for a staff to work out the details was not allocated until 1994. Officials at the National Organic Standards Board, the group of experts assigned to the issue, are still working away at a set of proposals to present to the governmental powers-that-be. Once a proposal has been made, it will likely be critiqued and revised before finally being set in stone—a process that could easily take another year or two.

Not in my backyard

Most people think farmers are the only people who need to take responsibility for pesticide use, but many suburbanites regularly dabble with lawn and garden chemicals that affect the environment as well. In fact, 64 million pounds of pesticides were spread on lawns and golf courses last year—amounting to 10 percent of all pesticides used in the United States. Keeping lawns green also wreaks havoc with the environment in other ways. Running a power lawn mower for one hour spews as much smog as driving a car 50 miles. And watering lawns regularly can contribute to water shortages.

Homeowners who want to care for their lawns in an eco-friendly manner can apply some of the same integrated pest management techniques currently used by farmers. The Environmental Protection Agency offers an excellent, free 18-page primer on the subject: *Healthy Lawn, Healthy Environment*. Write or call the National Center for Environmental Publications and Information, P.O. Box 42419, Cincinnati, OH 45242-2419; phone: (513) 489-8190.

While you're at it, you also might want to request another free publication, the *Citizen's Guide to Pest Control and Pesticide Safety*. This comprehensive 49-page resource covers everything from steps to control pests in and around your home; alternatives to chemical pesticides available to homeowners; ways to use, store, and dispose of pesticides safely; how to choose a pest control company; and what to do if someone is accidentally poisoned by pesticide exposure. Since pesticides are in everything from kitchen and bath disinfectants to pet collars to swimming pool chemicals, it's a booklet worth having.

New Scientific Review Reaffirms Safety of MSG

An independent review of scientific research has reaffirmed the safety of monosodium glutamate (MSG) for the general population.

The Food and Drug Administration (FDA) commissioned the review as part of its ongoing safety evaluations of Generally Recognized as Safe (GRAS) food ingredients. MSG was also found safe in FDA-sponsored reviews conducted in 1978 and 1980.

The Federation of American Societies for Experimental Biology (FASEB) conducted the latest review, which examined the results of nearly 600 studies on MSG. According to law, GRAS status may be determined only by qualified experts with scientific training and experience to evaluate the safety of substances directly or indirectly added to food. MSG has been on FDA's list of GRAS ingredients since 1958.

"This review clearly emphasizes that MSG is safe for both adults and children," said Daryl Altman, M.D., a food allergist in Hewlett, N.Y. "MSG has been extensively researched over many years, and nothing in this current review led FASEB to believe it was anything but safe."

MSG is the sodium salt of glutamic acid, commonly referred to as glutamate. An amino acid, glutamate is one of the most abundant and important components of proteins. Virtually every protein-containing food contains glutamate, including meat, fish, milk and many vegetables. Glutamate is also produced by the human body and is an essential part of human metabolism.

The flavor enhancer MSG is produced by a natural fermentation of starch, corn sugar or molasses from sugar cane or sugar beets. It only enhances flavors when it appears in its "free" form, not bound together with other amino acids in a protein. Free glutamate levels in foods vary greatly, but are especially high in tomatoes, peas and parmesan cheese.

Sensitivity to MSG

The FASEB panel found no link between the consumption of normal levels of MSG and any adverse reactions. The average person consumes about 10 grams of bound glutamate and 1 gram of free glutamate daily from meals. The added intake of MSG from processed foods is less than one gram per day.

The report also states that some presumably healthy individuals may be sensitive to MSG when more than three grams of MSG are consumed in a single dose or meal on an empty

To Label or Not to Label...

Under current federal regulations, MSG must be identified on the ingredient label of any food to which it has been added. When glutamate is a natural component of foods, such as tomatoes or peas, or part of other ingredients, such as autolyzed yeast or soy sauce, MSG is not required to be listed separately on the food label.

FDA intends to propose changing the regulations to indicate the glutamate content on the ingredient label of foods when their glutamate levels reach a threshold amount. The agency has not yet specified the intended threshold level to trigger labeling.

But some scientists say the anticipated labeling regulations are unjustified. "It doesn't make sense to label a substance that occurs naturally throughout the food supply," said Steve Taylor, Ph.D., the University of Nebraska's top food scientist.

stomach. Such symptoms usually develop within one hour of exposure and are mild and temporary, according to FASEB experts.

"Adverse reactions to MSG are difficult to study given their transient nature," said Steve Taylor, Ph.D., professor of food science and technology at the University of Nebraska. "In more than 500 challenges of individuals who thought that they were sensitive to MSG, none experienced reactions that could be clearly linked to MSG. Some study participants who believed they reacted to MSG developed the same reactions when administered placebos."

Since the body does not distinguish between added glutamate in food and naturally occurring free glutamate, one cannot have a reaction just to added MSG.

"It's important to realize," Taylor added, "that the FASEB reviewers found no evidence to suggest any long-term, serious health consequences from consuming MSG."

Additional Research

The FASEB report calls for continued research on whether high consumption of MSG may affect a small proportion of the general population with medical problems, such as severe asthma.

One study in Australia suggested that MSG exacerbates asthma, though such findings have not been confirmed in clinical studies of asthmatics at the National Institutes of Health, Beth Israel Hospital or the Scripps Clinic.

"For 15 years, we have evaluated asthmatic patients for MSG sensitivity and have not found any reactions to challenges with MSG in double-blind, placebo-controlled tests," said Ronald A. Simon, M.D., head of the Division of Allergy, Asthma and Immunology, Scripps Clinic and Research Foundation.

Additional studies on potential adverse reactions are now being conducted at Harvard University, Northwestern University and the University of California at Los Angeles, among other institutions.

The 1995 FASEB report joins independent reviews by the World Health Organization, the American Medical Association, the Institute of Food Technologists and the Scientific Committee of the European Community, which all concluded that MSG is safe for the general public.

"If you believe you're sensitive to MSG, see an allergist and be tested," said Altman. "It's clear from the research that people who believe they are having a reaction to MSG are really having a problem with some other food or some other medical condition."

From *Food Insight,* September/October 1995, p. 6. © 1995 by the International Food Information Council (IFIC) Foundation. Reprinted by permission.

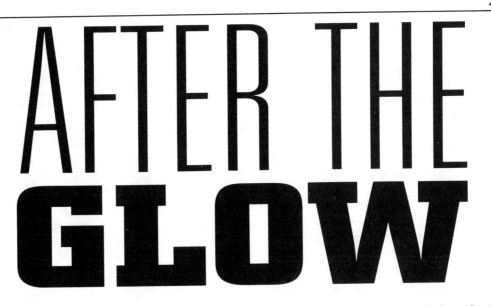

AFTER THE GLOW

Irradiation is gaining new acceptance as a possible defense against foodborne contaminants like E. coli

A L A N   M O R T O N

THIRTY NATIONS HAVE BANNED IT. CHAINS LIKE McDonald's and Boston Chicken won't have anything to do with it. Respected consumer-advocacy groups have blasted it as a serious health hazard and nutritional menace.

Yet concerns about food safety have kindled new interest in irradiation, the little-used process that kills foodborne pathogens with a burst of radiation. Proponents are touting the technology as one more safeguard against food contaminants, particularly the deadly E. coli bacterium. And their argument seems to be winning guarded support from regulators, foodservice suppliers and industry trade groups.

Influential opponents are still convinced the side effects of irradiation may be harmful even if the process itself is not. Still, advocates say the question is no longer whether food should be irradiated, but how it should be done. "It's inevitable," says Roy Martin, vice president of science and technology for the National Fisheries Institute.

That's good news for restaurants, says Robert Harrington, director of technical services for the National Restaurant Association. "We'd like to see irradiation added to the list of things available to be used" against food pathogens, he notes.

Consumers' demand for a more wholesome food supply has been repeatedly chronicled in repeated media flashbacks to the deaths two years ago of four children in the northwest U.S. who are fast-food hamburgers tainted with E. coli. One result: a petition for government approval for the irradiation of ground beef, with an estimated annual consumption of 7 billion pounds.

The public has already reacted favorably to the marketing of some irradiated foods, notably chicken treated to combat salmonella contamination. And some legislators who led efforts to ban the sale of irradiated products in their states are now rethinking their positions, particularly with the advent of new technology that would use electricity—rather than radioactive isotopes—to produce the irradiation.

But, Harrington is quick to point out, "it's definitely not a panacea." Health authorities stress that even irradiated foods can be contaminated through subsequent mishandling. "Food irradiation, like pasteurization of milk, can prevent countless infections," Dr. Phillip R. Lee, director of the U.S. Public Health Service, wrote last summer in the *Journal of the American Medical Association*. Yet "irradiation would neither replace good manufacturing practices nor provide the sole answer to foodborne illnesses."

A new push for safety at the point of production came in October when the U.S. Department of Agriculture reclassified E. coli O157:H7 as an illegal adulterant instead of a natural contaminant. Meat suppliers would be subject to hefty penalties if the bacteria were found in their products, and the USDA said it would conduct 5,000 sampling tests a year to enforce the regulation.

The American Meat Institute and other associations went to court to stop the USDA, claiming that the agency didn't have the authority to promulgate such a rule. But their request for an injunction was denied.

And so, says Dr. Joe Borsa, head of radiation applications for AECL Research in Canada, "The pressure is building" to make irradiation more widespread. "As far as I know there's only one effective technique for cleaning up meat with pathogens and that's irradiation," Borsa says.

The USDA's plan carries heavy economic implications for meat processors because E. coli O157:H7 is hard to detect without a comprehensive and costly effort. But even a few of the bacteria can be deadly if the screening isn't thorough.

"It takes millions of, say, salmonella organisms to cause disease," says Dennis Olson, meat irradiation researcher at Iowa State University, "but it takes just 10 of O157:H7 to cause illness and death."

Cooking to the well-done stage—at least 155°F.—kills E. coli, though some consumers stubbornly insist on having

Regulators are already considering proposals to permit the irradiation of ground beef and seafood

their meat cooked rare. But if other stringent safety measures are in place, the risk of contamination may be insignificant for most beef cuts.

Hamburger is another story. As a recent TV news report noted, a ground-beef patty could contain meat from 100 animals, any one of which may have harbored the deadly bacterium. Because irradiation would be used on whole patties prior to shipping, an E. coli bug would be destroyed regardless of its source.

So even though the American Meat Institute opposes USDA meat-sampling plans, the AMI is throwing its weight behind research to develop irradiation techniques to produce disease-free ground beef with acceptable taste and odor.

OR STARTERS, THE AMI IS SUPPORTING A PETItion that the Food and Drug Administration approve the sale of irradiated ground beef and other meat products. The petition was written by a well-known irradiation consultant, Dr. George Giddings, and presented on July 6 by Isomedix, a New Jersey-based company with a string of irradiation plants dedicated mainly to sterilizing medical supplies.

In November the petition appeared well on the road to approval although the FDA itself, as is its practice, would not predict a date for it. "We're in touch with the FDA every couple of weeks," says Isomedix senior vice president George R. Dietz, who was hoping for clearance early in 1995.

The Isomedix irradiation facilities use gamma rays produced by radioactive cobalt-60 or cesium-137. The radioactive rods are typically kept in 20-ft. pools of water that absorb the rays when out of use; the rods are raised to treat products.

The AMI is also backing research into the irradiation of meat using electron beams, instead of radioactive rods. A French-made machine of this type at Iowa State University in Ames has been irradiating ground beef patties, pork and other meat cuts since March 1993.

Project director Dennis Olson says the emphasis of the experiment is to preserve the quality of the meat patties. He says irradiation initially triggers an unusual odor, but taste is unaffected.

"We came across a similar situation when we first started vacuum-packing 25 years ago," says Olson. "You got an odor that dissipates quickly."

AMI also has been negotiating with Sandia National Laboratories in Albuquerque to adapt the labs' Repetitive High Energy Pulsed Power (RHEPP) electron-beam accelerator—originally created to test the radiation-resistance of components in nuclear missiles—as an irradiation device. Sandia senior researcher Ronald J. Kaye says commercial application "could be two to three years away."

The AMI sees a variety of advantages in electron-beam accelerators, which can be used to produce X-rays by slamming the electrons into plates of metal such as tungsten. Unlike the cobalt-60 devices, the electron beams can be switched on and off, and could be placed right on the meat-processing line.

And perhaps most significantly, an electronic device is much easier to sell to the public than a radioactive one. As AMI spokesperson James Marsden puts it: "It has much less emotional baggage."

The big difference between Iowa State's machine and Sandia's version is that the latter emits powerful pulses—up to 120 a second—instead of a continuous stream of electrons. The RHEPP's high power is useful in the inherently inefficient process of converting the electron beam to X-rays—which are necessary for the effective irradiation of products in boxes or on pallets.

About 40 cobalt-60 irradiation plants already exist in the country and are mostly used for sterilizing medical products. However, Andrew Welt, vice president of a New Jersey accelerator-design company, Alpha Omega Technology Inc., points out that most existing plants are already operating near capacity and could not handle the increase in volume that could come with the sudden mass irradiation of food. Alpha Omega is one of two companies petitioning the FDA for approval to irradiate fish.

Welt also says that the existing plants are not all that adaptable. Many are designed to punch high doses of radiation into things like cotton balls and cosmetics at close range, perhaps a few centimeters. Doses for food would have to be much smaller, with delivery at ranges of up to 15 feet.

The cost of opening an irradiation plant, whether electronic or radioactive, runs about $4 million, says Welt. On top of that, the cobalt-60 has to be replenished: In a typical plant, an initial 2 million curies (a measure of radioactivity) at $1.65 a curie decays at 12.3% a year—more than $400,000 worth—and delivers progressively less irradiation.

On the other hand, electron-beam plants run up some hefty costs in the form of heavy utility bills. These economic factors stand in the way of any rush to irradiate food on a mass scale.

As for existing projects, Mulberry, Fla.'s Food TECHnology Service Inc. irradiated its first product —strawberries, to extend shelf life—three years ago and has since added other produce, seafood and chicken. The company uses a cobalt-60 source but is exploring the use of electron-beam machines, which is one reason the firm changed its name from Vindicator, says safety director Fred Harris.

In operation, the plant's procedures are as varied as the products it contracts to handle. While much of the fruit and vegetables it irradiates are for the U.S. market, Harris says, the seafood—notably shrimp—is for export only, pending government clearance for domestic sales.

HE ADDED COST FOR IRRADIATED FOOD, HE says, is only pennies per pound. "As far as the consumer is concerned, we think the average serving" of irradiated chicken "in a fast-food restaurant is going to cost one-quarter cent more," Harris says. "That cost may be negligible because of the benefit they're going to derive from having a safer product," thus avoiding potential medical bills for consumers and food spoilage for restaurants.

Harris says his company is discussing plans for new plants in the Midwest, "closer to the beef and poultry producers." If they go ahead, he says, "our plant here [in Florida] would be more of a training site."

A number of restaurant chains have promised customers or shareholders that they would not serve irradiated food. McDonald's, for instance, was pressured to take the vow by some institutional investors.

Proponents say the cost of irradiating a fast-food chicken sandwich should be well below a penny

And even if they wanted to do so, irradiated products are not currently available in sufficient quantities. "Our plant is the only USDA-approved facility [for chicken] at this point," Harris says.

But Food TECHnology has found no problem with public acceptance of irradiated products, he says. A frozen chicken irradiated by the concern goes to a variety of outlets, including the Carrot Top produce market in McDonald's hometown of Oak Brook, Ill. Irradiated chicken is the only type that the store currently carries.

"The product is selling very well," says Carrot Top owner James Corrigan. But, he adds, customers clearly prefer fresh chicken to frozen.

Corrigan says he's negotiating with his neighbor for possible expansion of his 5,000-sq.-ft. store. And he's in talks with Isomedix to have locally produced chicken processed at its nearby Martin Grove irradiation facility for sale fresh, not frozen. Although FDA approval would be needed, he says, local chicken producers are solidly behind him.

Meanwhile, irradiation is getting a boost from other quarters. Irradiation of fruits and vegetables, in use since 1986 to control insects and ripening, is in line for expansion. Methyl bromide, used for years to fumigate warehoused produce, has been ordered phased out by the year 2000 because it contributes to ozone depletion. Something is going to have to take its place, and irradiation is a prime prospect.

Meanwhile, the FDA is examining two petitions for irradiation of seafood. Alpha Omega submitted one in late 1990, according to Welt. And United States Harvest Technologies Inc. of Baltimore was cleared to submit its petition in April 1991 and has been working on it since, according to chairman and CEO William L. Robinson Jr.

"We would like to see both petitions adopted by the FDA," says the National Fisheries Institute's Martin. "But we think it will take a while."

The FDA's interest in the proposals is whetted by the current concern over contamination of shellfish from the Gulf of Mexico, especially by an organism called vibrio vunificus. The microbe could be eliminated with irradiation.

But foes of irradiation remain active. Organizations such as the Center for Science in the Public Interest, the International Organization of Consumer Unions and Food and Water Inc. oppose the technology on several grounds—ranging from the possible danger associated with the transportation of radioactive cobalt, to concern that irradiation can reduce the nutritional value of food, to fears that the process will create disease-causing or carcinogenic agents within the treated products.

Even STOP—Safe Tables Our Priority, a food-safety group created in the wake of fast-food hamburger deaths by parents and acquaintances of the school-aged victims—opposes irradiation. It worries that the meat industry will use it as a substitute for safe meat-handling practices.

And the opponents have achieved results: Some 30 countries have laws against selling irradiated food, as do the states of New York and Maine.

Yet irradiation proponents can count some heavyweights within their ranks: Close to 40 countries permit food irradiation with France, the Netherlands and South Africa making extensive use of it. The practice also has the strong support of the World Health Organization, not to mention the American Medical Association.

Other domestic powerhouses are clearly warming to the idea. "The science that we've seen does not support concern about irradiation," says Jerry Redding, national communication coordinator of the USDA.

Even some locales that initially opposed irradiation are now reconsidering its use. New Jersey, for example, allowed its moratorium on the sale of irradiated food to expire a couple of years ago.

And New York's legislature is taking a new look at the law that currently bans sale of all irradiated foods except spices and special sterilized diet items for certain hospital patients.

Yet the bill's author, state Sen. William Sears, also introduced a bill that would consider ramifications of the law's repeal in view of what a spokesman called "a lot of evidence on both sides."

Among those watching the development is the Institute of Food Technologists, whose official stance on irradiation sums up the ongoing battle:

"Extension of the ban of food irradiation in New York State is not justified on any scientific basis nor is it in the public's best interest," the Institute says. "When provided factual information about the process, consumers will choose irradiated foods with confidence."

Not enough processing facilities are open in the U.S. to meet the demand for widespread irradiation of food

Naturally Occurring Toxins: Part of a Balanced Diet?

Tina Prow

Tina Prow, science writer, Agricultural Experiment Station

Nature brings a variety of chemicals to the table—by some estimates, many times more than humans could add to foods. Consider typical morning beverages: Coffee drinkers are exposed to more than 800 chemicals that occur naturally in coffee. At least 16 of the 21 chemicals tested to date are carcinogens. Researchers expect a typical cup of coffee to contain about 10 milligrams of rodent carcinogens.

If comfrey is your cup of tea, you consume pyrrolizidine alkaloids that cause cancer in rats. If you reach for orange juice, count on getting valuable vitamin C, but also D-limonene, a rodent carcinogen. Scientists estimate 125 compounds occur naturally in apple juice; of the five tested, three are carcinogens.

Americans eat about 1.5 grams of natural pesticides per day —10,000 times more than manufactured pesticides, according to Bruce Ames, a professor of biochemistry and molecular biology at the University of California, Berkeley. One of the most outspoken researchers investigating plant toxicants, Ames contends that Americans eat 5,000 to 10,000 different natural pesticides and their breakdown products.

These naturally occurring chemicals are necessary for plant survival. They help plants withstand and fend off fungi, viruses, insects, and animal predators. Although researchers have tested only a few plant toxins for carcinogenicity, the mounting evidence prompted Ames to

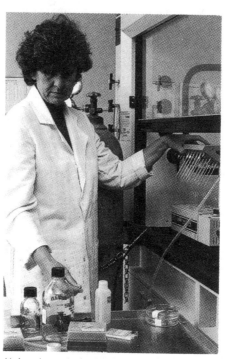

University toxicologist Elizabeth Jeffery prepares samples for analysis in her lab at the UI Institute for Environmental Studies.

write in a 1990 journal article that "it is probable that almost every fruit and vegetable in the supermarket contains natural plant pesticides that are rodent carcinogens."

Dining Dilemmas

Anise, apples, bananas, basil, black pepper, broccoli, brussels sprouts, cabbage, cantaloupe, carrots, cauliflower, celery, cinnamon, cloves, cocoa, coffee, cooked meats, fennel, grapefruit juice, honeydew melon, horseradish, kale, let-tuce, lima beans, mangos, mushrooms, mustard, nutmeg, orange juice, parsley, parsnips, peaches, pineapples, potatoes, radishes, raspberries, strawberries, tarragon, tea, and turnips are just a few of the beverages, spices, and foods known to have naturally occurring carcinogens.

Far from making a meal a dubious dining experience, however, many of these and other foods that likely have toxins are important to a balanced diet, according to Clare M. Hasler, coordinator for the University of Illinois Functional Foods for Health (FFH) program. One component of FFH is focused on how plant chemicals that protect plants from viruses and pests affect human health.

In fact, if health is a motivating factor in food choice, the diet change many people should make is to eat even more fruits and vegetables, she advises. Although these foods have naturally occurring toxins, researchers are finding that they also have disease-preventing and health-promoting benefits. For instance, small doses of certain toxicants also appear to act as antioxidants in the body. Antioxidants have been shown to protect against cancer by preventing cell damage that can lead to cancer.

Also, the human body has mechanisms for "detoxification" of natural or synthetic chemicals, Hasler adds. For instance, cells in the mouth, esophagus, stomach, intestine, colon, skin, lungs, and other areas that are exposed to toxins shed continuously.

From *Illinois Research*, Fall 1993, pp. 8-11. Reprinted by permission of the Illinois Agricultural Experiment Station at the University of Illinois, College of Agriculture.

In addition, the liver and intestinal cells have enzyme systems that become active when exposed to foreign compounds. These enzyme systems metabolize the compounds and then excrete them in a nontoxic form.

DNA in the cell also acts as a defense mechanism when it repairs itself after exposure to certain chemicals, including those chemicals that are naturally present in fruits and vegetables.

Detoxification and antioxidants explain in part how a diet high in fruits and vegetables that contains naturally occurring toxicants can be associated with lower rates of cancer.

"While naturally occurring plant toxicants in fruits and vegetables have destructive properties, there is overwhelmingly strong evidence that [these foods] can be protective against disease, depending on the dose of the compound," Hasler says. "So some of the old nutrition advice is still the best advice: 'eat a variety of foods' and 'everything in moderation.' A wide variety of foods in the diet can aid in favorably altering the balance between naturally occurring toxicants and anti-toxicants."

The Dose Makes the Poison

The adage "the dose makes the poison" can apply to naturally occurring toxins in plants. A number of studies show that while a certain amount of a carcinogenic compound may have a killing effect on human cells, a smaller amount may have no effect or a protective effect.

For example, the naturally high levels of cyanohydroxybutene (CHB) found in such cruciferous vegetables as cabbage and brussels sprouts are toxic to cells in the pancreas and liver. CHB forces cells to go through a programmed cell death similar to normal cell death that occurs as the body revitalizes itself: as functions within the cell shut down, the cell shrinks and eventually is engulfed by other cells.

Intrigued by the way CHB kills cells, a UI team is studying the effect of low doses of the chemical compound on cancer cells. Preliminary laboratory data indicate that these cells are more susceptible to programmed cell death from CHB than are normal cells. If it's proved that CHB provides significant chemoprotection against cancer, a possible future step might be for geneticists to increase CHB in vegetables.

> *It is probable that almost every fruit and vegetable in the supermarket contains natural plant pesticides.*

"What's happening in foods research is very exciting," says team member Elizabeth Jeffery, a toxicologist with joint appointments at the UI Institute for Environmental Studies, Veterinary Biosciences, Nutrition Program, and College of Medicine. "Beyond answering nutritional needs, foods have other nonnutritional components that have effects on the body. In the case of CHB, we started with something that looks toxic, but found something that possibly protects against pancreatic cancer."

Normally, no one would eat the high amount of vegetables necessary to take in toxic amounts of CHB, Jeffery notes. Neither would they eat the amount that would give them the beneficial "low" CHB dose used in UI studies—about one pound of brussels sprouts per day, every day. Furthermore, she suggests, those who dislike brussels sprouts should not force themselves to eat an extraordinary amount of it, or any other food, solely to prevent cancer.

"If you don't like brussels sprouts, don't torture yourself by eating them just for cancer prevention. You can't eat enough for that purpose," she advises. "The key to cancer prevention is unlikely to be in the one single food that makes headlines on one particular day—that's a simplistic approach to a very complex problem. Instead, the best strategy is to have a balanced, sensible, varied diet. That way, the likelihood of reaching toxicity levels from food becomes small."

That diet choices can be important is borne out in a study Jeffery is conducting on the interaction of caffeine and acetaminophen, a pain reliever. Considered a safe product at recommended doses, acetaminophen can have a fatal effect on the liver at about 70 tablets per day. Jeffery's study indicates that caffeine greatly aggravates the toxic effect of acetaminophen so that smaller doses become toxic. The results raise questions about whether there are other nonnutritive food components that have the same effect.

"This study shows that it's important to look at interactions," Jeffery says. Future research in her laboratory may focus on toxicity of acetaminophen in combination with some chemicals found in fruits and vegetables.

Redefining Cancer Risk

Knowing more about foods and the risk they pose is a concern of Robert J. Scheuplein, a toxicologist with the Food and Drug Administration. Although laws passed in 1958 require the FDA to approve food and color additives prior to marketing, the agency has virtually no authority to approve "traditional" foods or to test for naturally occurring toxins, he says.

"Ordinary, wholesome food was always considered perfectly safe. It was those things that were 'bad'—meaning additives, residues, and contaminants—that we had to watch for, and that's what the laws address," he says. "Now we're finding out that there are more natural toxins in food than we might ever think of adding. They've always been there and probably don't constitute a hazard to most people under most circumstances, but we know that diet can be a factor in exacerbating potential for carcinogenicity."

One issue Scheuplein grapples with is risk from synthetic chemical residues and additives compared to risk from naturally occurring toxins. A celery variety developed in the late 1980s focused attention

UI Researchers Target Aflatoxin

University of Illinois scientists Don White and Jack Widholm are using naturally resistant corn hybrids and genetic engineering to prevent aflatoxin from forming on corn. Aflatoxin, one of the most carcinogenic compounds yet discovered, is found on the seeds of crops such as corn or peanuts when the fungus *Aspergillus flavus* is present. When the aflatoxin is ingested by animals or by humans, it can be activated so that it binds to the host DNA to exert its carcinogenic properties. It can also cause liver damage.

Problem levels of aflatoxin do not often occur in Illinois except in years of weather-induced stress such as drought. If conditions are right, the toxin can develop both before harvest and after the grain is in storage. When aflatoxin does affect a crop, it is a dangerous and costly problem. Because it is so dangerous, corn used as food for animals and humans is always monitored closely for its presence. If levels above 20 parts per billion are found, the grain cannot be sold to grain elevators. Corn with somewhat higher levels can be fed to breeding and feeder cattle and swine.

The first approach being used by White to eliminate aflatoxin from corn involves identifying corn lines that are naturally resistant to the *Aspergillus* fungus. Many different corn hybrids are being screened by damaging the kernels with pins and injecting *Aspergillus* under the husk. Hybrids that had very little fungal growth have been identified. None of the naturally resistant lines are commercial hybrids, but the natural resistance can be transferred into commercial inbred lines, which can then be used to make commercial hybrids.

Researchers are also using genetic engineering to prevent *Aspergillus* growth on corn kernels. Genes that code for two different fungus-destroying enzymes have been isolated. The genes are modified so that they will be expressed at high levels in the seed and then placed back into the corn. To do this, a particle bombardment technique is being used. Very small metal particles, coated with DNA carrying the modified genes, are propelled at a high rate of speed by either a gunpowder charge or high-pressure gas acceleration. After the particles have penetrated the corn tissue culture cells, transformed cells can be identified by a marker gene that is also on the DNA. High levels of the enzymes should be toxic to *Aspergillus*, preventing growth and aflatoxin formation. These enzymes may also be effective in eliminating the fungus in stored grain. — *Jack Widholm, plant physiologist, Department of Agronomy*

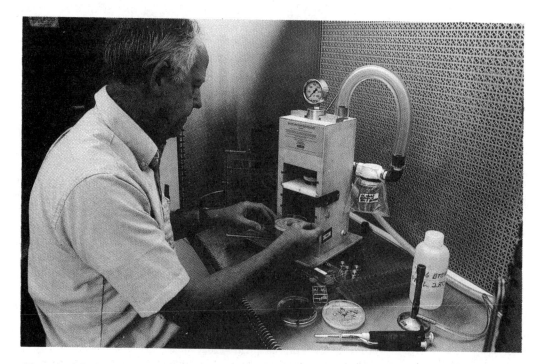

Plant physiologist Jack Widholm uses a "gene gun" to propel modified genetic material into corn tissue culture cells. The genes should help prevent the growth of Aspergillus flavus, *the fungus causing aflatoxin.*

on the question of whether natural pesticides are "safer" than synthetic pesticides. The new, highly insect-resistant celery variety reduced the need for chemical pest control. Considered a plus by those worried about use of synthetic chemicals on foods, the celery raised a red flag among those concerned about naturally occurring toxins in foods. Bruce Ames reported that the new variety had 6,200 parts per billion of carcinogenic psoralens, compared with 800 ppb found in other celery varieties.

The light-sensitive "natural" pesticide caused rashes and burns on celery handlers when they went out into sunlight. Those problems could be solved through handling procedures, but the incident represented a dilemma that remains: Should scientists breed plants with higher natural pesticides to eliminate any need for synthetic chemicals, or should they instead turn their efforts toward reducing naturally occurring toxicants in plants that then would be treated with synthetic chemicals if pest problems developed?

Scheuplein suggests that, although important, the ongoing debate over the merits and dangers from synthetic versus naturally occurring pesticides is secondary to the related problem of opportunity for exposure.

"The sheer volume of toxins in foods is so great that there really is no question that we should be looking at the broad pattern of food intake," he says. "When we consider exposure, synthetic pesticide residues is probably not where the human health risk from toxins is.

"What the risk argument brings into focus is that risk assessment really needs to be improved. It seems evident that we're going to find carcinogens in whatever we check, so finding them is not necessarily a useful process."

In fact, he adds, standard risk assessment yields questionable results when applied to fruits and vegetables. "The amount of one chemical in lettuce presents a one in 1,000 risk for cancer. I do

Scientists Debate Method for Identifying Human Carcinogens

If a substance is found to cause cancer in rodents, can one assume that it will also cause cancer in humans? Not necessarily.

A number of factors affect the reliability of tests to identify carcinogens. In rodents, chemicals are tested at the "maximum-tolerated dose," which gives no information about the effects of these compounds at low-dose exposure, as would typically be the case in humans. In addition, laboratory animals are relatively homogenous and are studied under strictly controlled conditions, whereas humans are quite heterogenous, varying from person to person with respect to genetic constitution, diet, lifestyle, and so on. Furthermore, the rodent assay was developed based on observations made with extremely potent chemicals (for example, aflatoxin and radiation) that damage DNA and therefore do cause cancer at low doses. We know that there are many agents that can cause cancer at high doses but do not damage DNA and therefore probably do not pose a risk at low-dose exposure.

It's a complex issue, particularly given today's technology and our current understanding of mechanisms of carcinogenesis. Unfortunately, though there are a number of problems with the use of the rodent bioassay for predicting human cancer risk, there is as yet no satisfactory substitute for the long-term testing of chemicals. Scientists are currently reevaluating much of the existing rodent carcinogenicity data, taking into consideration low-dose exposure and mechanistic factors in order to more realistically estimate human risk from rodent carcinogens.

—*Clare M. Hasler, visiting assistant professor, Department of Food Science, UIUC, and the departments of Nutrition and Medical Dietetics and Medicinal Chemistry and Pharmacognosy, UIC*

not believe that number," he says. "It hasn't changed my salad-eating habits."

Changing eating habits as more is known about cancer and foods is one way to reduce the cancer deaths attributable to diet. UI researchers Richard Doll and Richard Peto linked diet to approximately 35 percent of cancer deaths in a risk table published in 1981 and considered valid today, according to Scheuplein.

"We don't know how to 'avoid' natu-

rally occurring toxins. Basically, we know that macronutrients, like fat, can modify the expression of cancer, so we need to learn more about how the factors modulate the expression of cancer," Scheuplein says. "The research that would allow us to do that has not been done. But even small increases in knowledge that become behavior changes in the way people eat could have long-term beneficial effects on the quality of life and health."

Health Claims

Quackery has no such friend as credulity.

—C. Simmons

In ancient Rome, Cato the elder prescribed cabbages to cure "everything that ails you" and continued to do so even though his wife died from the "fevers." London pharmacists, in 1632, believed that bananas were so important to health that only trained druggists should administer them. Early in the history of this country, Elisha Perkins promoted vinegar as the cure for yellow fever, yet he died of this disease. All were sincere but wrong. Yet, almost any product, device, or regimen that promises the moon and five miles more will develop a following of users and believers.

Quackery is misinformation about health, according to the Food and Drug Administration (FDA). Certain fallacious statements have been made repeatedly by promoters for years, among them: "The American food supply is worthless because it is grown on depleted soil," "Everybody needs vitamin supplements for insurance," "Sugar from honey is healthier than table sugar," and "Natural is better." Such misinformation may be easier to find than facts. For example, popular talk show hosts provide a good promotional forum for misinformation, since their need to capture a large audience employs sensationalism. Nutritionists have often despaired of counteracting the exaggeration and blatantly false information frequently distributed through the popular information media.

But we can assume that anyone interested enough to read *this* book, much less take a nutrition course, also is able to avoid being taken in by misinformation and quackery. Right? Probably not! Will Rogers said, "Everybody is ignorant, only on different subjects," and it takes a great deal of knowledge and consciousness to effectively counteract promoters. Perpetrators of quackery have changed with the times, but their characteristics and goals are the same. At one time or another, most of us—perhaps all of us—have been victims. For this reason, it is critical to understand how manipulators adroitly influence the buying of both ideas and products. Only then will consumers be armed to defend themselves. Toward that end the articles in this unit were chosen.

The first article, "How Quackery Sells," will help you understand the strategies of promoters who have fine-tuned the art of selling to an exquisitely high level. They know how to influence the emotions of the vulnerable, easily convinced customer so that he or she will buy even though some small inner voice advises against it.

The next three articles are concerned with accurate reporting in the media, an important issue since surveys have shown the media to be the primary source of nutrition and food-safety information. "Confessions of a Former Women's Magazine Writer" describes how a long-time writer of nutrition articles wrote mainly to make advertisers happy, conscientiously avoiding the use of any information unflattering to the advertisers. By the time she had also manipulated content to conform to the art director's specifications and had ensured (following the publisher's directives) that the reader would not be intellectually challenged, little of substance was left. It is good news, then, that "Changing Channels" gives reason to be more encouraged by the quality of news reporting, although an inappropriate fixation on individual foods and reducing dietary fat, rather than on a healthful diet, continues. Even more heartening is the article describing the most recent review of popular magazines by the American Council on Science and Health. Twenty popular magazines were rated by nutrition experts for accuracy, presentation style, and recommendations. Only minor errors were found in *Better Homes and Gardens, Consumer Reports*, and *Parents,* resulting in very high scores. Twelve others were rated as "good," and *Cosmopolitan* alone was found to be "very poor."

It is sad that a question that must be raised about accurate reporting concerns the questionable behavior and ethics of nutrition professionals, the sources of journalists' information. When the Food and Nutrition Science Alliance (FNSA) released a list of ten red flags to help consumers recognize junk science, reporters refused to accept all of the blame. In counterpoint they provided evidence that, at the very least, overstatements and exaggerations are made by professionals and researchers to gain prestige, increase chances for scarce research funds, increase visibility, and bolster organizational membership roles. Pogo said, "We have met the enemy, and he is us!"

When nutrition advice seems to be constantly changing and contradictory, it may also confuse and discourage the consumer. The article "Why Do Those #&*?@! 'Experts' Keep Changing Their Minds?" deals with this issue, explaining that finding the truth is a process, not an event. Thus, recommendations will forever be altered as science becomes more sophisticated and increasingly able to build on prior knowledge. It pays to remain somewhat skeptical, and it certainly pays to wait for general acceptance of theories and information by the experts before jumping on a bandwagon.

Several articles on supplements of various kinds are included in this edition. Victor Herbert's article "Vitamin Pushers and Food Quacks" turns to the large cadre of dedicated vitamin pushers and supplement promoters found in health food stores and health spas, as well as home salesmen and others, even some who are considered health professionals. That a 1993 article remains appropriate is testimony to the continued overpromotion of the concept that supplements are desirable, even necessary. It also did not help that the Dietary Supplement Health and Education Act (DSHEA) was passed. Well orchestrated by the supplement industry, passage of this bill clearly permits the sale of questionable products, as the manufacturer is not required to prove effectiveness. Furthermore, the FDA must now prove that a product is unsafe before it can be removed from the market. By contrast, drugs require the manufacturer's proof of safety and efficacy before they can be sold.

A discussion of athletes and supplements is included in this unit because, in their search for the competitive edge, athletes are extremely vulnerable to supplement promotionals. However, the place to look is within themselves, not in a bottle or box.

In a similar vein, advertising now tries to convince lots of us that we need the same specialty products originally developed for use by the weak and the ill in nursing homes and hospitals. It can be argued that, appropriately used, they are a good addition to the choices available. However, as insurance against deficiencies, they make little sense for most of us and may promote the notion that a complete and healthful diet is unlikely or impossible. This is simply untrue.

The final topic selected for this unit is herbals, which are increasingly popular and currently account for about $1 billion in annual sales. Classified as food supplements by the FDA, they fall under the DSHEA discussed above. Given that herbals have medicinal qualities, questions of safety and efficacy must be raised. Some argue that this is a nonissue because herbs are natural. That can be refuted easily by pointing out that the amanita mushroom, fer-de-lance (a large pit viper) venom, and hurricanes are also quite natural. It is true, however, that about one-third of modern drugs are derived from herbs and other plants. Examples include digitalis (for heart conditions) from foxglove, and salicin (aspirin) from the bark of the white willow tree. Many rain forest plants and herbs used in traditional medicine are currently under investigation, some of which undoubtedly will be used to advance the modern medical arsenal against disease. But there is a clear distinction between pharmaceuticals and herbals, even when the active ingredients are the same. With pharmaceuticals, the active ingredients are purified and the doses carefully controlled. The amounts of active ingredients in herbals vary widely, depending on many conditions such as how they are grown, harvested, and stored. Some herbals are known to be safe and useful for treating minor ailments. The available literature on most herbals, however, is still grounded in folklore and tradition, not in scientific research. There are no guarantees of safety, and the consumer must decide if the risk is appropriate. Caveat emptor.

From time to time it becomes clear that a specific herbal is problematic, and the one most recently in the news is ephedra (ma huang), sold under such names as Cloud 9, Herbal Ecstacy, and Ultimate Xphoria. Watch for an FDA crackdown, as ephedra has been documented to cause heart attacks, strokes, psychiatric disorders, and at least 17 deaths. It is a stimulant and claims to improve strength and health, produce weight loss, and provide a herbal high similar to that of cocaine.

Victor Herbert has said that consumers with misinformation about nutrition typically fall into two categories: the deceived and the deluded. The deceived, he says, will respond to education, while the deluded are adamant—even fanatical—about their beliefs and will refuse to consider good scientific data or a logical presentation. This unit is offered to readers who are either already informed or are among the deceived searching for answers.

Looking Ahead: Challenge Questions

Why do you think people are so vulnerable to quackery? When have you been a victim?

Identify three current fallacies that you believe are the most dangerous to nutritional health. Why are they fallacies?

Make a list of characteristics you would look for in a *reliable* information source. Use them to evaluate nutrition articles in your local newspaper or a nutrition-oriented talk show.

What provisions would you change or add to the Dietary Supplement Health and Education Act of 1994 to increase its effectiveness?

Decide if there are any herbals you could safely use right now and which ones should wait for scientific testing and judgment. What criteria did you use?

HOW QUACKERY SELLS

William T. Jarvis, Ph.D.
Stephen Barrett, M.D.

Dr. Jarvis is a professor in the Department of Preventive Medicine at Loma Linda University and president of the National Council Against Health Fraud.

Dr. Barrett, who practices psychiatry in Allentown, Pennsylvania, is a board member of the National Council Against Health Fraud. In 1984 he received the FDA Commissioner's Special Citation Award for Public Service in fighting nutrition quackery.

Modern health quacks are supersalesmen. They play on fear. They cater to hope. And once they have you, they'll keep you coming back for more . . . and more . . . and more. Seldom do their victims realize how often or how skillfully they are cheated. Does the mother who feels good as she hands her child a vitamin think to ask herself whether he really needs it? Do subscribers to "health food" publications realize that articles are slanted to stimulate business for their advertisers? Not usually.

Most people think that quackery is easy to spot, but it is not. Its promoters wear the cloak of science. They use scientific terms and quote (or misquote) scientific references. On talk shows, they may be introduced as "scientists ahead of their time." The very word "quack" helps their camouflage by making us think of an outlandish character selling snake oil from the back of a covered wagon—and, of course, no intelligent people would buy snake oil nowadays, would they?

Well, maybe snake oil isn't selling so well, lately. But acupuncture? "Organic" foods? Mouthwash? Hair analysis? The latest diet book? Megavitamins? "Stress" formulas? Cholesterol-lowering teas? Homeopathic remedies? Nutritional "cures" for AIDS? Or shots to pep you up? Business is booming for health quacks. Their annual take is in the *billions!* Spot reducers, "immune boosters," water purifiers, "ergogenic aids," systems to "balance body chemistry," special diets for arthritis. Their product list is endless.

What sells is not the quality of their products but their ability to influence their audience. To those in pain, they promise relief. To the incurable, they offer hope. To the nutrition-conscious, they say, "Make sure you have enough." To a public worried about pollution, they say, "Buy natural." To one and all, they promise better health and a longer life. Modern quacks can reach people emotionally, on the level that counts the most. This article shows how they do it.

Appeals to Vanity

An attractive young airline stewardess once told a physician that she was taking more than 20 vitamin pills a day. "I used to feel run-down all the time," she said, "but now I feel really great!"

"Yes," the doctor replied, "but there is no scientific evidence that extra vitamins can do that. Why not take the pills one month on, one month off, to see whether they really help you or whether it's just a coincidence. After all, $300 a year is a lot of money to be wasting."

"Look, doctor," she said. "I don't care what you say. I KNOW the pills are helping me."

How was this bright young woman converted into a true believer? First, an appeal to her curiosity persuaded her to try and see. Then an appeal to her vanity convinced her to disregard scientific evidence in favor of personal experience—to *think for herself.* Supplementation is encouraged by a distorted concept of *biochemical individuality*—that everyone is unique enough to disregard the Recommended Dietary Allowances (RDAs). Quacks will not tell you that scientists deliberately set the RDAs high enough to allow for individual differences. A more dangerous appeal of this type is the suggestion that although a remedy for a serious disease has not been shown to work for other people, *it still might work for you. (You are extraordinary!)*

A more subtle appeal to your vanity underlies the message of the TV ad quack: *Do it yourself—be your own doctor.* "Anyone out there have 'tired blood'?" he used to wonder. (Don't bother to find out what's wrong with you, however. Just try my tonic.) "Troubled with irregularity?" he asks. (Pay no attention to the doctors who say you don't need a daily movement. Just use my laxative.) "Want to kill germs on contact?" (Never mind that mouthwash doesn't prevent colds.) "Trouble sleeping?" (Don't bother to solve the underlying problem. Just try my sedative.)

Turning Customers Into Salespeople

Most people who think they have been helped by an unorthodox method enjoy sharing their success stories with their

From *Nutrition Forum* newsletter, March/April 1991, pp. 9-13. Reprinted by permission of *Nutrition Forum* newsletter, now published by Prometheus Books, 59 John Glenn Drive, Amherst, NY 14228.

friends. People who give such *testimonials* are usually motivated by a sincere wish to *help their fellow humans*. Rarely do they realize how difficult it is to evaluate a "health" product on the basis of personal experience. Like the airline stewardess, the average person who feels better after taking a product will not be able to rule out coincidence— or the placebo effect (feeling better because he thinks he has taken a positive step). Since we tend to believe what others tell us of personal experiences, testimonials can be powerful persuaders. Despite their unreliability, they are the cornerstone of the quack's success.

Multilevel companies that sell nutritional products systematically turn their customers into salespeople. "When you share our products," says the sales manual of one such company, "you're not just selling. You're passing on news about products you believe in to people you care about. Make a list of people you know; you'll be surprised how long it will be. This list is your first source of potential customers." A sales leader from another company suggests, "Answer all objections with *testimonials*. That's the secret to *motivating* people!"

Don't be surprised if one of your friends or neighbors tries to sell you vitamins. More than a million Americans have signed up as multilevel distributors. Like many drug addicts, they become suppliers to support their habit. A typical sales pitch goes like this: "How would you like to look better, feel better and have more energy? Try my vitamins for a few weeks." People normally have ups and downs, and a friend's interest or suggestion, or the thought of taking a positive step, may actually make a person feel better. Many who try the vitamins will mistakenly think they have been helped—and continue to buy them, usually at inflated prices.

Faked endorsements are being used to promote anti-aging products and other nostrums sold by mail. The literature, which resembles a newspaper page with an ad on one side and news on the other, contains what appears to be a handwritten note from a friend (identified by first initial). "Dear Anne," it might say, "This really works. Try it! B." Although both the product and the "newspaper page" are fakes, many recipients wonder who among their acquaintances might have signed the note.

The Use of Fear

The sale of vitamins has become so profitable that some otherwise reputable manufacturers are promoting them with misleading claims. For example, for many years, Lederle Laboratories (makers of *Stresstabs*) and Hoffmann-La Roche advertised in major magazines that stress "robs" the body of vitamins and creates significant danger of vitamin deficiencies. Another slick way for quackery to attract customers is the *invented disease*. Virtually everyone has symptoms of one sort or another—minor aches or pains, reactions to stress or hormone variations, effects of aging, etc. Labeling these ups and downs of life as symptoms of disease enables the quack to provide "treatment."

Reactive hypoglycemia" is one such diagnosis. For decades, talk show "experts" and misguided physicians have preached that anxiety, headaches, weakness, dizziness, stomach upset, and other common reactions are often caused by "low blood sugar." But the facts are otherwise. Hypoglycemia is rare. Proper administration of blood sugar tests is required to make the diagnosis. A study of people who thought they had hypoglycemia showed that half of them had symptoms during a glucose tolerance test even though their blood sugar levels remained normal.

"Yeast allergy" is another favorite quack diagnosis. Here the symptoms are blamed on a "hidden" infection that is treated with antifungal drugs, special diets, and vitamin concoctions.

Food safety and environmental protection are important issues in our society. But rather than approach them logically, the food quacks exaggerate and oversimplify. To promote "organic" foods, they lump all additives into one class and attack them as "poisonous." They never mention that natural toxicants are prevented or destroyed by modern food technology. Nor do they let on that many additives are naturally occurring substances.

Sugar has been subject to particularly vicious attacks, being (falsely) blamed for most of the world's ailments. But quacks do more than warn about imaginary ailments. They sell "antidotes" for real ones. Care for some vitamin C to reduce the danger of smoking? Or some vitamin E to combat air pollutants? See your local supersalesman.

Quackery's most serious form of fear-mongering has been its attack on water fluoridation. Although fluoridation's safety is established beyond scientific doubt, well-planned scare campaigns have persuaded thousands of communities not to adjust the fluoride content of their water to prevent cavities. Millions of innocent children have suffered as a result.

Hope for Sale

Since ancient times, people have sought at least four different magic potions: the love potion, the fountain of youth, the cure-all, and the athletic superpill. Quackery always has been willing to cater to these desires. It used to offer unicorn horn, special elixirs, amulets, and magical brews. Today's products are vitamins, bee pollen, ginseng, *Gerovital*, "glandular extracts," and many more. Even reputable products are promoted as though they are potions. Toothpastes and colognes will improve our love life. Hair preparations and skin products will make us look "younger than our years." And Olympic athletes tell us that breakfast cereals will make us champions.

False hope for the seriously ill is the cruelest form of quackery because it can lure victims away from effective treatment. Even when death is inevitable, however, false hope can do great damage. Experts who study the dying process tell us that while the initial reaction is shock and disbelief, most terminally ill patients will adjust very well as long as they do not feel abandoned. People who accept the reality of their fate not only die psychologically prepared, but also can put their affairs in order. On the other hand, those who buy false hope can get stuck in an attitude of denial. They waste financial resources and, worse yet, their remaining time.

The choice offered by the quack is not between hope and despair but between false hope and a chance to adjust to reality. Yet hope springs eternal. The late Jerry Walsh was a severe arthritic who crusaded coast-to-coast debunking arthritis quackery on behalf of the Arthritis Foundation. After a television appearance early in his career, he received 5,700 letters. One hundred congratulated him for blasting the quacks, but 4,500 were from arthritis victims who asked where they could obtain the very fakes he was exposing!

Clinical Tricks

The most important characteristic to which the success of quacks can be attributed is probably their ability to exude confidence. Even when they admit that a method is unproven, they can attempt to minimize this by mentioning how difficult and expensive it is to get something proven to the satisfaction of the FDA these days. If they exude *self-confidence* and enthusiasm, it is likely to be contagious and spread to patients and their loved ones.

Because people like the idea of making choices, quacks often refer to their methods as *"alternatives."* Correctly used, it can refer to aspirin and Tylenol as alternatives for the treatment of minor aches and pains. Both are proven safe and effective for the same purpose. Lumpectomy can be an alternative to radical mastectomy for breast cancer. Both have verifiable records of safety and effectiveness from which judgments can be drawn. Can a method that is unsafe, ineffective or unproven be a genuine alternative to one that is proven? Obviously not.

Quacks don't always limit themselves to phony treatment. Sometimes they offer legitimate treatment as well—the quackery is promoted as *something extra*. One example is the "ortho-molecular" treatment of mental disorders with high dosages of vitamins in addition to orthodox forms of treatment. Patients who receive the "extra" treatment often become convinced that they need to take vitamins for the rest of their life. Such an outcome is inconsistent with the goal of good medical care, which should be to discourage unnecessary treatment.

The *one-sided coin* is a related ploy. When patients on combined (orthodox and quack) treatment improve, the quack remedy (e.g., laetrile) gets the credit. If things go badly, the patient is told that he arrived too late, and conventional treatment gets the blame. Some quacks who mix proven and unproven treatment call their approach *complementary therapy*.

Quacks also capitalize on the natural healing powers of the body by *taking credit* whenever possible for improvement in a patient's condition. One multilevel company—anxious to avoid legal difficulty in marketing its herbal concoction—makes no health claims whatsoever. "You take the product," a spokesperson suggests on the company's introductory videotape, "and tell me what it does for you." An opposite tack—*shifting blame*—is used by many cancer quacks. If their treatment doesn't work, it's because radiation and/or chemotherapy have "knocked out the immune system."

To promote their ideas, quacks often use a trick where they bypass an all-important basic question and *ask a second question* which, by itself, is not valid. An example of a "second question" is "Why don't the people of Hunza get cancer?" The quack's answer is "because they eat apricot pits" (or some other claim). The first question should have been "Do the people of Hunza get cancer?" The answer is "Yes!" Every group of people on earth gets cancer. So do all animals (vegetarians and meat-eaters alike) and plants. Another common gambit is the question, "Do you believe in vitamins?" The real question should be, "Does the average person eating a well balanced diet need to take supplements?" The answer is no.

Another selling trick is the use of *weasel words*. Quacks often use this technique in suggesting that one or more items on a list is reason to suspect that you *may* have a vitamin deficiency, a yeast infection, or whatever else they are offering to fix.

The *money-back guarantee* is a favorite trick of mail-order quacks. Most have no intention of returning any money—but even those who are willing know that few people will bother to return the product.

Another powerful persuader—*something for nothing*—is standard in advertisements promising effortless weight loss. It is also the hook of the telemarketer who promises a "valuable free prize" as a bonus for buying a water purifier, a 6-month supply of vitamins, or some other health or nutrition product. Those who bite receive either nothing or items worth far less than their cost. Credit card customers may also find unauthorized charges to their account.

The willingness to believe that a stranger can supply unique and valuable "inside" information—such as a tip on a horse race or the stock market—seems to be a universal human quirk. Quacks take full advantage of this trait in their promotion of *secret cures*. True scientists don't keep their breakthroughs secret. They share them with all mankind. If this were not so, we would still be going to private clinics for the vaccines and other medications used to conquer smallpox, polio, tuberculosis, and many other serious diseases.

Seductive Tactics

The practice of healing involves both art and science. The art includes all that is done for the patient psychologically. The science involves what is done about the disease itself. If a disease is psychosomatic, art may be all that is needed. The old-time doctor did not have much science in his little black bag, so he relied more upon the art (called his "bedside manner") and everyone loved him. Today, there is a great deal of science in the bag, but the art has been relatively neglected.

In a contest for patient satisfaction, art will beat science nearly every time. Quacks are masters at the art of delivering health care. The secret to this art is to make the patient believe that he is cared about as a person. To do this, quacks *lather love lavishly*. One way this is done is by having receptionists make notes on the patients' interests and concerns in order to recall them during future visits. This makes each patient feel special in a very personal sort of way. Some quacks even send birthday cards to every patient. Although seductive tactics may give patients a powerful psychological lift, they may also encourage over-reliance on an inappropriate therapy.

Handling the Opposition

Quacks are involved in a constant struggle with legitimate health care providers, mainstream scientists, government regulatory agencies, and consumer protection groups. Despite the strength of this orthodox opposition, quackery manages to flourish. To maintain their credibility, quacks use a variety of clever propaganda ploys. Here are some favorites:

"They persecuted Galileo!" The history of science is laced with instances where great pioneers and their discoveries were met with resistance. Harvey (nature of blood circulation), Lister (antiseptic technique), and Pasteur (germ theory) are notable examples. Today's quack boldly asserts that he is another

example of someone ahead of his time. Close examination, however, will show how unlikely this is. First of all, the early pioneers who were persecuted lived during times that were much less scientific. In some cases, opposition to their ideas stemmed from religious forces. Second, it is a basic principle of the scientific method that the burden of proof belongs to the proponent of a claim. The ideas of Galileo, Harvey, Lister, and Pasteur overcame their opposition because their soundness could be demonstrated.

A related ploy, which is a favorite with cancer quacks, is the charge of *"conspiracy."* How can we be sure that the AMA, the FDA, the American Cancer Society, and others are not involved in some monstrous plot to withhold a cancer cure from the public? To begin with, history reveals no such practice in the past. The elimination of serious diseases is not a threat to the medical profession—doctors prosper by curing diseases, not by keeping people sick. It should also be apparent that modern medical technology has not altered the zeal of scientists to eliminate disease. When polio was conquered, iron lungs became virtually obsolete, but nobody resisted this advancement because it would force hospitals to change. Neither will medical scientists mourn the eventual defeat of cancer.

Moreover, how could a conspiracy to withhold a cancer cure hope to be successful? Many physicians die of cancer each year. Do you believe that the vast majority of doctors would conspire to withhold a cure for a disease that affects them, their colleagues, and their loved ones? To be effective, a conspiracy would have to be worldwide. If laetrile, for example, really worked, many other nations' scientists would soon realize it.

Organized quackery poses its opposition to medical science as a philosophical conflict rather than a conflict about proven versus unproven or fraudulent methods. This creates the illusion of a "holy war" rather than a conflict that could be resolved by examining the facts.

Quacks like to charge that *"Science doesn't have all the answers."* That's true, but it doesn't claim to have them. Rather, it is a rational and responsible process that can answer many questions—including whether procedures are safe and effective for their intended purpose. It is quackery that constantly claims to have answers for incurable diseases. The idea that people should turn to quack remedies when frustrated by science's inability to control a disease is irrational. Science may not have all the answers, but quackery has no answers at all! It will take your money and break your heart.

Many treatments advanced by the scientific community are later shown to be unsafe or worthless. Such failures become grist for organized quackery's public relations mill in its ongoing attack on science. Actually, "failures" reflect a key element of science: its willingness to test its methods and beliefs and abandon those shown to be invalid. True medical scientists have no philosophical commitment to particular treatment approaches, only a commitment to develop and use methods that are safe and effective for an intended purpose.

When a quack remedy flunks a scientific test, its proponents merely reject the test. Science writer John J. Fried provides a classic description of this in his book, *Vitamin Politics:*

Because vitamin enthusiasts believe in publicity more than they believe in accurate scientific investigation, they use the media to perpetuate their faulty ideas without ever having to face up to the fallacies of their nonsensical theories. They announce to the world that horse manure, liberally rubbed into the scalp, will

cure, oh, brain tumors. Researchers from the establishment side, under pressure to verify the claims, will run experiments and find that the claim is wrong. The enthusiasts will not retire to their laboratories to rethink their position. Not at all. They will announce to the world that the establishment wasn't using enough horse manure, or that it didn't use the horse manure long enough, or that it used horse manure from the wrong kind of horses. The process is never-ending. . . . The public is the ultimate loser in this charade.

Promoters of laetrile were notorious for shifting their claims. First they claimed that laetrile could cure cancer. Then they said it could not cure but could prevent or control cancer. Then they claimed laetrile was a vitamin and that cancer was a disease caused by a vitamin deficiency. Today they say that laetrile alone is not enough—it is part of "metabolic therapy," which includes special diet, supplement concoctions, and other modalities that vary from practitioner to practitioner.

The *disclaimer* is a related tactic. Instead of promising to cure your specific disease, some quacks will offer to "cleanse" or "detoxify" your body, balance its chemistry, release its "nerve energy," bring it in harmony with nature, or do other things to "help the body to heal itself." This type of disclaimer serves two purposes. Since it is impossible to measure the processes the quack describes, it is difficult to prove him wrong. In addition, if the quack is not a physician, the use of nonmedical terminology may help to avoid prosecution for practicing medicine without a license.

Books espousing unscientific practices typically suggest that the reader consult a doctor before following their advice. This disclaimer is intended to protect the author and publisher from legal responsibility for any dangerous ideas contained in the book. Both author and publisher know full well, however, that most people will not ask their doctor. If they wanted their doctor's advice, they probably would not be reading the book in the first place. Sometimes the quack will say, "You may have come to me too late, but I will try my best to help you." That way, if the treatment fails, you have only yourself to blame. Patients who see the light and abandon quack treatment may also be blamed for stopping too soon.

"Health Freedom"

If quacks cannot win by playing according to the rules, they try to change the rules by switching from the scientific to the political arena. In science, a medical claim is treated as false until proven beyond a reasonable doubt. But in politics, a medical claim may be accepted until proven false or harmful beyond a reasonable doubt. This is why proponents of laetrile, chiropractic, orthomolecular psychiatry, chelation therapy, and the like, take their case to legislators rather than to scientific groups.

Quacks use the concept of *"health freedom"* to divert attention away from themselves and toward victims of disease with whom we are naturally sympathetic. "These poor folks should have the freedom to choose whatever treatments they want," cry the quacks—with crocodile tears. They want us to overlook two things. First, no one wants to be cheated, especially in matters of life and health. Victims of disease do not demand quack treatments because they want to exercise their "rights," but because they have been deceived into thinking that they offer hope. Second, the laws against worthless nostrums are not directed against the victims of disease but at the promoters who attempt to exploit them.

Any threat to freedom strikes deeply into American cultural values. But we must also realize that complete freedom is appropriate only in a society in which everyone is perfectly trustworthy—and no such society exists. Experience has taught us that quackery can even lead people to poison themselves, their children, and their friends.

It is because of the vulnerability of the desperately ill that consumer protection laws have been passed. These laws simply require that products offered in the health marketplace be both safe and effective. If only safety were required, any substance that would not kill you on the spot could be hawked to the gullible.

Some people claim we have too much government regulation. But the issue should be one of quality, not quantity. We can always use good regulatory laws. Our opposition should be toward bad regulations that stifle our economy or cramp our lifestyles unnecessarily. Consumer protection laws need to be preserved.

Unfortunately, some politicians seem oblivious to these basic principles and expound the "health freedom" concept as though they are doing their constituents a favor. In reality, "health freedom" constitutes a hunting license for quackery, with open season declared on the sick, the frightened, the alienated, and the desperate. It represents a return to the law of the jungle in which the strong feed upon the weak.

How to Avoid Being Tricked

The best way to avoid being tricked is to stay away from tricksters. Unfortunately, in health matters, this is no simple task. Quackery is not sold with a warning label. Moreover, the dividing line between what is quackery and what is not is by no means sharp. A product that is effective in one situation may be part of a quack scheme in another. (Quackery lies in the promise, not the product). Practitioners who use effective methods may also use ineffective ones. For example, they may mix valuable advice to stop smoking with unsound advice to take vitamins. Even outright quacks may relieve some psycho-somatic ailments with their reassuring manner.

This article illustrates how adept quacks are at selling themselves. Sad to say, in most contests between quacks and ordinary people, the quacks still are likely to win.

Changing Channels

*How the media report on
food safety and nutrition*

American consumers rely on the news media for most of their information about nutrition and food safety, surveys show. Given the central role media play in shaping the public's dietary outlook, what sort of job are the media doing? In the first study of its kind, the International Food Information Council (IFIC) Foundation commissioned a content analysis of food and nutrition reporting in the media nationally over a three-month period in 1995.

"As part of an ongoing dialogue among media who report on nutrition and food safety, and opinion leaders who are sources of information—including health professionals, research institutes, consumer advocates, the food industry and government—it's important to consider carefully what the consumer is hearing," said IFIC Foundation President Sylvia Rowe. "This study provides us a snapshot."

"The media research shows many positive developments in food and nutrition reporting," Rowe said. "It also shows there are many ways that journalists and all involved in the communication process can work together to better meet the challenge of keeping consumers informed." The study's major findings show:

■ Media seldom provide the context needed to understand overall nutrition recommendations in news reports about individual foods.

■ Media reports on scientific research often lack details that would allow consumers to judge a study's relevance to their own diets.

■ The need to reduce dietary fat is the top story in food news, getting twice the coverage of any other nutrition topic and relegating other dietary recommendations to virtual obscurity.

■ Local newspapers and news broadcasts deliver substantially more food safety and nutrition reports than national news outlets, but are less likely to accent positive messages.

"More and more journalists are getting better at reporting on these issues. That's the good news," said Jeanne Goldberg, Ph.D., R.D., associate professor, School of Nutrition Science and Policy at Tufts University. "But this research shows us the media still tend to focus too much on the benefits and harms of individual foods. In reality, consumers need to know how to put together a variety of foods to build a healthful diet."

"The good news on nutrition and food safety is that the media are covering it and bringing that information to the public," said Sharon M. Friedman, Iacocca professor and director, Science and Environmental Writing Program, Lehigh University. "There are many issues related to public health in other areas that are never discussed because the media pay no attention."

> ## "More and more reporters are getting better at reporting on these issues."
>
> **JEANNE GOLDBERG, PH.D., R.D.**
> **TUFTS UNIVERSITY**

"Traditionally if you look at news coverage of risk issues, the negatives are the things that the media will go for." Friedman said. "It's useful that media are covering good and bad aspects of food in fairly equal proportions. It's a good sign also that a variety of sources, including industry, are getting quoted in these stories."

Sheer Volume of Food News. There can be no doubt that food safety and nutrition make big news. The research sample is characterized by sheer volume. During three months, almost 1,000 food and nutrition reports filling over 10,000 column inches and 11 hours of broadcast airtime were collected and analyzed from 53 separate news outlets, including national and local newspapers and TV news programs, two wire services, syndicated TV talk shows and national magazines.

Local newspapers and evening news broadcasts devoted twice the attention to food safety and nutri-

From *Food Insight*, Spring 1996, pp. 1, 4-5. © 1996 by the International Food Information Council (IFIC) Foundation. Reprinted by permission.

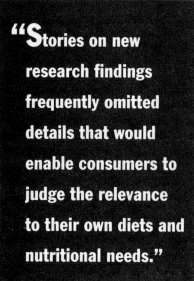

"**S**tories on new research findings frequently omitted details that would enable consumers to judge the relevance to their own diets and nutritional needs."

tion as their national counterparts. At the networks, food news appeared on morning news programs more often than evening broadcasts. Among national magazines, the women's publications dominated coverage over general news magazines and even *American Health*. Overall, newspapers carried a majority or 60 percent of the food news reports in the total study sample.

Reporters drew upon diverse sources of information, citing with greatest frequency the federal government and the food industry as represented by small food producers, chefs and restaurateurs, rather than trade associations. When stories focused on food additives and contaminants, environmental and health activists were cited five times as often as industry, showing their strong influence in driving food safety reports.

Dietary Fat Is Top Story. The study found the media lavishing attention on dietary fat. Nearly half of all the news reports mentioned the need to reduce fat consumption, giving fat twice the coverage of any other nutritional topic. Reporters also covered dietary fat in greater depth, with more than half of fat-related stories providing "extensive discussions" defined as more than 20 seconds on air or two paragraphs in print.

The media may accurately reflect scientific consensus that lowering fat intake is a leading priority in reducing

the risk of many chronic diseases. Yet the overriding focus on fat obscures other important dietary recommendations such as increasing fiber intake and eating more grains, fruits and vegetables. When discussing any food, fat content was the attribute most often mentioned followed by overall vitamin and mineral content, and flavor.

In fact, media are reporting an "inverted pyramid" but not the one they teach in journalism school. The research found media mentions of various foods flipped the Food Guide Pyramid on end, with the least attention to grains, breads and cereals, which normally form the pyramid's base and the largest recommended part of a balanced diet.

Magic Bullets Shoot Context. Second only to fat were reports on the diet's role in disease prevention. Some packaged overall nutrition advice in terms of disease prevention, but many of these stories focused on individual foods as "magic bullets." Most of these stories overlooked the benefits of a balanced and varied diet in favor of discussion of a single food.

The media analysis found a tendency of food news reporting to move from one research finding or press release to another, without presenting a broader look at diet and health. Context was the missing ingredient of many food news reports and that was the greatest overall failing by media, the study found.

While media reports were full of advice on what to eat or what to avoid, the research revealed that readers and viewers would have a difficult time finding out how, or even if, that advice applied to them.

For example, fewer than one of three statements about the risks and benefits of dietary choices mentioned how much one needed to eat, and only one in 14 discussed how often. Only one in six statements identified to whom the advice might be particularly important, such as athletes, the elderly, children or pregnant women.

"The media can get caught up in the story of the day, reporting on what's 'hot' even if that story

doesn't change the nutrition advice we give people about what constitutes a healthful diet," observed Nancy Wellman, Ph.D., R.D., professor, dietetics and nutrition, Florida International University in Miami and past president of The American Dietetic Association. Although Wellman believes reporters are increasingly putting food stories into context, that information often ends up too late in the story to be read or absorbed.

Getting context into a story not only helps consumers make better food choices but can motivate them to stay with the changes they've already made. "People can get information fatigue," observed Goldberg of Tufts University. "There's a limit on how much new 'news' any of us can absorb."

"Putting the latest advice into context and making a story more personally relevant reassures people that it's been worth the effort to change their behavior and that they'll continue to reap the rewards of dietary change," Goldberg said.

News Omits Key Details. Just as discussions of food choices often lacked context, stories on new research findings frequently omitted details that would enable consumers to judge the relevance of the results to their own diets and nutritional needs.

Only a minority of the reports on new studies described the samples on which research conclusions were based. Questions of statistical significance and causal inference were almost never addressed. One out of four news reports failed to mention such basic details of the study as its research design.

Because many dietary recommendations appearing in media are associated with new research findings, consumers need information to size up the studies behind any such advice. Part of the challenge may be that not every new scientific study lends itself easily to news coverage for non-technical audiences.

"Many scientific studies are simply not for public consumption. They repre-

Notable Quotables (Sources of Information)

Food Industry & Trade Associations	**346**
Food producers	134
Chefs/Restaurateurs	101
Trade associations	63
Federal Government	**341**
Department of Agriculture	69
Centers for Disease Control	61
U.S. Congress	61
Food and Drug Administration	47
National Institutes of Health	36
Environmental Protection Agency	25
National Academy of Sciences	6
Independent Experts/Researchers	**288**
Environmental /Consumer Groups	**150**
Center for Science in the Public Interest	44
Natural Resources Defense Council	21
Environmental Working Group	19
Medical Sources	**131**
State Government	**42**
Voluntary Health Groups	**30**
Local Government	**27**

sent scientists talking to scientists," said Delia Hammock, R.D., director and editor of nutrition at *Good Housekeeping*.

Sources Provide Context. "Providing context is the job of the nutrition educator," said Wellman. "For every 'new and improved' piece of nutrition advice that appears on TV or in the newspaper, we need to talk about how much more or less, and how often to eat or not eat a food. If a finding looks negative for a particular food category, explain to the reporter what moderation means to you. Talk about how much of a food could be too much and for whom."

"Use a reporter's inquiry as an opportunity for an impromptu backgrounding session," said Lehigh University's Sharon Friedman. "When there is no story and no deadline, reporters are far less likely to take the time for a briefing."

Ask first about the reporter's background and make judgments about how much background information would be useful to provide. A general assignment reporter may have very little experience with the subject, unlike regular science, health or food reporters. "It's important for information sources to orient the reporter to the larger perspective. Even if all the information doesn't get into the story, help the reporter understand the issues," Friedman said.

"As a rule, information from sources should be unbiased and provide all sides to the story," Friedman observed. "I give that advice to anyone speaking to reporters, whether from industry, academia or consumer organizations."

"The only way to have any credibility as an information resource is to serve as an educator to the reporter and provide full perspective on the issues," Friedman said.

The media research commissioned by the IFIC Foundation was conducted by the Center for Media and Public Affairs, a non-profit media research organization based in Washington, D.C. and appears in a report entitled, "Food for Thought." You may request a free copy of the executive summary from the IFIC Foundation or purchase a copy of the full report using the order form on page 7. The executive summary is also available from IFIC Foundation On-line.

CONFESSIONS OF A FORMER WOMEN'S MAGAZINE WRITER

Marilynn Larkin

Ms. Larkin is a freelance writer in New York City. In 1985, she received a first-place award for consumer journalism from the National Press Club. Her most recent work is *What You Can Do About Anemia* [Dell Publishing, 1993].

Writing about "hot" nutrition topics still has impact. During the decade or so that I wrote for women's magazines, I received much positive feedback from readers.

In 1989, at the height of oat bran's popularity as a panacea to lower cholesterol, the president and chief operating officer of a leading cereal manufacturer estimated that sales of oat-bran cereals would grow to nearly $600 million annually. I wrote five oat-bran stories that year for various women's magazines. A year later, when a study called oat bran's health-promoting properties into question, sales plummeted 50 percent within a week; at that point, I couldn't give away an article on oat bran.

I also covered other "hot" nutrition topics. But although they appeared on the nutrition page, these articles tended to be either "food-of-the-month" stories (the grapefruit diet, carrot power) or quasi-entertainment pieces that positioned foods as medicine: to fight cancer, strengthen the immune system, lower blood pressure, cut cholesterol, stave off heart attacks, prevent osteoporosis, reduce stress, or improve your sex life.

Earning a living this way was quick, easy, and—for a while at least—fun. I readily recycled material from publication to publication, since all were prone to hopping on the same bandwagons. And editors who saw my work in one magazine often asked me to "do a story like this for *our* audience." It never dawned on me that I might be misleading the public by promoting "food-as-magic-bullet" mythology. I labored under the illusion that by carefully executing assignments according to the editors' parameters, I was informing the public and being a good writer.

What I was really doing was helping to sell magazines by presenting a lopsided point of view: the world according to women's magazine editors. Their world (and my assignments) was shaped primarily by two considerations: providing a "nice environment" for advertisers and making sure readers were not challenged by anything more than simple tips for healthy living.

(The word *healthful* does not exist in women's magazine stylesheets.)

Elizabeth Whelan, Sc.D., M.P.H., president of the American Council on Science and Health, thinks women's magazines are shirking responsibility by focusing on trivia and ignoring the devastating effects of cigarette smoking. In a recent op-ed piece in *The New York Times,* she said, "What advice do the magazines offer on how to stay healthy? Here is a sampling: Eat lots of broccoli to ward off cancer . . . take vitamins E and C and beta-carotene; eat garlic to fight colds and flu . . . and eat active-culture yogurt to live longer."

Conflicting views are seldom presented in women's magazines. After all, the "logic" goes, readers might become confused if they actually have to weigh more than one side of a story. Instead, editors usually decide in advance what readers should think, infantilizing readers in the process. This condescending philosophy was a major reason why I decided to get out of the whole business and into writing for physicians. Today, more than two years after making the transition, I savor the fact that I am writing for grown-ups.

How Articles Evolve

One reason why trivial and/or incorrect nutrition advice appear so often is the desire to please the magazines' lifeline: advertisers. Most marketing executives view women's magazines as "products" or "vehicles" that are part of a "marketing package" for their wares. That's where the "nice environment" comes in. Before agreeing to buy space, advertisers want to know what kinds of articles will appear in the magazine—and, particularly, what copy will appear near the ad. "Negative" stories—topics that may upset readers or otherwise interfere with a "feel-good" atmosphere—are routinely rejected. Unfortunately, this means that manuscripts that tell the truth (for example, that the link between specific foods and specific health effects is largely hype) seldom get published.

"Women's magazines are controlled by advertisers in ways that other magazines aren't," *Ms.* co-founder Gloria Steinem told a gathering of writers from the American Society of Journal-

From *Nutrition Forum* newsletter, May/June 1993, pp. 17-20. Reprinted by permission of *Nutrition Forum* newsletter, now published by Prometheus Books, 59 John Glenn Drive, Amherst, NY 14228.

ists and Authors in 1991. She described how women's magazines began as catalogs, with short stories woven in between the ads. The link between advertising and editorial has remained, she said, creating a situation wherein "85 percent of women's magazine copy is really 'unmarked advertorial.'" A few months later, co-founder Patricia Carbine talked about "Advertising and Editorial—The Uneasy Coexistence" to a group of advertising, marketing, and public relations professionals attending a forum on business ethics. "Advertisers are insisting on concessions from women's service magazines that they wouldn't insist on from *Time* or *Newsweek*," she said. According to Ms. Carbine, declining circulation has put even greater pressure on women's publications to continually cross the line between advertising and editorial. Examples include presenting a certain number of recipes that use soup as an ingredient to satisfy a soup advertiser, or refusing to run results of "taste tests" that could offend an advertiser whose product appears at the bottom of the heap.

When I wrote regular nutrition columns for women's magazines, my topics were determined in most cases by advertisements already commissioned or those the publication hoped to bring in. "[A major cereal manufacturer] is advertising in September. Why don't you do a fiber story for that issue?" one editor suggested. "We'd love to get an ad from [a leading manufacturer of lowfat dairy products]. We want you to do a story on foods that are low in fat and high in calcium," said another.

Michael Hoyt, associate editor of *Columbia Journalism Review*, has expressed concern about the blurred boundaries between advertising and editorial content. In the March/April 1990 issue, in an article called "When The Walls Come Tumbling Down," he stated:

> From a reader's perspective this confluence of advertising and editorial is confusing: Where does the sales pitch end? Where does the editor take over? ... Magazines of all stripes are suddenly competing to give advertisers something extra—"value added" in ad-world lingo—in return for their business. Many of these extras are perfectly legitimate and have little or nothing to do with editorial content; others fall into a gray and foggy area; still others involve the selling of pieces of editorial integrity, from slivers to chunks to truckloads.

When it comes to nutrition information, the "confusion" Hoyt alludes to is rampant. In a recent interview (*not* for a women's magazine), Richard Rivlin, M.D., of New York Hospital told me: "The public is enormously confused. They need a better understanding of the role nutrition plays with respect to disease. We haven't been doing a very good job of putting things in perspective." Writing in the *Journal of the American Medical Association*, Dr. Rivlin stressed that it is more realistic to think that good nutrition can help delay the onset or reduce the effects of such illnesses as heart disease, stroke, cancer, and diabetes—not that nutrition can prevent or eliminate these disorders entirely. He added that proper nutrition won't do much to protect an individual who continues to smoke cigarettes, drinks excessively, or leads a sedentary lifestyle.

But that type of moderate message seldom makes its way into magazines where "food as medicine" themes are regarded as an essential editorial ingredient. During my tenure as a health and nutrition writer, I wrote everything from the "diet that can save your life" to the "fertility diet" and the "brain power diet." I also wrote about diets to calm your kids, boost their I.Q., and keep them from becoming overweight adults.

The Ingredients of a "Good" Nutrition Article

The other force that drives the editorial content of women's magazines is the desire to grab attention to boost sales. The quickest, surest way to sell article ideas to a women's magazine is to come up with a great cover line. Once I learned this secret, getting assignments was a snap. Whereas some writers labored long and hard over query letters, I would think up titles and bullet them on a page, fleshing out the "story" with one or two sentences. Examples include: "16 Great Food Finds," "20 Hunger-Fighting Foods," "6 Myths That Keep You Fat," and "What Your Snacks Say About You." At least 75% of the topics I proposed in this way ended up as assignments.

Of course, the process also worked in reverse. Editors would call me and say, "We want such-and-such story (naming a provocative headline). You figure out what to put in the article." Although all this smacks of deception, I did have scruples. Despite the jazzy-sounding titles, in most instances I merely repackaged basic nutrition advice into my articles, slipping in qualifiers ("there's no proof as yet") for spurious speculations and liberally peppering my articles with "may" and "they speculate." Does this excuse me? Not really. What astounds me in retrospect is how many "experts" were willing to go along with this charade.

Another essential ingredient in good articles is the voice of authority. As a women's magazine writer, I needed "experts" to validate my editor's point of view. Many "experts" who regularly appear in women's magazines are willing to trade scientific credibility for the opportunity to have their name in print. Some would give me quotes even when the premise of a story made little sense. For example, one women's magazine editor asked me to do a feature article called "Ten Foods to Make You Prettier." I balked, saying that unless an "expert" would corroborate that such a story could include some substance, I wouldn't do it. I was given the name of an "authority" at the school of public health of a major university. *She* convinced *me* it could be done and provided me with additional sources. I not only wrote the article but recycled it to other women's publications under such titles as "Eat Your Way to Perfect Skin" and "Beauty Is More Than Skin Deep."

Some "experts" I had quoted once were only too pleased to appear in subsequent articles—but not just the spin-offs. In some cases, they "trusted me" to put quotes in their mouths without even doing another interview or clearing the information with them. At one point, I had a psychiatrist, a psychologist, several nutritionists, an eating disorder specialist, and a dietitian that I could pull out of my hat (by making up quotes based on past interviews) whenever an editor wanted a particular viewpoint point substantiated. In other words, I had "instant sources."

I won't speculate on the reasons why people with M.D.s and Ph.D.s (the ones most coveted as sources by women's magazines), who presumably know better, permit themselves to be used in that way. The fact is, many do. Of course, not all have been manipulated. But I'll bet that most are not challenged, either by the writer who interviews them or by others who are quoted.

"Hiring" of Writers

A little-publicized, unethical practice that is more common than writers would like to admit can directly affect what "expert" information gets into a women's magazine and what doesn't. On several occasions, people from public relations agencies representing weight-loss centers and other clients have called me with a proposition. They would "hire" me to write a nutrition story that quoted their client if I would "place" it in a women's magazine. (I was never asked to place a piece in a more "reputable" type of magazine. I guess it was assumed that only women's magazines, and their writers, could be bought.) For an unscrupulous writer, this is an opportunity to be paid twice for the same article. I have consistently refused such work, telling callers that if their client's views were appropriate for something I am writing, they would be used without charge.

In another typical women's magazine scenario, the writer is required to skip attribution altogether—the rationale being that "we want the magazine to be the authority." The result of this abuse of power is that the magazine gives itself a free hand to say whatever it wants, merely by having the writer pepper the article with convenient phrases such as "experts agree," "scientists have found," and "experts say." What experts? The writer and editor, of course.

Style over Substance

Another practice that makes it easier for writers to write for women's magazines than for many other publications—and that has the potential of leaving readers seriously misinformed—is lack of fact-checking. Although some women's magazines call sources to check quotes for accuracy and require writers to provide backup material for statistics, many (I would venture to guess most) don't. I wrote weekly nutrition columns for one women's magazine that preferred to be the authority (in other words, no experts were to be quoted). In more than a year and a half, no one on the magazine's staff ever asked where I got my information. Each column was composed of an article that provided a good headline, a Q&A that I had made up (including a name and city for the supposed writer), and a "fast fact" pertaining to nutrition (for example, that 40% of consumers eat vanilla ice cream). No one ever asked where my "fast facts" came from. [*Editor's note:* Fact-checking can improve accuracy, but does not guarantee it. When checkers limit their contact to people mentioned in the article, errors originating from inaccurate or misleading sources may go undetected. The only way to ensure accuracy is expert prepublication review—a process few media outlets utilize.]

In addition to a catchy headline and good sources, the article must "lay out well" on the page. Typically this means using sidebars and boxes, with cute little quizzes ("What's Your Nutrition IQ?"; "Are You An Emotional Eater?"), fascinating

facts ("Did You Know..."), or 2-day "starter menus" for special diet stories. It's a plus if the article itself can be done up in an easy-to-swallow format, such as "Your A-Z Guide To Fighting Fat," "Seven Secrets Every Thin Person Knows," or "Nutrition Myths That Keep You Fat." Editors seem to assume that straightforward stories won't be read, that readers must be entertained, and that "text-heavy" pages will intimidate them.

The women's magazine writer must also understand an editor's mandate to "work with the art director." In many cases, this means the writer must include points in the text to validate the accompanying photos. For example, if the art director thinks a story on summer fruit would "look great" accompanied by a photo of bananas, grapefruit, and kiwi fruit, then the writer must make sure these fruits are mentioned in the article. Sometimes the photography is planned or even executed before the article is written.

The power of the art director was carried *ad absurdum* in one article I wrote on eating "mini-meals." I had paid a registered dietitian to plan meals that would meet all the Recommended Dietary Allowances for adult women. Imagine my shock when my editor called to demand that a meal be changed to include the foods that the art director thought would "look good on the page." "Luscious strawberries" and "juicy orange slices" would have to replace raisins and bananas!

The final ingredient in a "good" nutrition story is the writing style. Three tones are permitted:

1. Bouncy two-year-old: "Don't wait! Start now on our power-packed, energy-boosting diet."

2. Concerned parent: "Eclairs are tempting, so have one—very occasionally . . . If you do have one, make it your only indulgence that day"; "If you must use white sauce, remember: the thinner the sauce, the thinner *you'll* stay."

3. Pseudosophisticated "friend": "Of course you can diet and lose weight. You've done it before . . . and before that . . . but each time the pounds you shed creep back, causing you to groan with disappointment when you step on the scale. Yet we all know women whose weight rarely fluctuates more than a pound or two and former fatties who managed to lose weight and *keep it off* for good . . . Now, we bring you the *real* secrets behind their success."

Once a writer has these chatty tones down pat, she simply asks which style the editor wants, and bingo! Another successful assignment!

No Journalistic Skills Required

What probably helped me most in becoming a successful women's magazine writer was the fact that I had no journalism training whatsoever. I have never taken a writing course in my life.

In 1980, I went into business for myself as a freelance public relations person for various agencies in New York City. The skills I acquired made it easy to shift from press kits into women's magazine writing. These included: (1) the ability to write headlines and opening paragraphs that were punchy and attention-grabbing; (2) an unquestioning attitude towards "experts"; and (3) the ability to produce unfailingly upbeat, inoffensive copy.

Writing press kits for new diet pills, migraine medicines, and blood pressure drugs, for example, required me to digest complex information and spew it back in easy-to-swallow, bite-size pieces, rarely using words of more than one syllable and remaining as one-dimensional as possible (sound familiar?). Snappy headlines and subheads were more important than hard information—after all, my primary responsibility was to help ensure that our material wasn't hurled immediately into the "circular file."

I made my first women's magazine contacts when pitching editors with story ideas that would include whatever clients I happened to be handling at the time. If the editors wanted more, I would send a press kit or bulleted list of article ideas that could be built around the client. Some of the "low-end" women's magazines willingly take articles provided by public relations firms, which I promptly produced for them. Several even gave me bylines—a joy to someone starting out in the field.

These assignments, paid for by the public relations agencies I worked for, provided me with "clips" which I then used to approach larger publications. Soon editors of women's magazines were asking me to write for them on assignment. Within a year, I had so much magazine work that I stopped doing public relations work altogether.

After a number of years playing at this kind of writing, I grew incredibly bored. Women's magazines like to pigeonhole writers (e.g., "health writer," "travel writer," "money writer"). Even though I managed somewhat to defy definition by writing in all three of these categories, editors who gave me "regular work" really wanted me to write the same stories issue after issue, year after year: How to shed five pounds in five days; Think yourself thin; De-stress yourself; Eat right over the holidays; Get in shape for summer; How to stick to your diet while eating out; Why your food diary is your best friend, etc, etc. These are women's magazine "staples"—the stories readers presumably want to read over and over.

Perhaps it's true. Maybe all those women out there really do want to read that stuff. But if that's the case, at least I have the satisfaction of knowing I no longer contribute to the propaganda that feeds such a mindset. And I can't help but believe that women's magazine readers are capable of taking in a healthy dose of hard information, meaningful speculation, and controversy—about food, nutrition, health, life—if their favorite magazines would only make the effort, and take the risk, of presenting them.

This article is based on my experiences in writing for more than a dozen women's magazines and talking with fellow journalists. There is no question that some women's magazines have more editorial "depth" than others. Those that cater to "educated" women generally offer less simplistic-sounding articles than those catering to "the secretary in Middle America." And magazines with bigger editorial budgets are apt to subject articles to more scrutiny than those with small budgets and little money for editorial content. Nevertheless, all operate under pressure from the market forces I have described.

FOOD FOR THOUGHT: CAN YOU TRUST YOUR FAVORITE MAGAZINE TO TELL YOU WHAT TO EAT?

DIANE WOZNICKI AND DR. RUTH KAVA

Popular magazines—*Reader's Digest, Good Housekeeping, McCall's* and the like—used to be America's number-one source of nutrition information. Today, magazines take a back seat to TV; but according to the American Dietetics Association, a solid 39 percent of the American public still gets most of its nutrition news from magazines. Those readers need to know that the information they get from their favorite magazines is both accurate and reliable.

Since 1982 the American Council on Science and Health has been conducting a biennial survey of the nutrition coverage in popular magazines. ACSH recently wrapped up its sixth such survey, and there's good news: Fifteen of the 20 magazines studied were found to be "excellent" or "good" sources of nutrition information. Furthermore, for the first time in the 14-

> **For the first time in the 14-year history of the survey, a strong majority . . . of the magazines reviewed earned ratings in the top two categories.**

year history of the survey, a strong majority—75 percent—of the magazines reviewed earned ratings in the top two categories. This reflects a heartening new trend—a trend toward real quality—in magazine nutrition reporting.

Three magazines—*Consumer Reports, Better Homes and Gardens* and *Parents*—were rated as "excellent" sources of nutrition information. Twelve magazines—*Cooking Light, Glamour, Reader's Digest, Mademoiselle, American Health, Prevention, Self, Woman's Day, Good Housekeeping, McCall's, Redbook* and *Health*—were rated as "good." Four magazines—*Men's Health, New Woman, Vogue* and *Runner's World*—were rated as "fair." Only one magazine—*Cosmopolitan*—was rated as a "poor" source of nutrition information.

How the Survey Was Conducted

Using *Advertising Age* circulation figures, ACSH identified 20 best-selling American magazines that regularly feature nutrition articles. We chose magazines whose target audiences differed in order to sample articles aimed at a variety of consumers. Eight articles per magazine were randomly selected for evaluation; to prevent judging bias, the selected articles were scanned and reset in a uniform format with magazine and author names deleted.

Four experts in nutrition and food science judged each article's accuracy in three areas: providing factual information, presenting information objectively and making sound recommendations. For each article, the judges were presented with comments such as, "The article documented the source of the information," "The headline was an accurate reflection of the article's content" and, "The recommendations were supported by information from the article."

The judges were instructed to say whether they "strongly agreed," "somewhat agreed," "were neutral," "somewhat disagreed" or "strongly disagreed" with the sample comments. These response categories corresponded to numerical scores ranging from a high of five ("strongly agreed") to a low of one ("strongly disagreed"). A composite score for each article was determined by averaging the judges' scores; the overall score for each magazine was derived by averaging the composite scores of each magazine's articles.

An independent statistician tabulated the results and ranked the magazines. The highest rating was set at 100 percent, and categories were assigned as follows: "excellent," 90% to 100%; "good," 80% to 89%; "fair," 70% to 79%; and "poor," below 70%.

Using the composite score for each article, the statistician evaluated individual article performance with respect to factual accuracy, presentation style and recommendations. Generally, articles with high composite scores were found to reflect consistently good scores in all three categories; similarly, articles with poor composites were found deficient in all three categories. The "excellent" and "good" magazines had many articles earning high composite scores, but no single magazine lacked articles whose composite scores were either mediocre or low. Thus, even in the best ranked magazines room was found for improvement.

Reprinted with permission from *Priorities,* Vol. 8, No. 2, 1996, pp. 42-46. © 1996 by the American Council on Science and Health, Inc., 1995 Broadway, 2nd Floor, New York, NY 10023-5860.

The 'Excellent' Three

Articles in *Consumer Reports*, *Better Homes and Gardens* and *Parents* were consistently reliable (some minor errors resulted in small point losses).

Consumer Reports' high-scoring, hallmark product-analysis articles provided readers with factual overviews of their subject matter. Data were translated into easy-to-grasp concepts, and specific foods were not labeled "bad" or "good." Instead, *CR*'s authors recommended reasonable alternatives.

Better Homes and Gardens articles promoted lifestyle change rather than food restriction and suggested novel substitutions—such as halving the number of walnuts in a Waldorf salad but toasting them first to enhance their flavor—to lower a meal's fat content. *Better Homes and Gardens* lost a few points for articles such as "Our Food Police," which overstated the role of advocacy groups in monitoring the nation's food supply.

Parents magazine handled new research smoothly. The magazine used well-documented sources, and its recommendations echoed expert scientific opinion. According to one judge, a *Parents* article on milk did a good job of explaining why people are hearing so much controversy over milk, but the judge also noted that the article's implication that consumers are being served antibiotic-tainted milk from treated cows was an overstatement.

There's a Good Deal of 'Good' Out There

Cooking Light led the "good" category. One article cautioned against restricting calories in the high-growth adolescent years. But another piece recommended eating 100 grams of carbohydrate after heavy exercise and following that up with an additional 100 grams every two to four hours. A judge who is also a sports nutritionist noted that that quantity is appropriate for a 200-pound person—and is about double what the average female would need.

Glamour also received a rating. One judge commented that a *Glamour* piece on caffeine presented "the latest on a complex issue" and "did an excellent job of documenting the source and identifying researchers doing the work on caffeine." Overall, *Glamour*'s discussions were balanced, its sources were recognizably expert and the magazine was not afraid to tackle new research; it didn't just stay on safe ground rehashing the same old stuff.

In an article on food poisoning, "good" *Reader's Digest* advised its readers to make sure their meat is cooked beyond the pink stage. It also told restaurant patrons to request a new plate when returning undercooked meat, since raw meat juices contaminate. A piece called "Attacked by a Killer Egg Roll" satirized low-fat mania, but that article lost points for labeling eggs, mayonnaise and other foods "bad."

Mademoiselle's "Before You Go on Another Diet, Read This" sensibly quoted a variety of experts to point out mainstream thinking on weight issues. An article on herbal products (called "Natural Wonders?") was basically sound, but while it started with an overview of the dangers of herbal products marketed as diet aids, it ended by saying, "It's

> **One . . . article, "Fantastic Folic Acid," received a nearly perfect score from the judges. The article served to educate a vulnerable segment of the population and exemplified nutrition reporting at its finest.**

up to you to decide if the risk is really worth the weight loss," thus implying that herbal aids are effective. The judges would have preferred a strong condemnation of these unproved products.

American Health is a magazine known for addressing new research. One *American Health* article, "Fantastic Folic Acid," received a nearly perfect score from the judges. The article served to educate a vulnerable segment of the population and exemplified nutrition reporting at its finest. But a piece on antioxidants relied on the unconventional views of a medical researcher who offered unreasonable criticism of both the Recommended Dietary Allowances (RDA) and the Food and Drug Administration (FDA)'s ruling prohibiting antioxidant health claims on product labels. And an article on "Safer Supplements" cited a supplement trade association, whose representatives downplayed the risk of hepatitis from the use of chaparral as a sleep aid and said that the FDA is biased against supplements. The judges noted that quoting a critic of "establishment" nutrition is certainly acceptable, but not providing a counter quote from the FDA presents an unbalanced picture.

On the whole, *Prevention*'s efforts to maintain objectivity were commendable; they earned it its "good." But *Prevention* ran an article on beta-carotene whose title suggested that science already knows this nutrient will provide protection against skin cancer, while the article itself presented the research as preliminary, not proved. An article on "40-Plus Eating" stated that fats should not exceed 25 percent of calorie intake, but the statement wasn't illustrated in a way that would allow the reader to follow through. The article also stated that "Fat calories are the primary source of calories in most people's diets"; according to the United States Department of Agriculture, however, carbohydrates currently contribute the majority of the calories in the average diet.

Self earned its "good" rating with high-scoring articles like "From Twinkies to Tofu," a piece about eating trends. But major point loss occurred with an article that falsely attributed long-known behavior modification techniques to someone with a Ph.D. in psychology but no apparent credentials in nutrition. The article's "me" versus "them" summary of what works to shed pounds lacked objectivity, and the article did not acknowledge that many of the behavioral principles espoused by the profiled practitioner are part of other modern weight-loss strategies.

Woman's Day articles written by nutrition experts contributed to that magazine's "good" rating. *Woman's Day*'s "Best Ever One Week Diet" made expert use of the Food Guide Pyramid. A few articles lost minor points for saying "according to experts" instead of documenting their sources, and a "No Time to Diet Diet" failed to provide enough calories.

Good Housekeeping's nutrition coverage, while rated "good" overall, was uneven. An article on frozen yogurt did a competent job of comparing the nutrient profiles of yogurt products, but a September '93 "Eating Right" column sacrificed accuracy for brevity. A reader asked, "Is breast milk really better for my newborn?"; and a physician responded that although breast milk is optimal, "you aren't putting her at any risk by choosing formula." The judges felt that this brief answer failed to provide a complete picture of breast-feeding's benefits.

Redbook's "Hottest Diet Advice in America" was actually based on long-known information, as repackaged by a popular diet guru. The judges found nothing wrong with the article's advice (exercise and eat well), but they didn't find it particularly new or "hot." A piece entitled "The Morning After Diet" explained the physiology of weight loss using experts' quotes. But breakfasts of pancakes, eggs and bacon and chicken and biscuits were called high-carbohydrate meals when in fact both are high in fat.

McCall's well-rated "25 Ways to Eat Chocolate and Not Gain Weight" gave readers permission to indulge as long as portion size was respected. But

in "Lose Three Pounds in One Weekend!" a health spa worker with no nutrition credentials made two statements—"Holiday weight is mostly caused by water retention" and "Avoid alcohol . . . [it] weakens your diet resolve"—that are not necessarily true. Also, the article erroneously referred to olives and hummus as being "low fat."

Health was one of the lower rated magazines in the "good" group. One article, "The Bran News About Rice," was particularly well rated; but when it came to scientific interpretation, *Health* occasionally struggled to present balanced reports.

The 'Fair' Four

On the whole, *New Woman*'s message seems rather inconsistent. "Have Yourself a Fat Christmas" erred in its throw-in-the-towel, holiday-weight-gain-is-inevitable stance. But *New Woman* had previously run an article ("Getting Over Overeating") with a conflicting message. The earlier piece was an interesting take on emotional connections to overeating and according to one judge was as objective and balanced as preliminary-research reporting can be. It lost credibility only for implying that sugar was a mood-altering culprit for all individuals.

Men's Health's "Burn Fat Faster" was a summary of fat-burning techniques that work. It was generally balanced and thorough but lost points for failing to document its sources. A piece that purported to be a "Guide to Vitamin and Mineral Supplements" recommended antioxidant supplements to prevent wrinkles and disease, advice the scientific consensus does not support for all individuals.

Vogue ran a well-researched report on "The Death of Dieting" that included the author's own personal testimonial about the shortcomings of commercial weight-loss programs. The article received an almost flawless rating. But *Vogue*'s "Dieting to Extremes: Tipping the Scales" was a major source of point loss. The low-carbohydrate diet described in the article was based on unproved assumptions such as, "Eat all you want but only the right foods and in the right combinations," and, "Exercise is irrelevant."

Runner's World was plagued by problems of oversimplification of complex issues and failure to cite sources. The magazine also singled out certain foods and promoted nutrient supplementation as keys to running faster and living longer. One article said that eating guava lowers cholesterol levels. How much guava, what other dietary or lifestyle changes were necessary and the source of the research were all undocumented.

'Poor' Cosmo!

Cosmopolitan was the only magazine ranked as "poor." While *Cosmo* seemed to run fewer fad diets than in previous years, no other magazine was as conspicuously lax about its credibility quotient. An article called "Do You or Don't You Need Vitamins and Minerals?" was blatantly unscientific; it was written by a physician to promote nutrient cure-alls. The author admonished readers to supplement 15 different vitamins and minerals, stating that young, active women "need them all." The article's misguided advice to take 100 milligrams of vitamin B_6 daily to alleviate PMS has not been clinically proved—and that amount could even be toxic if taken over long periods of time. *Cosmopolitan*'s articles, consistently poorly rated as they were, suggest a strong need for real improvement under the magazine's new editor.

How the Magazines Stack Up by Target Audience

As a group, the "consumer-focused" *Consumer Reports*, *Parents* and *Reader's Digest* scored highest, racking up a 91 percent score overall. ACSH concluded that these magazines' factual approach triumphed over the fluffier approaches common to the lower scoring titles.

The second-highest rated group—the "home-focused" magazines—consisted of *Better Homes and Gardens*, *Cooking Light* and *Good Housekeeping*. Their group score was 88. Within this group, however, the first two outscored *Good Housekeeping* to a statistically significant extent.

"Health-focused" and "women's" magazines, taken as groups, were significantly less accurate from a statistical standpoint than either the consumer-focused or home-focused groups.

American Health and *Prevention* led the health-focused magazines with similar ratings; they were statistically better than the health-focused *Health*, *Men's Health* and *Runner's World*. On the whole, the magazines in this group (which scored 82 overall) tended to publish the highest volume of nutrition information.

Glamour was the highest scoring women's magazine, followed by *Mademoiselle*, *Self*, *Woman's Day*, *Redbook* and *McCall's*. According to the survey's statistician, the low-ranking *New Woman*, *Vogue* and *Cosmopolitan* scored significantly worse than any of the other women's titles and so pulled the women's magazines down as a group. The group score was 82.

Some Advice to the Magazines—and to Consumers

This latest survey found that the accuracy of nutrition reporting in magazines has definitely improved. Dr. Manfred Kroger has served as a judge in every ACSH survey so far, and he attributes the improvement to the fact that "Reporters, writers and editors [are] doing a better job because they recognize [that] ACSH and the public are watching them and their work." Dr. Kroger adds that "The media are increasingly relying on experts to scrutinize their output before going public, a welcome trend."

On the whole, the nutrition reporting in popular magazines is becoming increasingly sophisticated. Outlandish claims, endorsements of fad diets and gross misinterpretations of scientific research —all commonly seen in earlier surveys—have for the most part been replaced by balanced, science-based reports designed to promote nutrition literacy. New research findings are showing up, and the magazines are moving toward providing more hands-on information. Writers are telling readers how to fix poor eating habits and how to make needed lifestyle changes in accord with public health policy.

ACSH commends those magazines whose nutrition reporting was rated "excellent" or "good" and encourages the editors at those magazines rated "fair" or "poor" to assign nutrition topics to writers and researchers who understand science. All magazines should strive to achieve better consistency and better quality in their nutrition articles, with the ultimate goal of educating their readers and stemming the spread of misinformation.

DIANE WOZNICKI, M.S., R.D., IS AN ADJUNCT NUTRITION INSTRUCTOR AT THE UNIVERSITY OF PENNSYLVANIA. RUTH KAVA, PH.D., R.D., IS DIRECTOR OF NUTRITION AT THE AMERICAN COUNCIL ON SCIENCE AND HEALTH. THE ARTICLES FOR THE *SPECIAL REPORT* WERE COMPILED BY RENA SELYA, M.A., A RESEARCH INTERN AT ACSH.

THE SURVEY WAS JUDGED BY:
IRENE BERMAN-LEVINE, PH.D., R.D., ADJUNCT NUTRITION INSTRUCTOR AT THE UNIVERSITY OF PENNSYLVANIA AND NUTRITION CONSULTANT IN PRIVATE PRACTICE IN HARRISBURG, PA.

F.J. FRANCIS, PH.D., PROFESSOR OF FOOD SCIENCE, UNIVERSITY OF MASSACHUSETTS, AMHERST.

KATHRYN M. KOLASA, PH.D., R.D., L.D./N., SECTION HEAD AND PROFESSOR OF NUTRITION, DEPARTMENT OF FAMILY MEDICINE, EAST CAROLINA UNIVERSITY, GREENVILLE, NC.

MANFRED KROGER, PH.D., PROFESSOR OF FOOD SCIENCE AND PROFESSOR OF SCIENCE, TECHNOLOGY AND SOCIETY, THE PENNSYLVANIA STATE UNIVERSITY, UNIVERSITY PARK, PA.

STATISTICAL ANALYSIS BY:
JEROME LEE, PH.D., ASSOCIATE PROFESSOR OF PSYCHOLOGY, ALBRIGHT COLLEGE, READING, PA.

Why do those #&*?@! "experts" keep changing their minds?

Let's say that for the last five years you've been paying close attention to health news as reported on TV and in newspapers. Perhaps you learned about antioxidants (notably vitamins E and C and beta carotene), which you can get both from foods and supplements. These antioxidants may help lower the risk of heart disease, cancer, cataracts, and other ills. The scientist who had told you this on the *Today* show was a handsome fellow in a good-looking suit (no rumpled Einstein he). He had led the groundbreaking study that had just appeared in *The Impeccable Journal of Medicine*. Not only was the evidence "very exciting," but he was taking hefty amounts of antioxidant supplements himself. So you started taking the pills. Next thing, you read that a study conducted in Finland showed that not only was beta carotene *not* protective against lung cancer, it actually seemed to increase the risk of getting it. Feeling deceived, you stopped taking your supplements and even gave up your daily carrot. You were tired of carrots anyway.

You may have seen something similar happen with oat bran (good one week, outmoded the next), margarine (you switched to this supposed health food a few years ago, and now it's been tagged as an artery-clogger), DDT and breast cancer (first linked, then not), hot dogs and childhood leukemia (a headline-maker that soon pooped out, since even the researchers had a hard time explaining their findings), and household electricity (cancer again—but by then you had gotten bored). Do these folks just not know what they are talking about?

In fact, the experts don't change their minds as often as it may seem. This newsletter, for example, never told you that margarine was a health food or that oat bran would solve your cholesterol problems. Both these foods were hyped by the media and by manufacturers—but most nutritionists never thought or said there was anything magic about them. A few researchers and journalists eagerly spread the idea that your power line and your electric toaster and clock could give you cancer. Most experts thought all along that the evidence was pretty thin. Headline writers change their minds more often than scientists.

Science is a process, not a product, a work in progress rather than a book of rules. Scientific evidence accumulates bit by bit. This doesn't mean scientists are bumblers (though perhaps a few are), but that they are trying to accumulate enough data to get at the truth, which is always a difficult job. Within the circle of qualified, well-informed scientists, there is bound to be disagreement, too. The same data look different to different people. A good scientist is often his/her own severest critic.

The search for truth in a democracy is also complicated by
- Intense public interest in health
- Hunger for quick solutions
- Journalists trying to make a routine story sound exciting
- Publishers and TV producers looking for audiences
- Scientists looking for fame and grants
- Medical journals thirsting for prestige
- Entrepreneurs thirsting for profits.

It pays to keep your wits about you as you listen, watch, and read.

The search for evidence

In general, there are three ways to look for evidence about health:

■ **Basic research** is conducted in a laboratory, involving "test tube" or "in vitro" (within glass) experiments, or experiments with animals such as mice. Such work is vital for many reasons. For one, it can confirm observations or hunches and provide what scientists call plausible mechanisms for a theory. If a link between heart disease and smoking is suspected, laboratory experiments might show how nicotine affects blood vessels.

The beauty of lab research is that it can be tightly controlled. Its limitation is that what happens in a test tube or a laboratory rat may not happen in a free-living human being.

■ **Clinical or interventional trials** are founded on observation and treatment of human beings. As with basic research, the "gold standard" clinical trial can and must be rigorously controlled. There'll be an experimental group or groups (receiving a bona-fide drug or treatment) and a control group (receiving a placebo, or dummy, treatment). A valid experiment must also be "blinded," meaning that no subject knows whether he/she is in the experimental or the control group. In a double-blind trial, the researchers don't know either.

But clinical trials have their limitations, too. The researchers must not knowingly endanger human life and health—there are ethics committees these days to make sure of this. Also, selection criteria must be set up. If the research is about heart disease, maybe the researchers will include only men, since middle-aged men are more prone to heart disease than women the same age. Or maybe they'll include only nurses, because nurses can be reliably tracked and are also good reporters. But these groups are not representative of the whole population. It may or may not be possible to generalize the findings. The study that determined aspirin's efficacy against heart attacks, for instance, was a well-designed interventional trial. But, for various reasons, nearly all the participants were middle-aged white men. No one is sure that aspirin works the same way for other people.

■ **Epidemiologic studies.** These generate the most news because so many of them have potential public appeal. An indispensable arm of research, epidemiology looks at the distribution of disease ("epidemics") and risk factors for disease in a human population in an attempt to find disease determinants. Compared with clinical trials or basic research, epidemiology is beset with pitfalls. That's because it deals with people in the real world and with situations that are hard to control.

The two most common types of epidemiologic research are:

Case control studies. Let's say you're studying lung cancer. You select a group of lung cancer patients and match them (by age, gender, and other criteria) with a group of healthy people. You try to identify which factors distinguish the healthy subjects (the "controls") from those who got sick.

Cohort studies. You select a group and question them about their habits, exposures, nutritional intake, and so forth. Then you see how many of your subjects actually develop lung cancer (or whatever you are studying) over the years, and you try to identify the factors associated with lung cancer.

Pitfalls and dead ends

Epidemiologic studies cannot usually prove cause and effect, but can identify associations and risk factors. Furthermore, epidemiology is best at identifying very powerful risk factors—smoking for lung cancer, for example. It is less good at risk assessment when associations are weak—between radon gas in homes and lung cancer, for example.

No matter how well done, any epidemiologic study may be open to criticism. Here are just a few of the problems:

■ People may not reliably report their eating and exercise habits. (How many carrots did you eat each month as an adolescent? How many last month? Few of us could say.) People aware of the benefits of eating vegetables may unconsciously exaggerate their vegetable consumption on a questionnaire. That's known as "recall bias."

■ Hidden variables or "confounders" may cloud results. A study might indicate that eating broccoli reduces the risk of heart disease. But broccoli eaters may be health-conscious and get a lot of exercise. Was it the broccoli or the exercise?

■ Those included in a study may seem to be a randomly selected, unbiased sample and then turn out not to be. For example, searching for a control group in one study, a re-

---

Words for the wise

✓ **"May"**: does *not* mean "will."

✓ **"Contributes to," "is linked to,"** or **"is associated with"**: does *not* mean "causes."

✓ **"Proves"**: scientific studies gather evidence in a systematic way, but one study, taken alone, seldom proves anything.

✓ **"Breakthrough"**: this happens only now and then—for example, the discovery of penicillin or the polio vaccine. But today the word is so overworked as to be meaningless.

✓ **"Doubles the risk"** or **"triples the risk"**: may or may not be meaningful. Do you know what the risk was in the first place? If the risk was 1 in a million, and you double it, that's still only 1 in 500,000. If the risk was 1 in 100 and doubles, that's a big increase.

✓ **"Significant"**: a result is "statistically significant" when the association between two factors has been found to be greater than might occur at random (this is worked out by a mathematical formula). But people often take "significant" to mean "major" or "important."

---

searcher picked numbers out of the telephone book at random and called his subjects in the daytime. But people who stay home during the day may not be a representative sample. Those at home in the daytime might tend to be very young or very old, ill, or recovering from illness.

Some commonsense pointers

✓ **Don't jump to conclusions.** A single study is no reason for changing your health habits. Distinguish between an interesting finding and a broad-based public health recommendation.

✓ **Always look for context.** A good reporter—and a responsible scientist—will always place findings in the context of other research. Yet the typical news report seldom alludes to other scientific work.

✓ **If it was an animal study or some other kind of lab study, be cautious about generalizing.** Years ago lab studies suggested that saccharin caused cancer in rats, but epidemiologic studies later showed it didn't cause cancer in humans.

✓ **Beware of press conferences** and other hype. Scientists, not to mention the editors of medical journals, love to make the front page of major newspapers and hear their studies mentioned on the evening news. The fact that the study in question may have been flawed or inconclusive or old news may not seem worth mentioning. This doesn't mean you shouldn't believe anything. Truth, too, may be accompanied by hype.

✓ **Notice the number of study participants and the study's length.** The smaller the number of subjects and the shorter the time, the greater the possibility that the findings are erroneous.

✓ **Perhaps the most blatantly hyped research of late has been genetic.** But the treatment of human illness by altering human genes is still at a very early stage.

---

6. HEALTH CLAIMS

■ Health effects, especially where cancer is concerned, may take 20 years or more to show up. It's not always financially or humanly possible to keep a study running that long.

Reading health news in an imperfect world

And this is only the half of it. Sometimes the flaws lie in the study, sometimes in the way it has been promoted and reported. Science reporters may be deluged with data. Many are expected to cover all science, from physics and astronomy to the health effects of hair dyes. Sometimes health reporters may not even have read the studies in question or may not understand the statistics.

Many medical organizations issue press releases. Some of these are excellent, and some aren't. Some deliberately try to manipulate the press, overstating the case, failing to provide context, and so forth. Researchers, institutions, and corporations often hire public relations people to promote their work. These people may actually know less than the enterprising reporter who calls to interview them.

Finally, people tend to draw their own conclusions, no matter what the article says.

However, the bottom line is pretty good...

None of this means epidemiology doesn't work. *One study may not prove anything, but a body of research, in which evidence accumulates bit by bit, can uncover the truth.* Research into human health has made enormous strides and is still making them. There may be no such thing as a perfect study, but here is only the briefest list of discoveries that came out of epidemiologic research:

■ Smoking is the leading cause of premature death in developed countries.

■ High blood cholesterol is a major cause of coronary artery disease and heart attack.

■ Exercise is important for good health.

■ Good nutrition offers protection against cancer; or, conversely, poor nutrition is a factor in the development of cancer.

■ Obesity is a risk factor for heart disease, cancer, and diabetes.

The list could go on and on. We suggest that you retain a spirit of inquiry and a healthy skepticism, but not lapse into cynicism. *The "flip-flops" you perceive are often not flip-flops at all, except in the mind of some headline writer.*

There is a great deal of good reporting, and it's an interesting challenge to follow health news. You don't believe everything you read or see on TV about politics, business, or foreign relations, so it's no surprise that you shouldn't believe some health news. Luckily, there are many sources for health news—none infallible, but some a lot better than others.

VITAMIN PUSHERS AND FOOD QUACKS

Victor Herbert, M.D., J.D.

Victor Herbert, M.D., J.D., is professor of medicine at Mt. Sinai School of Medicine in New York City and chief of the Hematology and Nutrition Laboratory at the Sinai-affiliated Bronx VA Medical Center. He is a board member of the National Council Against Health Fraud and a member of the American Cancer Society's Committee on Questionable Methods. He has served on the Food and Nutrition Board of the National Academy of Sciences and its Recommended Dietary Allowances (RDA) Committee. He has written more than 650 scientific articles and received several national awards for his nutrition research. His books include *The Mount Sinai School of Medicine Complete Book of Nutrition* and *Genetic Nutrition: Designing a Diet Based on Your Family Medical History.*

We still are in the midst of a vitamin craze. Nutrition hustlers are cleaning up by stoking our fears and stroking our hopes. With their deceptive credentials, they dominate air waves and publications. Talk show hosts love them because their false promises of superhealth draw huge audiences. The situation now appears even worse than it was more than twenty-five years ago, when FDA Commissioner George P. Larrick stated:

> The most widespread and expensive type of quackery in the United States today is the promotion of vitamin products, special dietary foods, and food supplements. Millions of consumers are being misled concerning the need for such products. Complicating this problem is a vast and growing "folklore" or "mythology" of nutrition which is being built up by pseudoscientific literature in books, pamphlets and periodicals. As a result, millions of people are attempting self-medication for imaginary and real illnesses with a multitude of more or less irrational food items. Food quackery today can only be compared to the patent medicine craze which reached its height in the last century.

"Health food" rackets cost Americans billions of dollars a year. The major victims of this waste are the elderly, the pregnant, the sick, and the poor.

The Fundamentals of Good Nutrition

Have you been brainwashed by vitamin pushers? Do you believe you should supplement your diet with extra nutrients? Do you believe that, "If some is good, more is better"? Do you believe extra nutrients can't hurt"? Or that they provide "nutrition insurance"? If you believe any of these things, you have been misled.

The fundamentals of good nutrition are simple: To get the amounts and kinds of nutrients your body needs, eat moderate amounts of food from each of the food groups designated by the U.S. Department of Agriculture's Daily Food Guide, choosing a wide variety within each category. (For detailed instructions send $1 for USDA's *Food Guide Pyramid* booklet [Publication No. HG 249] to the Consumer Information Center, Pueblo, CO 81009.) This food plan provides for adequate quantities of all vitamins, minerals, and protein components. Actually, normal people eating a balanced variety of foods are likely to consume *more* nutrients than they need. Of course, health hucksters won't tell you this because their income depends upon withholding that truth. Unlike responsible practitioners, they do not make their living by trying to keep you healthy, but rather by tempting you with false claims. These claims raise their personal appearance fees, sell their books and magazine articles, and sell the products of companies in which (unknown to you) they may have a financial interest.

The Dangers of Excess Vitamins

When on the defensive, quacks are quick to demand, "How do you know it doesn't help?" The reply to this is "How do you know it doesn't *harm?*" Many substances that are harmless in small or moderate doses can be harmful either in large doses or by gradual build-up over many years. Just because a substance (such as a vitamin) is found naturally in food does not mean it is harmless in large doses.

When scientists speak of "excess" vitamins, they mean dosages in excess of the "Recommended Dietary Allowances (RDAs)" set by the Food and Nutrition Board of the National Research Council, National Academy of Sciences. The RDAs are the "levels of intake of essential nutrients considered, in the judgment of the Food and Nutrition Board on the basis of available scientific knowledge, to be adequate to meet the known nutritional needs of practically all healthy persons." RDAs should not be confused with "requirements." They are more than most people require. They are set not only to meet body needs, but to allow substantial storage to cover periods of reduced intake or increased need. Amounts higher than the RDAs serve no vitamin function in the body. They should be considered *drugs* and can be an invitation to trouble.

There are two situations in which the use of vitamins in excess of the RDAs is legitimate. The first is the treatment of

From *Nutrition Forum* newsletter, March/April 1993, pp. 9-15. Reprinted by permission of *Nutrition Forum* newsletter, now published by Prometheus Books, 59 John Glenn Drive, Amherst, NY 14228.

medically diagnosed deficiency states—conditions that are rare except among alcoholics, persons with intestinal malabsorption defects, and the poor, especially those who are pregnant or elderly. The other use is in the treatment of certain conditions in which vitamins are used for their chemical (non-vitamin) actions. None of these situations is suitable for self-treatment.

How can vitamin pushers and food quacks be identified? The following behavior should make you suspicious.

They use anecdotes and testimonials to support their claims.

We all tend to believe what others tell us about personal experiences. But separating cause and effect from coincidence can be difficult. If people tell you that product X has cured their cancer, arthritis, or whatever, be skeptical. They may not actually have had the condition. If they did, their recovery most likely would have occurred without the help of product X. Most single episodes of disease recover with just the passage of time, and most chronic ailments have symptom-free periods. Establishing medical truths requires careful and repeated investigation—with well-designed experiments, not reports of coincidences misperceived as cause-and-effect. That's why testimonial evidence is forbidden in scientific articles and usually is inadmissible in court.

Never underestimate the extent to which people can be fooled by a worthless remedy. During the early 1940s, many thousands of people became convinced that "glyoxylide" could cure cancer. Yet analysis showed it was simply distilled water!

Symptoms that are psychosomatic (bodily reactions to tension) are often relieved by anything taken with a suggestion that it will work. Tiredness and other minor aches and pains may respond to any enthusiastically recommended nostrum. For these problems, even physicians may prescribe a placebo. A placebo is a substance that has no pharmacological effect on the condition for which it is used, but is given to satisfy a patient who supposes it to be a medicine. Vitamins (such as B_{12}) are commonly used in this way.

Placebos act by suggestion. Unfortunately, some doctors swallow the advertising hype or become confused by their own observations and "believe in vitamins" beyond those supplied by a good diet. Those who share such false beliefs do so because they confuse coincidence or placebo action with cause and effect. Homeopathic believers make the same error.

Talk show hosts give quacks a boost when they ask "What do all the vitamins you take do for you personally?" Then thousands or even millions of viewers are treated to the quack's talk of improved health, vigor and vitality—with the implicit point: "It did this for me. It will do the same for you." A most revealing testimonial experience was described during a major network show that hosted several of the world's most prominent promoters of nutritional faddism. While the host was boasting that his new eating program had cured his "hypoglycemia," he mentioned in passing that he was no longer drinking twenty to thirty cups of coffee a day. Neither the host nor any of his "experts" had the good sense to tell their audience how dangerous it can be to drink so much coffee. Nor did any of them recognize that the host's original symptoms were probably caused by excess caffeine.

They promise quick, dramatic, miraculous cures.

The promises are usually subtle or couched in "weasel words"—so they can deny making them when the feds close in. Such promises are the quacks' most immoral practice. They don't seem to care how many people they break financially or in spirit—by elation over their claims of quick cure followed by deep depression when the claims prove false. Nor do quacks keep count—while they fill their bank accounts—of how many people they lure away from effective medical care into disability or death.

They use disclaimers couched in pseudomedical jargon.

Instead of promising to cure your disease, some quacks will promise to "detoxify" your body, "balance" its chemistry, release its "nerve energy," bring it in harmony with nature, "stimulate" or "strengthen" your immune system, or "support" various organs in your body. (Of course they never identify or make valid before-and-after measurements of any of these processes.) These disclaimers serve two purposes. Since it is impossible to measure the processes they allege, it may be difficult to prove them wrong. Moreover, if a quack is not a physician, the use of nonmedical terminology may help to avoid prosecution for practicing medicine without a license—although it shouldn't.

They display credentials not recognized by responsible scientists or educators.

The backbone of educational integrity in America is a system of accreditation by agencies recognized by the U.S. Secretary of Education and/or the Council on Postsecondary Accreditation. "Degrees" from unaccredited schools are rarely worth the paper they are printed on. In the health field, there is no such thing as a reliable school that is not accredited. Since quacks operate outside of the scientific community, they also tend to form their own "professional" organizations.

In some cases, the only membership requirement is payment of a fee. My office wall displays fancy "professional member" certificates for Charlie Herbert (a cat) and Sassafras Herbert (a dog). Each was acquired simply by submitting the animal's name, our address, and a check for $50. Don't assume that all groups with scientific-sounding names are respectable. Find out whether their views are scientifically based.

Unfortunately, possession of an accredited degree does not guarantee reliability. Some schools that teach unscientific methods (chiropractic, naturopathy, and acupuncture) have achieved accreditation. Worse yet, a small percentage of individuals trained in reputable institutions (such as medical or dental schools or accredited universities) have strayed from scientific thought.

Some quacks are promoted with superlatives like "the world's foremost nutritionist" or "America's leading nutrition expert." There is no law against this tactic, just as there is none against calling oneself the "World's Foremost Lover." However, the scientific community recognizes no such title.

They encourage patients to lend political support to their treatment methods.

A century ago, before scientific methodology was generally accepted, valid new ideas were hard to evaluate and were sometimes rejected by a majority of the medical community, only to be upheld later. But today, treatments demonstrated as effective are welcomed by scientific practitioners and do not need a group to crusade for them. *Quacks seek political endorsement because they can't prove that their methods work.* Instead, they may seek to legalize their treatment and force insurance companies to pay for it. Judges and legislators who believe in caveat emptor (let the buyer beware) are natural allies for quacks.

They say that most disease is due to faulty diet and can be treated with "nutritional" methods.

This simply isn't so. Consult your doctor or any recognized textbook of medicine. They will tell you that although diet is a factor in some diseases (most notably coronary heart disease), most diseases have little or nothing to do with diet. Common symptoms like malaise (feeling poorly), tiredness, lack of pep, aches (including headaches) or pains, insomnia and similar complaints are usually the body's reaction to emotional stress. The persistence of such symptoms is a signal to see a doctor to be evaluated for possible physical illness. It is not a reason to take vitamin pills.

Some quacks seem to specialize in the diagnosis and treatment of problems considered rare or even nonexistent by responsible practitioners. Years ago hypothyroidism and adrenal insufficiency were in vogue. Today's "fad" diagnoses are "hypoglycemia," "mercury amalgam toxicity," "candidiasis hypersensitivity," and "environmental illness." Quacks are also jumping on the allergy bandwagon, falsely claiming that huge numbers of Americans are suffering from undiagnosed allergies, "diagnosing" them with worthless tests, and prescribing worthless "nutritional" treatments.

They recommend a wide variety of substances similar to those found in your body

The underlying idea—like the wishful thinking of primitive tribes—is that taking these substances will strengthen or rejuvenate the corresponding body parts. For example, according to a health food store brochure:

Raw glandular therapy, or "cellular therapy" . . . seems almost too simple to be true. It consists of giving in supplement form (intravenous or oral) those specific tissues from animals that correspond to the "weakened" areas of the human body. In other words, if a person has a weak pancreas, give him raw pancreas substance; if the heart is weak, give raw heart, etc.

Vitamins and other nutrients may be added to the various preparations to make them more marketable. When taken by mouth, such concoctions are no better than placebos. They usually don't do direct harm, but their allure may steer people away from competent professional care. Injections of raw animal tissues, however, can cause severe allergic reactions to their proteins. Some preparations have also caused serious infections.

Proponents of "tissue salts" allege that the basic cause of disease is mineral deficiency—correction of which will enable the body to heal itself. Thus, they claim, one or more of twelve salts are useful against a wide variety of diseases, including appendicitis (ruptured or not), baldness, deafness, insomnia, and worms. Development of this method is attributed to a nineteenth-century physician named W.H. Schuessler.

Enzymes for oral use are another rip-off. They supposedly aid digestion and "support" many other functions within the body. The fact is, however, that enzymes taken by mouth are digested into their component amino acids by the stomach and intestines and therefore don't function as enzymes within the body. Oral pancreatic enzymes have legitimate medical use in diseases involving decreased secretion of one's own pancreatic enzymes. Anyone who actually has a pancreatic enzyme deficiency probably has a serious underlying disease requiring competent medical diagnosis and treatment.

When talking about nutrients, they tell only part of the story.

They tell you all the wonderful things that vitamins and minerals do in your body and/or all the horrible things that can happen if you don't get enough. But they conveniently neglect to tell you that a balanced diet can provide all the nutrients you need, and that the USDA Pyramid Food Guide system makes balancing your diet simple. Unfortunately, it is legal to lie in a publication or lecture or on a talk show as long as the claims are not connected to selling a specific product. Many supplement manufacturers use subtle approaches. Some simply say "Buy our product X . . . It contains nutrients that help promote healthy eyes (or hair, or whatever organ you happen to be concerned about)." Others distribute charts saying what each nutrient does and the signs and symptoms of deficiency disease. This encourages supplementation with the hope of enhancing body functions and/or avoiding the troubles described.

Another type of fraudulent concealment is the promotion of "supplements" and herbal extracts based on incomplete information. Many health food industry products are marketed with claims based on faulty extrapolations of animal research and/or unconfirmed studies on humans. The most notorious such product was L-tryptophan, an amino acid. For many years it was promoted for insomnia, depression, premenstrual syndrome and overweight, even though it had not been proven safe or effective for any of these purposes. In 1989, it triggered an outbreak of eosinophilia-myalgia syndrome, a rare disorder characterized by severe muscle and joint pain, weakness, swelling of the arms and legs, fever, skin rash, and an increase of eosinophils (certain white blood cells) in the blood. Over the next year, more than 1,500 cases and 28 deaths were reported.

The out-break was traced to a manufacturing problem at the plant of a wholesale supplier. The naked truth is that L-tryptophan should not have been marketed to the public in the first place because—like most single-ingredient amino acids—it had not been proven safe for medicinal use. In fact, the FDA had issued a ban during the mid-1970s, but had not enforced it.

They claim that most Americans are poorly nourished.

This is an appeal to fear that is not only untrue, but ignores the fact that the main forms of bad nourishment in the United States are undernourishment among the poverty-stricken and overweight in the population at large, particularly the poor. Poor people can ill afford to waste money on unnecessary vitamin pills. Their food money should be spent for nourishing food. With one exception, food-group diets contain all the nutrients that people need. The exception involves the mineral iron. The average American diet contains barely enough iron to meet the needs of infants, fertile women, and, especially, pregnant women. This problem can be solved simply by cooking in a "Dutch oven" or any iron pot or eating iron-rich foods such as soy beans, liver, and veal muscle.

It is falsely alleged that Americans are so addicted to "junk" foods that an adequate diet is exceptional rather than usual. It is true that some snack foods are mainly "naked calories" (sugars and/or fats without other nutrients). But it is not necessary for every morsel of food we eat to be loaded with nutrients. No normal person following the USDA's food group system is in any danger of vitamin deficiency.

They tell you that if you eat badly, you'll be OK if you take supplements.

This is the "Nutrition Insurance Gambit." The statement is not only untrue but encourages careless eating habits. The remedy for eating badly is a well balanced diet. If in doubt about the adequacy of your diet, write down what you eat for several days and see whether your daily average is in line with the USDA's guidelines. If you can't do this yourself, your doctor or a registered dietitian can do it for you.

They allege that modern processing methods and storage remove all nutritive value from our food.

It is true that food processing can change the nutrient content of foods. But the changes are not so drastic as the quack, who wants you to buy supplements, would like you to believe. While some processing methods destroy some nutrients, others add them. A balanced variety of foods will provide all the nourishment you need.

Quacks distort and oversimplify. When they say that milling removes B-vitamins, they don't bother to tell you that enrichment puts them back. When they tell you that cooking destroys nutrients, they omit the fact that only a few nutrients are sensitive to heat. Nor do they tell you that these few nutrients are easily obtained from a portion of fresh uncooked fruit, vegetable, or fresh or frozen fruit juice each day.

They claim that fluoridation is dangerous.

Curiously, quacks are not always interested in real deficiencies. Fluoride is necessary to build decay-resistant teeth and strong bones. The best way to obtain adequate amounts of this essential nutrient is to augment community water supplies so their fluoride concentration is about one part fluoride for every million parts of water. But quacks are usually opposed to water fluoridation, and some advocate water filters that remove fluoride. It seems that when they cannot profit from something, they may try to make money by opposing it.

They oppose pasteurization of milk.

One of the strangest aspects of nutrition quackery is its embrace of "raw" (unpasteurized) milk. Public health authorities advocate pasteurization to destroy any disease-producing bacteria that may be present. Health faddists and quacks claim that it destroys essential nutrients. Although about 10 percent of the heat-sensitive vitamins (vitamin C and thiamine) are destroyed during pasteurization, milk would not be a significant source of these nutrients anyway. Raw milk, whether "certified" or not, can be a source of harmful bacteria that cause dysentery and tuberculosis. The FDA has banned the interstate sale of raw milk and raw-milk products packaged for human consumption. In 1989, a California Superior Court judge ordered the nation's largest raw milk producer to stop advertising that its raw milk products are safe and healthier than pasteurized milk and to label its products with a conspicuous warning.

They claim that soil depletion and the use of "chemical" fertilizers result in less nourishing food.

These claims are used to promote the sale of so-called "organically grown" foods. If a nutrient is missing from the soil, a plant just does not grow. Chemical fertilizers counteract the effects of soil depletion. Plant vary in mineral content, but this is not significant in the American diet. Quacks also lie when they claim that plants grown with natural fertilizers (such as manure) are nutritionally superior to those grown with synthetic fertilizers. Before they can use them, plants convert natural fertilizers into the same chemicals that synthetic fertilizers supply.

They claim that under stress, and in certain diseases, your need for nutrients is increased.

Many vitamin manufacturers have advertised that "stress robs the body of vitamins." One company has asserted that, "if you smoke, diet, or happen to be sick, you may be robbing your body of vitamins." Another has warned that "stress can deplete your body of water-soluble vitamins ... and daily replacement is necessary." Other products are touted to fill the "special needs of athletes."

While it is true that the need for vitamins may rise slightly under physical stress and in certain diseases, this type of advertising is fraudulent. The average American—stressed or not—is not in danger of vitamin deficiency. The increased needs to which the ads refer almost never rise above the RDAs and can be met by proper eating. Someone who is really in danger of deficiency as a result of illness would be a very ill person who needs medical care, probably in a hospital. But these promotions are aimed at average Americans who certainly don't need vitamin supplements to survive the common cold, a round of golf, or a jog around the neighborhood! Athletes get more than enough vitamins when they eat the food needed to meet their caloric requirements.

Many vitamin pushers suggest that smokers need vitamin C supplements. While it is true that smokers in North America have somewhat lower blood levels of this vitamin, these levels are still far above deficiency levels. In America, cigarette smoking is the leading cause of death preventable by self-discipline. Rather than seeking false comfort by taking vitamin C, smokers who are concerned about their health should stop smoking. Moreover, since doses of vitamin C high enough to acidify the urine speed up excretion of nicotine, they may even cause some smokers to smoke more to avoid symptoms of nicotine withdrawal. Suggestions that "stress vitamins" are helpful against emotional stress are also fraudulent.

They claim you are in danger of being "poisoned" by ordinary food additives and preservatives.

This is a scare tactic designed to undermine your confidence in food scientists and government protection agencies. Quacks want you to think they are out to protect you. They hope that if you trust them, you will buy what they recommend. The fact is that the tiny amounts of additives used in food pose no threat to human health. Some actually protect our health by preventing spoilage, rancidity, and mold growth.

Two examples illustrate how ridiculous quacks can get about food additives, especially those found naturally in food. Calcium propionate is used to preserve bread and occurs naturally in Swiss cheese. Quacks who would steer you toward (higher-priced) bread made without preservatives are careful not to tell you that a one-ounce slice of "natural" Swiss cheese contains the same amount of calcium propionate used to retard spoilage in two one-pound loaves of bread. Similarly, those who warn about monosodium glutamate (MSG) don't tell you that the wheat germ they hustle as a "health food" is a major natural source of this substance.

Also curious is their failure to warn that many plant substances sold in health food stores are potentially toxic and can cause disability or death. The April 6, 1979, *Medical Letter* listed more than thirty such products, most of them used for making herbal teas.

They claim that "natural" vitamins are better than "synthetic" ones.

This claim is a flat lie. Each vitamin is a chain of atoms strung together as a molecule. Molecules made in the "factories" of nature are identical to those made in the factories of chemical companies. Does it make sense to pay extra for vitamins extracted from foods when you can get all you need from the foods themselves?

They claim that sugar is a deadly poison.

Many vitamin pushers would have us believe that sugar is "the killer on the breakfast table" and is the underlying cause of everything from heart disease to hypoglycemia. The fact is, however, that when sugar is used in moderation as part of a normal, balanced diet, it is a perfectly safe source of calories and eating pleasure. In fact, if you ate no sugar, your liver would make it from protein and fat because your brain needs it.

They recommend that everybody take vitamins or "health foods" or both.

Food quacks belittle normal foods and ridicule the food-group systems of good nutrition. They may not tell you that they earn their living from such pronouncements—via public appearance fees, product endorsements, sale of publications, or financial interests in vitamin companies, health food stores, or organic farms.

The very term "health food" is a deceptive slogan. All food is health food in moderation; any food is junk food in excess. Did you ever stop to think that your corner grocery, fruit market, meat market, and supermarket are also health food stores? They are—and they generally charge less than stores that use the slogan.

Many vitamin pushers make misleading claims for bioflavonoids, rutin, inositol, paraaminobenzoic acid (PABA), and other such food substances. These substances are not needed in the diet, and the FDA forbids nutritional claims for them on product labels.

By the way, have you ever wondered why people who eat lots of "health foods" still feel they must load themselves up with vitamin supplements?

They suggest that hair analysis can be used to determine the body's nutritional state.

"Health food" stores and various unscientific practitioners suggest this test. For $25 to $50 plus a lock of your hair, you can get an elaborate computer printout of vitamins and minerals you supposedly need. Hair analysis has limited value (mainly in forensic medicine) in the diagnosis of heavy metal poisoning, but it is worthless as a screening device to detect nutritional problems. In fact, a deficiency in the body may be accompanied by an *elevated* hair level. If a hair analysis laboratory recommends supplements, you can be sure that its computers are programmed to recommend them to everyone.

Several years ago Dr. Stephen Barrett sent hair samples from two healthy teenagers under different assumed names to thirteen commercial hair analysis laboratories. The reported levels of most minerals varied considerably between identical samples sent to the same laboratory and from laboratory to laboratory. The labs also disagreed about what was "normal" or "usual" for many of the minerals. So even if hair analysis could be useful in nutritional practice, there's no assurance that commercial laboratories perform it accurately.

They suggest that a questionnaire can be used to indicate whether you need dietary supplements.

No questionnaire can do this. A few entrepreneurs have devised lengthy computer-scored questionnaires with questions about symptoms that could be present if a vitamin deficiency exists. But such symptoms occur much more frequently in conditions unrelated to nutrition. Even when a deficiency actually exists, the tests don't provide enough information to discover the cause so that suitable treatment can be recommended. That requires a physical examination and appropriate laboratory tests. Many responsible nutritionists use a computer to help evaluate their clients' diet. But this is done to make *dietary* recommendations, such as reducing fat content or increasing fiber content. Supplements are seldom useful unless the person is unable (or unwilling) to consume an adequate diet.

Be wary, too, of brief questionnaires purported to provide a basis for determining whether supplements may be needed. Responsible questionnaires compare the individual's average daily consumption with the recommended numbers of servings from each food group. The safest and best way to get nutrients is generally from food, not pills. So even if a diet is deficient, the most prudent action is usually diet modification rather than supplementation with pills.

They tell you it is easy to lose weight.

Diet quacks would like you to believe that special pills or food combinations can cause "effortless" weight loss. But the only way to lose weight is to burn off more calories than you eat. This requires self-discipline: eating less, exercising more, or preferably doing both. There are 3,500 calories in a pound of body weight. To lose one pound a week (a safe amount), you must eat an average of 500 fewer calories per day than you burn up. The most sensible diet for losing weight is one that is nutritionally balanced in carbohydrates, fats and proteins. Most fad diets "work" by producing temporary weight loss—as a result of calorie restriction. But they are invariably too monotonous and are often too dangerous for long-term use. Unless a dieter develops and maintains better eating and exercise habits, weight lost on a diet will soon return.

They offer phony "vitamins."

With vitamins so popular, why not invent some new ones. Ernst T. Krebs, M.D., and his son Ernst T. Krebs, Jr., invented two of them. In 1949 they patented a substance that they later named pangamate and trade-named "vitamin B-15." The Krebs' also developed the quack cancer remedy, laetrile, which was marketed as "vitamin B-17."

To be properly called a vitamin, a substance must be an organic nutrient that is necessary in the diet, and deficiency of the substance must be shown to cause a specific disease. Neither pangamate nor laetrile is a vitamin. Pangamate is not even a single substance. Different sellers put different synthetic ingredients in the bottle. Laetrile contains six percent of cyanide by weight and has poisoned people.

They warn you not to trust your doctor.

Quacks, who want you to trust them, suggest that most doctors are "butchers" and "poisoners." For the same reason, quacks also claim that doctors are nutrition illiterates. This, too, is untrue.

The principles of nutrition are those of human biochemistry and physiology, courses required in every medical school. Some medical schools don't teach a separate required course labeled "nutrition" because the subject is folded into other courses, at the points where it is most relevant. For example, nutrition in growth and development is taught in pediatrics, nutrition in wound healing is taught in surgery, and nutrition in pregnancy is covered in obstetrics. In addition, many medical schools do offer separate instruction in nutrition.

A physician's training, of course, does not end on the day of graduation from medical school or completion of specialty training. The medical profession advocates lifelong education, and some states require it for license renewal. Physicians can further their knowledge of nutrition by reading medical journals and textbooks, discussing cases with colleagues, and attending continuing education courses. Most doctors know what nutrients can and cannot do and can tell the difference between a real nutritional discovery and a piece of quack nonsense. Those who are unable to answer questions about dietetics (meal planning) can refer patients to someone who can—usually a registered dietitian.

Like all human beings, doctors sometimes make mistakes. However, quacks deliver mistreatment most of the time.

They claim they are being persecuted by orthodox medicine and that their work is being suppressed!

They may also claim that the American Medical Association is against them because their cures would cut into the incomes that doctors make by keeping people sick. Don't fall for such nonsense! Reputable physicians are plenty busy. Moreover, many doctors engaged in prepaid health plans, group practice, full-time teaching, and government service receive the same salary whether or not their patients are sick—so keeping their patients healthy reduces their workload, not their income.

Quacks claim there is a "controversy" about facts between themselves and "the bureaucrats," organized medicine, or "the establishment." They clamor for medical examination of their claims, but ignore any evidence that refutes them.

Any physician who found a vitamin or other preparation that could cure sterility, heart disease, arthritis, cancer, or the like, could make an enormous fortune. Patients would flock to such a doctor (as they now do to those who *falsely* claim to cure such problems), and colleagues would shower the doctor with awards—including the $700,000+ Nobel Prize! And don't forget, doctors get sick, too. Do you believe they would conspire to suppress cures for diseases that also afflict them and their loved ones?

The Bottom Line

Food quacks benefit only themselves, collecting large fees for public appearances, publications, or "consultant" status to vitamin and health food companies which they sometimes control. Their victims are not only milked financially (for billions of dollars each year), but may also suffer serious harm from vitamin overdosage and from seduction away from proper medical care.

There is nutritional deficiency in this country, but it is found primarily among the poor, particularly among those who are elderly, are pregnant or are small children. These groups need improved diets. Their problems will not be solved by the phony panaceas of hucksters, but by better dietary practices. The best way to get vitamins and minerals is in the packages provided by nature: foods that are contained in a balanced and varied diet. If humans needed to eat pills for nutrition, pills would grow on trees.

The basic rule of good nutrition is moderation in all things. Contrary to the claim that "It may help," the advice of food quacks may harm—both your health and your pocketbook. They will continue to cheat the American public, however, until the communications industries develop sufficient concern for the public interest to attack their quackery instead of promoting it. And if the media cannot develop adequate social conscience on their own, they should be forced to do so by stronger laws and more vigorous law enforcement.

I don't mean to imply that everyone who promotes quack ideas is deliberately trying to mislead people. One reason why quackery is so difficult to spot is that most people who spread health misinformation hold sincere beliefs. For them nutrition is not a science but a religion—with quacks as their gurus. But where health is concerned, sincerity is not enough!

Supplement Bill Passes

Stephen Barrett

Stephen Barrett, M.D., is the founder of *Nutrition Forum* and a board member of the National Council Against Health Fraud. The drive for DSHEA passage is described in more detail in *The Vitamin Pushers* (Prometheus Books, 1994), which was reviewed in the previous issue of *NF*. A copy of the Act plus the Congressional Research Service's 14-page report on DSHEA are available for $5 from LVCAHF, P.O. Box 1747, Allentown, PA 18105.

The Dietary Supplement Health and Education Act (DSHEA) of 1994, purported to "assure consumers access to all supplements on the market as long as they are not unsafe," was signed by President Clinton on October 25. Passage capped an aggressive three-year lobbying campaign by the health food industry, whose intention had been to cripple FDA regulation of its products. Senator Orrin Hatch (R-UT) had championed the bill, an early version of which *The New York Times* had described as "The 1993 Snake Oil Protection Act."

Three industry-related groups led the drive for passage: (1) the Nutritional Health Alliance (NHA), an umbrella organization formed early in 1992, which coordinated all segments of the supplement industry; (2) the National Nutritional Foods Association (NNFA), the major trade association of supplement manufacturers, distributors, and retailers; and (3) Citizens for Health (CFH), a "consumer" group organized by Alexander Schauss. The most active opposing force was the Center for Science in the Public Interest (CSPI), a consumer-protection group concerned with accurate labeling of nutritional products.

To support their legislative agenda, proponents generated mail and phone calls from manufacturers, retailers, and distributors of health foods; patrons of health food stores; customers of mail-order companies; multilevel-marketing distributors; "natural health" practitioners; and bodybuilding and fitness enthusiasts who use supplements. This outpouring of messages was represented as a grassroots effort by consumers who wished to preserve "freedom of choice." Most of the barrage, however, came from supplement sellers and their confused customers.

To mobilize their troops, NHA and its allies harped on two themes: (1) if sellers don't act, most of them will be put out of business; and (2) if consumers don't protest, the FDA will deprive them of their right to buy vitamins. To fire up consumers, the coalition portrayed the FDA as a Gestapo-like agency and urged supplement users to "write to Congress today or kiss your vitamins goodbye!" NHA even claimed, falsely, that "if the FDA has its way, you will have to go to a doctor for prescriptions for many supplements and then pay $80 for a supplement which presently costs $10 at a health food store." Many stores set up a "political action center" that displayed sample letters and stationery with which customers could write their own letters. Some stores offered discounts as an incentive to potential letter-writers. Many held a "blackout day," during which they exhibited empty shelves, draped "endangered" products in black and refused to sell them, or conducted other publicity stunts to reinforce their message. Virtually every periodical philosophically aligned with the health food industry published articles and editorials urging readers to write their legislators on this issue. Hundreds of radio talk shows, many with supplement companies among their sponsors, served as vehicles for health food industry propaganda. Several groups organized fax campaigns as well. As pressure from constituents mounted, a majority of Congressional representatives became co-sponsors of Hatch's bill or a similar one in the House.

The Senate passed a version of Hatch's bill on August 13, but Representative Henry Waxman (D-CA) prevented consideration by the House until Hatch agreed to make certain concessions. According to *Health Foods Business*, during the final two weeks of the Congressional session, CFH set up a toll-free number whereby members could call the Capitol switchboard. According to Alexander Schauss, House majority leader Richard Gephart received over ten thousand phone calls on the issue and "other Congressmen complained that constituents were jamming their confidential fax machines with letters imploring them to pass the bill." The final "compromise" still favors the supplement industry.

Pandora's Pillbox?

DSHEA defines the term "dietary supplement," places the burden of proof of safety on the FDA, sets standards for the distribution of third-party literature, allows statements regarding "nutritional support" under certain circumstances, gives specifications for label information on ingredients and nutrients, and requires good manufacturing practices. It also mandates the establishment of an advisory commission and an office

From *Nutrition Forum* newsletter, January/February 1995, pp. 9-11. Reprinted by permission of *Nutrition Forum* newsletter, now published by Prometheus Books, 59 Glenn Drive, Amherst, NY 14228.

within the National Institutes of Health (NIH), both of which are discussed below. DSHEA's main provisions are:

- DSHEA defines "dietary supplement" as any product except tobacco that contains at least one of the following: (1) a vitamin, (2) a mineral, (3) an herb or botanical, (4) an amino acid, (5) a dietary substance "for use to supplement the diet by increasing total dietary intake," or (6) any concentrate, metabolite, constituent, extract, or combination of any of the aforementioned ingredients. Products that meet this definition are excluded from regulation as a drug or food additive. (Drugs and food additives require premarket approval.) The 5th category apparently includes virtually any substance a manufacturer chooses to call a supplement. This provision is bad because it enables manufacturers to market large numbers of worthless substances as long as no direct health claims are made for them. (The claims, of course, will reach consumers through other channels.)

- The burden of proving safety is shifted from the manufacturers to the FDA. The FDA can object only if a product or ingredient presents a "significant and unreasonable risk of illness or injury" or poses an imminent safety hazard. DSHEA does not define "unreasonable risk"; defining it might require lengthy litigation. Before DSHEA, the FDA could ban worthless "dietary supplements" by regulating them as "unapproved food additives."

- Third-party literature can be used to promote supplements to consumers if: (1) they are not false or misleading; (2) they do not promote a particular manufacturer or brand; (3) they are presented with other items on the same subject, so as to provide "a balanced view of the available scientific information"; and (4) they are physically separated from supplement products when displayed in a store. In any proceeding to establish that such material is misleading, the FDA would bear the burden of proof. The terms "misleading" and "balanced" are not defined. Even if they were, there is no provision for enforcing the requirement that the information meet any standard. Nor does the FDA have the resources to monitor what takes place in individual stores. This provision greatly weakens the ability of the FDA to protect consumers from unsubstantiated claims used to sell products. In the past, promotional literature was considered a form of labeling, and therapeutic claims in such literature would render the product a "drug" subject to enforcement. If a dispute arose, it was the manufacturer's obligation to prove that experts generally considered the product safe and effective for its intended purposes.

- A claim may be made for a dietary supplement in the following forms: (1) a claim of benefit related to a classical nutrient deficiency that discloses the prevalence of such disease in the United States, (2) an accurate description of how a nutrient affects the structure or function of the human body, and (3) a general description of well-being resulting from consumption of a dietary ingredient. The statement must be truthful, not misleading, and accompanied by a prominently displayed disclaimer: "This statement has not been evaluated by the Food and Drug Administration. This product is not intended to diagnose, treat, cure, or prevent any disease." This provision may enable manufacturers to flood the market with misleading statements about the function of nutrients in the body. (For example, a statement about the role of vitamin A in eye function, even if it is literally true, would be misleading if it implies that taking vitamin A supplements improves the vision of well-nourished persons.) DSHEA requires that manufacturers submit "structure/function" statements to the FDA within 30 days after first using them for marketing, but substantiation is not required. The FDA probably won't have the resources to challenge misleading claims of this type, and even if misleading claims are withdrawn, they will have been permitted to influence consumer purchases for significant periods of time.

DSHEA requires an independent Commission on Dietary Supplement Labels, composed of seven members with expertise and experience in the manufacture, regulation, distribution, and use of dietary supplements. At least three members must be "qualified by scientific training and experience to evaluate the benefits to health of the use of dietary supplements." However, members and staff of the Commission must be "without bias in the issue of dietary supplements." According to DSHEA, the Commission will review claims and statements about dietary supplements and make nonbinding recommendations for regulating the claims and statements, including those in marketing literature. The Commission's report is due in two years, and subsequent rule-making must be completed within two years after the report is made. If it is not, the FDA dietary supplement regulations published on January 4, 1994, would be nullified.

DSHEA further calls for the establishment of an Office of Dietary Supplements within the NIH to: (1) explore the potential role of dietary supplements in the improvement of healthcare; (2) promote the scientific study of supplements for maintaining health and preventing chronic disease and other health-related conditions; (3) advise other federal agencies; (4) compile a database of scientific research related to dietary supplements and individual nutrients; and (5) coordinate NIH funding related to research on dietary supplements. The Act authorizes $5 million for fiscal year 1994 to enable the Office to carry out its functions. Proponents of alternative healthcare have trumpeted the establishment of the NIH Office of Alternative Medicine as "government and scientific recognition" of their methods. Undoubtedly, the NIH supplement office will be abused in the same way by supplement promoters. And it appears that Senators Hatch and Tom Harkin (D-IA) are planning to promote additional pro-quackery legislation when Congress reconvenes.

Supplements Are Unnecessary to Enhance Athletic Performance

Dr. Stephen Barrett

MORE THAN A HUNDRED companies are marketing phony "ergogenic aids" — combinations of various vitamins, minerals, amino acids and other "dietary supplements" — claimed to build muscles and/or enhance athletic performance. In 1991, researchers from the U.S. Centers for Disease Control and Prevention surveyed 12 popular health and bodybuilding magazines (one issue each) and found ads for 89 brands and 311 products with a total of 235 unique ingredients. *Health*

nent. (Actually, it is water.) These protein beliefs were further reinforced during the 1930s by Bob Hoffman (1899-1985) and later by Joe Weider (1923-), both of whom published magazines that catered to bodybuilders and weightlifters. They asserted that athletes have special protein needs, that protein supplements have special muscle-building and health-giving powers and that the most efficient way to get enough protein is by using supplements. The scientific facts are otherwise. Muscle-building is

misleading claims. In 1960, the company was charged with misbranding its *Energol Germ Oil Concentrate* because literature accompanying the oil falsely claimed that it could prevent or treat more than 120 diseases and conditions, including epilepsy, gallstones and arthritis. In 1961, 15 other York Barbell products were seized as misbranded. In 1968, a larger number of products came under attack by the government for similar reasons. In 1972, the FDA seized three types of York Barbell protein supplements, charging that they were misbranded with false and misleading bodybuilding claims. In 1974, the company was again charged with misbranding *Energol* and protein supplements. The oil had been claimed to be a special source of vigor and energy. False bodybuilding claims had been made for the protein supplements.

> **More than a hundred companies are marketing phony "ergogenic aids" — combinations of various vitamins, minerals, amino acids and other "dietary supplements" — claimed to build muscles and/or enhance athletic performance.**

Foods Business estimated that in 1993, total sales of such products through health-food stores exceeded $130 million. They are also sold through pharmacies and superstores.

Roots of "Ergogenic" Mythology

The notion that massive amounts of protein are necessary during training has evolved from the ancient belief that great strength could be obtained by eating the raw meat of lions, tigers or other animals that displayed great fighting strength. Today, although few athletes consume raw meat, the idea that "you are what you eat" is still widely promoted by food faddists.

During the early 1900s, when muscles were discovered to contain protein, athletes and coaches mistakenly concluded that protein was the principal compo-

not caused by eating extra protein. It is stimulated by increased muscular work. Once basic protein needs have been met, the small additional amount needed during intense training is easily obtainable from a balanced diet. Few Americans fail to consume adequate amounts of protein.

Hoffman marketed supplement products and bodybuilding equipment through his York Barbell Company of York, PA. A prolific writer, he published two magazines and more than 30 books on fitness and nutrition. For many years, York Barbell's nutritional products were promoted with false and

Despite his many brushes with the law, Hoffman achieved considerable professional prominence. During his athletic career, first as an oarsman and then as a weightlifter, he received over 600 trophies, certificates and awards. He was the Olympic weightlifting coach from 1936 to 1968 and was a founding member of the President's Council on Physical Fitness and Sports.

Weider began bodybuilding as a teenager and was 16 when he launched a newsletter called *Your Physique*. A few years later, he started a company that sold bodybuilding equipment and instructional booklets through the mail.

From *Priorities*, Vol. 6, No. 3, 1994, pp. 23-25. © 1994 by Stephen Barrett. Reprinted by permission.

In 1946, Joe's brother Ben joined the business and they set up the International Federation of Bodybuilders, which promotes the sport worldwide and sponsors competitions. According to press reports, their business empire, Weider Health & Fitness, now grosses over $500 million annually.

The company is the dominant player in the sports-supplement marketplace. It publishes four magazines, sells bodybuilding equipment, broadcasts "Muscle Magazine" on ESPN and sponsors many athletic and aerobic events throughout the year. The magazines are *Muscle & Fitness*, *Shape*, *Flex* and *Men's Fitness*. The supplements include *Anabolic Mega-Pak*, *Dynamic Life Essence*, *Dynamic Super Stress-End*, *Dynamic Power Source*, *Dynamic Driving Force*, *Dynamic Fat Burners*, *Dynamic Liver Concentrate Energizer*, *Dynamic Sustained Endurance*, *Dynamic Recupe*, *Dynamic Body Shaper* and *Dynamic Muscle Builder*. None of these products appears capable of doing what its name suggests, and none contains any nutrients not readily obtainable from a balanced diet.

In 1984, the FTC charged that ads for *Anabolic Mega-Pak* (containing amino acids, minerals, vitamins and herbs) and *Dynamic Life Essence* (an amino acid product) had been misleading. The FTC complaint was settled in 1985 when Weider and the company agreed not to falsely claim that these products can help build muscles or are effective substitutes for anabolic steroids. They also agreed to pay a minimum of $400,000 in refunds or (if refunds did not reach this figure) to fund research on the relationship of nutrition to muscle development. Although the forbidden claims no longer appear in Weider ads, similar messages appear in articles in the magazines and are implied by endorsements and pictures of muscular athletes as well as by the names of the products themselves. False and misleading claims also appear in a series of 18 booklets published in 1990 by Weider Health & Fitness and marketed through GNC stores.

The Marketplace Expands

During the 1970s, in addition to protein supplements and assorted vitamins, the main products touted to athletes were wheat germ oil and bee pollen (falsely claimed to boost energy and endurance). In the early 1980s, Weider Health & Fitness introduced an "Olympians" line said to have been developed by working closely with "Olympians and nutritional researchers." Most were sustained-release vitamin concoctions that included an exotic ingredient or two. As public interest in fitness grew, several drug companies began falsely claiming that multivitamin or "stress" supplements were just what active people needed.

Following the publication in 1982 of *Life Extension*, by Durk Pearson and Sandy Shaw, the authors appeared on hundreds of radio and television talk shows. The book claimed that supplements of certain amino acids would cause the body to release growth hormone, which would produce muscle growth and fat loss with little or no effort. These claims were based on faulty extrapolations of experiments in which animals were given large doses of these amino acids by injection. Swallowing amino acids does not cause humans to release growth hormone, but the massive publicity garnered by Pearson and Shaw inspired the health-food industry to market hundreds of new products for athletes and would-be dieters. Many of these products are falsely claimed to be "natural steroids" or "steroid substitutes." In the years since, scores of other useless ingredients have been marketed as "ergogenic aids."

Some manufacturers make no claims in their ads but imply them in product names. Many use pictures of athletes to convey their messages. Some make explicit claims in their ads or product literature, while other use simple puffery. Several have published charts suggesting which products are good for specific purposes. Some even market products for specific sports.

Calling the bodybuilding supplement industry "an economic hoax with unhealthy consequences," the New York City Department of Consumer Affairs urged the FDA and FTC to stop the "blatantly drug-like claims" and false advertising used to promote these products.

Simple Truths

Athletes who eat a balanced diet don't need extra protein or vitamins. In *The Complete Sports Medicine Book for Women*, sports medicine specialist Gabe Mirkin, M.D., and gynecologist Mona Shangold, M.D., explain why:

You don't need much extra protein even to enlarge your muscles. For example, one pound of muscle contains only about 100 grams of protein, since it is composed of more than 72 percent water. So if you are gaining one pound of muscle every week in an excellent strength training program, you are adding only about 100 grams of protein each week, or about 15 grams of protein each day. Two cups of corn and beans will meet this need

— far less than you would expect…. Requirements for only four vitamins increase with exercise: thiamin, niacin, riboflavin, and pantothenic acid. These vitamins are used up minimally in the breakdown of carbohydrates and, to a small degree, protein for energy. But you will find them abundantly in food…. Furthermore, deficiencies of these vitamins have never been reported in athletes.

What about other products? The most thorough investigation has been conducted by David Lightsey, an exercise physiologist and nutritionist who coordinates the National Council Against Health Fraud's Task Force on Ergogenic Aids. During the past four years, he has telephoned more than 80 companies that market "ergogenic aids." In a recent interview, Lightsey told me:

> In each case, I told a company representative that I had been asked to collect data on the company's product(s) and issue a formal report. After they described the alleged benefits, I would ask how data supporting these claims were collected. As my questions became more specific, their responses became more vague. Some said they could not be more specific because they did not wish to reveal trade secrets.
>
> I ended each interview with a request for written documentation. Fewer than half sent anything. Most of the studies they sent were poorly designed and proved nothing. The few that were well designed did not support product claims but were taken out of context. Some companies claimed that one team or another was using their products. In each such case, I contacted the team management and learned that although one or more players used the company's products, the management had neither endorsed the products nor encouraged their use.

Lightsey believes there are two reasons why many athletes believe that various products have helped them: (1) use of the product often coincides with natural improvement due to training, and (2) increased self-confidence or a placebo effect inspires greater performance. Any such "psychological benefit," however, should be weighed against the dangers of misinformation, wasted money, misplaced faith and adverse physical effects — both known and unknown — that can result from megadoses of nutrients. Moreover, how many people who are involved in fitness programs or recreational sports *need* a placebo for inspiration?

More Enforcement Action Is Needed

Little government effort has been made to protect consumers from wasting money on "sports nutrient" products. The FTC did take the action noted above against Weider Health & Fitness, the market leader. In 1986, the agency acted against A.H. Robins and its subsidiary, the Viobin Corporation, which had been making false claims for wheat germ oil products for more than 15 years. The case was settled with a consent agreement prohibiting claims that the oil could help consumers improve endurance, stamina, vigor or other aspects of athletic fitness; or that its active ingredient "octacosanol" is related in any way to body reaction time, oxygen uptake, oxygen debt or athletic performance.

In 1992, the New York City Department of Consumer Affairs (DCA) published a report called *Magic Muscle Pills!! Health and Fitness Quackery in Nutrition Supplements*. DCA investigators found that manufacturers they contacted for information about their products were unable to provide a single published report from a scientific journal to back the claims that their products could benefit athletes.

Along with its report, DCA issued "Notices of Violation" to six companies whose products it had investigated. It also warned consumers to beware of terms like "fat burner," "fat fighter," "fat metabolizer," "energy enhancer," "performance booster," "strength booster," "ergogenic aid," "anabolic optimizer" and "genetic optimizer." Calling the bodybuilding supplement industry "an economic hoax with unhealthy consequences," DCA officials urged the FDA and FTC to stop the "blatantly drug-like claims" and false advertising used to promote these products.

In 1994, the FTC reached a consent agreement under which General Nutrition, Inc.,* paid $2.4 million dollars to settle charges that it had falsely advertised 41 products, most of which had been packaged by other manufacturers. The products included Weider's *Super Fat Burners*, 11 other "muscle builders," and five other phony "ergogenic aids." No action was taken against the other manufacturers, but the FTC's staff is well aware that the "sports nutrition" marketplace needs cleaning up.

STEPHEN BARRETT, M.D., A RETIRED PSYCHIATRIST, IS CO-AUTHOR/EDITOR OF 36 BOOKS. HIS LATEST WORK, CO-AUTHORED BY VICTOR HERBERT, M.D., J.D., IS *THE VITAMIN PUSHERS: HOW THE HEALTH-FOOD INDUSTRY IS SELLING AMERICA A BILL OF GOODS*. IN 1984 HE RECEIVED THE FDA COMMISSIONER'S SPECIAL CITATION AWARD FOR PUBLIC SERVICE IN FIGHTING NUTRITION QUACKERY.

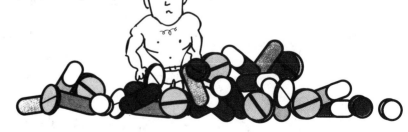

Nutrition Shortcut in a Can?

THE STORY

A recent barrage of advertising implies that we could all use a Boost to Ensure we're getting our dietary ReSources or meeting our daily Nutri-Needs. According to the high-profile ads, meals in a can with names like these will help keep us healthy and active and, by improving nutrition, will help ward off the ravages of aging. Here's an example: "Sustacal can't add years to your life, but it may add life to your years." Ads for Boost show fit fortysomethings drinking nutritional supplements to "fill in the blanks" because they skipped a meal or are working too hard.

Ensure, the granddaddy of nutrient supplements, was originally developed for use in hospitals and nursing homes for people who were too sick or too weak to eat. But thanks to an aggressive marketing campaign, it is now being sold in grocery stores and pharmacies. Skyrocketing demand has spawned a bevy of competitors. The *Wall Street Journal* reports that sales of these canned nutritional supplements grew 49 percent in both 1994 and 1995, topping $400 million last year.

Just what can you get from downing one of these supplements? As the table shows, they all contain protein, carbohydrates, vitamins, and minerals, and most contain some fat. A single can costs between $1 and $2. Drinking three cans of Ensure a day (that's what its label suggests) would cost about $1,500 per year.

We asked the chief of surgical nutrition at the New England Deaconess Hospital to discuss the pluses and minuses of meals in a can and to describe who really needs them.
— *The Editors*

THE PHYSICIAN'S PERSPECTIVE

George Blackburn, MD

Thirty years ago, it was not uncommon for cancer patients or people who had undergone surgery to starve to death in hospitals, either because they could not eat or because their illnesses obliterated their appetites. Medical researchers across the country were trying to determine the special nutritional needs of these patients, and whether it was best to deliver nutrients intravenously — into the bloodstream — or through small tubes directly into the stomach or intestines.

Back in 1974, some colleagues and I wrote an article for the *Journal of the American Medical Association* on the causes of malnutrition in hospitalized patients and the critical need for new treatments. Soon after it was published, I was invited to speak on this topic at Ross Laboratories, a leading baby-food maker. Ross researchers were then trying to make a complete "formula" for sick adults. They ultimately came up with Ensure. A person could drink it, or it could be delivered to the digestive system via a small tube.

Because this product was sold as a specialty food, it did not have to go through the extensive and expensive testing process the Food and Drug Administration requires for drugs. And it could also be marketed directly to consumers without the fine print that accompanies ads for prescription drugs.

In the beginning, Ensure and its competitors were sold primarily to hospitals and nursing homes. For people who could

WHAT'S IN THOSE CANS?					
	Boost	Sustacal HP	ReSource	Ensure	NutraStart
Calories	240	240	180	250	210
Total fat	4 g (6%)	6 g (9%)	0	9 g (14%)	2.5 g (4%)
Saturated fat	0.5 g (3%)	1 g (5%)	0	1.5 g (8%)	0.5 g (3%)
Sodium	130 mg (5%)	220 mg (9%)	55 mg (2%)	200 mg (8%)	350 mg (15%)
Total carbohydrates	40 g (13%)	33 g (11%)	36 g (12%)	34 g (11%)	38 g (13%)
Fiber	0	<1 g (<4%)	0	<1 g (<4%)	5 g (20%)
Protein	10 g (20%)	15 g (30%)	9 g (18%)	9 g (18%)	10 g (20%)
Vitamin A	15%	20%	15%	15%	50%
Vitamin C	100%	20%	60%	60%	100%
Vitamin D	25%	20%	15%	15%	25%
Vitamin E	100%	20%	20%	20%	100%
Folate	35%	20%	15%	25%	25%
Iron	20%	20%	15%	15%	20%
Calcium	30%	20%	15%	15%	50%

% = % of Recommended Dietary Allowance

not eat, these products were a godsend and saved thousands of lives. But, as hospital stays shortened, and more people began receiving medical care as outpatients or at home, the makers of nutritional supplements began selling them over the counter. People with AIDS turned to meal replacements in an effort to counter the severe wasting that accompanies this disease. In fact, the meal replacement called Advera is specially designed for people who are HIV positive.

In an effort to broaden their market, manufacturers are no longer limiting their sales pitch to people who are ill or who cannot eat. They are now targeting everyone from frail senior citizens to fit, healthy baby boomers.

Some people can clearly benefit from meal replacements:

◆ People over age 50 who have a chronic illness accompanied by weight loss, weakness, and fatigue, and who are eating fewer than three meals a day.

◆ People who have trouble swallowing or chewing.

◆ People eager to recover from an illness and regain their strength and stamina so they can get back to work or to their normal activities.

◆ People who eat alone, and thus often eat poorly, or those who don't have the money to buy the healthy food they need.

What about people who aren't sick? According to several national surveys, five out of six Americans do not eat three meals a day, and nine out of 10 don't eat breakfast. These meal replacement products actually do represent a reasonable choice for people on the go who skip meals or eat junk food in place of a healthy meal.

Spending $1.50 for a breakfast consisting of a canned meal replacement certainly makes better nutritional sense than spending $2.00 for a cafe latte. A can of Ensure offers 250 calories, nine grams of protein, nine grams of fat, and a dozen or so vitamins and minerals. The best thing is that it requires no preparation. To get the nutritional equivalent of a can of Ensure from food, you would have to eat a bowl of cereal with fruit and low-fat milk, plus a piece of toast, or a cup of yogurt with a piece of fruit and a whole-grain muffin. In each case, you'd have to take a multi-vitamin tablet too.

But real food has benefits the meal replacements just can't offer. Most don't include any fiber, which is known to help prevent colorectal cancer and may lower cholesterol levels (see *HN*, February 13 and March 26). And despite being fortified with several vitamins and minerals, meal replacements don't contain micronutrients such as isoflavones, carotenoids, and other plant-derived compounds that maintain health and prevent disease.

Certainly, drinking a canned supplement in place of the occasional skipped meal is better than eating junk food or fat-saturated fast food. But in the long run, there are no shortcuts to healthful eating — a can a day won't keep the doctor away. The smart consumer will design his or her own prescription for a healthy, realistic lifestyle, ideally in concert with a registered dietitian or certified nutritionist. In addition to a healthy diet, this lifestyle will include plenty of physical activity and several different strategies for managing stress.

Dr. Blackburn is director of nutrition support services at New England Deaconess Hospital and vice president-elect of the North American Society for the Study of Obesity.

HERBAL ROULETTE

The makers of these 'natural' remedies don't have to prove they work, and they don't have to prove they're safe. You have to be very careful.

The bottles, lined up neatly on a shelf, promise botanical wonders from around the world: Bilberry extract. The fruit of cayenne pepper. Korean ginseng. Valerian root. Yucca stalk. Nearby hangs a laminated card, describing the benefits of each—dong quai root to normalize women's systems, milk thistle extract for healthy liver function.

The shelf, despite what you might think, is not in the back aisle of a health-food store. The products are lined up right next to the vitamin C capsules and calcium tablets at a brightly lit CVS store, part of one of the country's largest drugstore chains. And you could find similar products at your local SavOn, Thrifty, or Eckerd. Roughly one drugstore in ten now carries a large line of herbs; others stock at least garlic and ginseng.

Encouraged by widespread interest and greatly relaxed Federal laws, sales of "natural" herbal remedies are growing by an estimated 15 percent a year, and now total $1.5-billion, almost half the amount spent on "regular" vitamins and minerals. These products now are classified as "dietary supplements," a grouping that includes plant extracts, enzymes, minerals, and at least one hormone—the very popular melatonin.

The products range from ground-up herbs you probably never heard of (Kava Kava root) to nationally advertised brands (*Ginsana* ginseng and *One-A-Day* garlic.) The pills can cost $20 a bottle. Some consist of a single traditional medicinal herb, like feverfew. But others mix a handful: The ingredients of a supplement called *Up Your Gas,* a supposed energy-booster, include ginseng, spirulina, bee pollen, royal jelly, ma huang, guarana, wheat grass, gotu kola, and cayenne pepper.

Many people have good reason to be interested in plant products that might improve their health. A number of studies have shown that certain herbs may help people with conditions ranging from headaches to high cholesterol (see "Herbs that Might Help"). Some supplements might even have the potential to become the next quinine, aspirin, or digitalis—all drugs that were originally derived from plants.

But if you do decide you want to give herbal medicine a try, you face a formidable obstacle: The supplement marketplace is a shambles. There is no guarantee that the pills are what they say they are—and in most cases no one really knows what will happen if you take them. You have no way to be sure:

□ Whether a plant's active ingredients, whatever they might be, have actually ended up in the herbal pills you buy.

□ Whether a supplement's ingredients are in a form your body can use.

□ Whether the dosage makes any sense.

□ What else is in the pills.

□ Whether the pills are safe.

□ Whether the next bottle of those same pills will have the same ingredients.

Even the manufacturers may not know those things; they're not required to do the testing or quality control that are routine for regular drugs. In this marketplace, its hard to know what to trust. Varro E. Tyler of Purdue University, a leading expert in plant medicines, has written that much of what surrounds herbal medicine in the U.S. is "a minefield of hyperbole and hoax."

An unregulated market

This throwback to the days before drug standards and regulation comes to you courtesy of Congress, whose efforts last year to loosen up the regulations for traditional herbs have opened up a loophole big enough to be exploited by anyone with a pill-making machine and an eye for clever marketing.

For years the U.S. Food and Drug Administration did not quite know what to do about products like these. While prescription and over-the-counter drugs must be proven safe and effective, and foods need to meet manufacturing standards and be safe to consume, there was no place in the rule book for most plant products that claim medicinal effects; they fell somewhere between foods and drugs. So for decades there was an uneasy standoff. The FDA sometimes seized supplements on the grounds that they were unapproved food additives or unapproved drugs. But in general, the agency tolerated quiet sales of herbal remedies as long as manufacturers labeled them only as nutritional supplements and didn't mention medicinal uses.

"If a brand simply listed a dosage or contraindictations on the label, it could trigger drug law," said John B. Cordaro, head of the Council for Responsible Nutrition, a trade group representing the larger vitamin and supplement companies. Some manufacturers avoided that problem by simply giving their products suggestive names like "Sleep and Get Trim" and "PMS."

To promote their products, many manufacturers counted on word of mouth or on pamphlets about the medicinal benefits of various supplements—displayed nearby in the health-food store.

Then, in mid-1993, fresh from overhauling the nation's food labels, the FDA decided to turn to supplements—in 11 dense pages in the Federal Register, an "advance notice of proposed rulemaking." It was dry bureaucratese—peppered with reports of deaths, poisonings, and medical mayhem attributed to vitamins, herbs, and other supplements. The subtext: Stricter regulation needed.

That touched off a multimillion-dollar industry campaign urging Americans to "Write to Congress today—or kiss your supplements good-bye!" The country's 10,000 health-food stores became beachheads in virtually every Congressional district—with handbills, petitions, and discounts offered to letter-writers. Almost half of Americans take supplements, at least occasionally, so Congress was deluged—with four million letters and faxes, by one count.

The result—the Dietary Supplement and Health Education Act of 1994—created a new category, distinct from food or drugs, that is nearly immune to the rules the FDA once used against questionable products. The new category is quite broad; it includes vitamins, minerals, herbs, amino acids, and practically anything else that had been sold as a "supplement" before October 15, 1994. There may be 20,000 such products; no one keeps count.

Here's what the law allows:

Products can go to market with no testing for efficacy. That skips the years-long, research-laden process that drugs are subjected to.

Companies don't have to prove that their products now on the market are safe. Before, a supplement maker had to prove its product safe if the FDA challenged it. Now the burden has shifted to the FDA, to prove the produce *unsafe*. The maker must merely provide "reasonable assurance" that no ingredient "present[s] a significant or unreasonable risk of illness or injury."

Supplements need not be manufactured according to any standards. Federal standards—even the basics of quality control—won't be introduced for at least two years.

Claims are permitted on the packages. Supplements still may not claim to cure or prevent a *disease*, but labels may detail how a supplement affects the body's "structure or function," as long as claims are "truthful and nonmisleading." Thus, saw palmetto, an herb, can't be sold with the promise that it will cure an enlarged prostate, but the label may say it will "improve urinary flow" in older men—or say simply that it's "for the prostate."

Label statements might not have much evidence behind them. The new law simply says that manufacturers must have "substantiation" in hand. (That hasn't been defined.) And they need not show their evidence unless their label claims are challenged by regulators.

FDA approval is not needed for package or marketing claims. The label does have to say that any claims have not been reviewed or approved by the FDA, but that caveat can be in rather small type.

Though the new law has trans-

GINSENG
MUCH ADO ABOUT NOTHING?

For an example of the triumph of mystique over medicine, it's hard to beat ginseng. This Asian root has, at one time or another, been credited with curing almost everything. In reality, studies of its effects on humans have found almost nothing.

What's more, our own tests of 10 brands of ginseng suggest that manufacturers haven't even agreed on what to put inside.

Ginseng sales are booming. The market leader alone, nationally advertised *Ginsana* brand, now sells Americans 120 million capsules a year. A *Ginsana* radio ad promises "an all-natural supplement shown to help build energy and endurance" and says ginseng will "help your body utilize oxygen."

Those are comparatively modest claims for a root whose botanical name—*Panax ginseng*—has the same origins as "panacea," a cure-all. Ginseng has been called beneficial for stress, hypertension, ulcers, diabetes, atherosclerosis, depression, edema, impaired memory, anemia, and menopause. It's been dubbed a tonic, restorative, aphrodisiac, and life extender.

In the marketplace, confusion about ginseng abounds. *Nature's Resource* bottles say ginseng has been used for over 2000 years. *Rite Aid* says it's been used for over 5000. (What's three millennia among friends?) Some products say they contain raw root powder; others are extracts claiming an optimal balance of "ginsenosides," the root's supposed active ingredients. Still other products contain Siberian ginseng, which is an entirely different plant.

But evidence for ginseng's usefulness is scant. Many studies show that ginseng, often in big doses, affects small animals in interesting ways, but there's little human research—and most is not well controlled. One review calls ginseng "a medical enigma with no proven efficacy for humans." What about *Ginsana's* claims? Thomas Peterson, an executive at the company that distributes *Ginsana*, told us the evidence is a secret. "It is not our policy to release any clinical support behind the product," he said.

But even if ginseng is good for your health, consumers face another hurdle: There's no way to be sure what's in a ginseng supplement. We measured the amount of six ginsenosides in 10 different brands of ginseng. We found a wide variation, from brand to brand, in the pills' total ginsenoside concentration. Some pills had 10 or 20 times as much as others, and one brand had very little ginsenoside.

The labels don't help you tell what's inside. A bottle of *Natural Brand Korean* labeled "648 mg." had 10 times as much ginsenoside per pill as a bottle of *Naturally Korean* that also was labeled "648 mg."

Ginsana did appear to be standardized—single packages from each of three lots had nearly identical ginsenoside profiles. For the other brands, we tested two bottles or packages of each from the same lot. The results may not represent each brand nationwide, but they do show the sort of brand-to-brand variation in content a shopper can expect to encounter.

Inside ginseng Our tests showed that the concentration of total "ginsenoside," the supposed active ingredient, varied greatly among 10 brands of ginseng. Similar variation has been found in other dietary supplements.

Product (listed alphabetically)	Ginseng per capsule [1]	Ginsenosides per capsule [2]	Concentration [2] (percentage ginsenoside)
American Ginseng	250 mg	12.8 mg	
Ginsana (extract)	100	3.0	
Herbal Choice Ginseng-7 (extract)	100	6.5	
KRG Korean Red Ginseng	518	11.5	
Natural Brand Korean Ginseng	648	23.2	
Naturally Korean Ginseng	648	2.3	
Nature's Resource Ginseng	560	10.7	
Rite Aid Imperial Ginseng	250	0.4	
Solgar Korean Ginseng (extract)	520	10.6	
Walgreen's Gin-zing (extract)	100	7.6	

0 1 2 3 4 5 6 7 8%

[1] According to label.
[2] Based on six major ginsenosides. Estimates for two other ginsenosides, if added, would boost totals only slightly and not change variation in concentrations.

formed the rules of the marketplace, few people know it. An analysis by the Congressional Research Service notes that consumers still believe "any product that appears in pill form has been reviewed for safety by the FDA, which is not true for supplements."

Even pharmacists may be confused. When our reporter asked the pharmacist at Duane Reade, a large local drugstore chain, about the value of St. John's wort (a nearby chart said it helped to fight depression), the pharmacist eyed the bottle, assured him, "It probably won't knock you out," and pronounced the contents safe. "It must be," she summed up: "If it's sold over-the-counter, it's FDA approved." Unfortunately, she was wrong.

Which herbs do what?

Marketing aside, it's difficult to find out which supplements even *ought* to help you. There is clear evidence supporting a few herbs and dismissing others. But in most cases the data are slim.

Many herbs have been promoted on the basis of anecdotal accounts, sometimes *centuries* of anecdotes—people attesting that a particular root, leaf, or berry has helped them. The problem with such accounts is that there is no way to tell what would have happened if the person had not taken the remedy. Most ailments are self-limiting. And many more cases are susceptible to the placebo effect: You may feel better as long as you *think* you've taken medicine.

To distinguish real efficacy from the placebo effect, FDA-approved drugs have to rely on the consensus findings of several proper clinical trials. The gold standard of such research is the randomized, double-blind trial. Participants are assigned either to take the drug under study or an ineffective placebo. The study is "blinded": Neither participants nor the researchers are told who got what until the study ends, to rule out any possibility that suggestion might influence the results.

Few supplements can meet that standard. There's little economic incentive for manufacturers to bankroll new studies—you can't patent an herb, to recoup the costs.

No matter how shaky the evidence, supplement makers and promoters often parlay suggestive results into miracle cures. A book on pycnogenol, a derivative of pine bark, is subtitled "the amazing antioxidant that fights arthritis, diabetes and stroke, and promotes prevention of heart disease and cancer." Another tome, titled "Sharks Don't Get Cancer," has helped move countless bottles of shark-cartilage capsules. But the book's thesis—that sharks possess a cancer-protective substance—remains unproved. Besides, sharks *do* get cancer, even in their cartilage.

What if you ask the clerk in the health-food store for advice? The FDA did just that in a 1993 study that sent staffers, under cover, to stores from coast to coast. Some inquired about "anything [for] my immune system." Others asked about "help for high blood pressure," or "something that works on cancer." They asked 129 times in all and got specific recommendations on what to buy 120 times. For cancer, the advice ranged from honeysuckle crystals (in a Sherman Oaks, Calif., store), to shark cartilage (Dearborn, Mich.), to co-enzyme Q10, garlic, and betacarotene (in Louisville, Ky.), to saw palmetto with vitamins (in Rocky Hill, Conn.).

Pharmacists are unlikely to give you such recommendations, but they're often clueless about the supplements sold in their drugstores. Schools of pharmacy usually don't teach courses about the uses of herbal remedies.

Consumers can still count on the Federal Trade Commission, at least, to check false advertising. An FTC lawyer told us the commission intends to go after supplement makers as vigorously as it had before the new supplement act. Last year, for example, the Commission got the corporate parent of GNC, the largest health-food chain in the country, to pay a $2.4-million civil penalty—without admitting any wrongdoing—to settle several years' worth of charges. According to the Commission, GNC had failed to substantiate disease-treatment, weight-loss, muscle-building, and endurance claims for more than 40 products.

What's in the pills?

Knowing what a supplement is supposed to do is just the first hurdle. The second is knowing whether any useful substance made it into the pills.

For starters, individual plants of the same species can differ appreciably in potency. Two such plants can be "as different as two people on a street," says James A. Duke, a U.S. Department of Agriculture botanist and specialist in medicinal plants. In extreme cases, says Duke, differences in some compounds could reach 10,000-fold. Growing conditions, storage, and handling also affect potency.

Some manufacturers are striving to standardize their products. While some companies merely put raw, ground-up plants into capsules, others—who usually identify themselves on their labels—aim for a more consistent product using pharmaceutical methods to make what are called standardized extracts. They remove extraneous matter, assay what's left for the chemicals thought responsible for the herb's action, and mix batches to achieve a consistent strength. They print labels giving details of their pills' composition and even list expiration dates (although it's not clear how they determine those dates).

But even with the best intentions, no one knows for sure the correct formulation for an herbal product. Medicinal plants typically contain a cocktail of compounds, and it's unclear whether it's individual chemicals, or particular combinations of

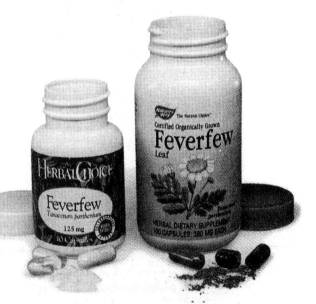

No consistency Herbal Choice feverfew capsules contain a tan powder said to contain 0.2 percent parthenolides, to combat migraine headaches. By contrast, Nature's Way capsules weigh three times as much and hold olive-colored ground-up leaves. Which contains more parthenolides? You can't tell.

WINNERS AND LOSERS IN THE WORLD OF PLANTS

HERBS THAT MIGHT HELP

Anyone who's soothed a toothache with oil of cloves or been jolted to life by coffee knows that plants offer powerful medicine. But with dubious claims being made for so many herbs, some proponents fear the truly promising herbs may be overlooked.

Here are 10 herbs for which there is reasonably strong evidence of beneficial physiological effects, and which appear to merit further study. The list is based on the work of two respected and prominent "pharmacognocists" (specialists in plant medicinals)—Varro Tyler of Purdue University and Norman Farnsworth of the University of Illinois—and on other published medical research.

This is not a recommendation that you buy and use these products. While some—like chamomile and ginger—are innocuous, others should not be relied on for regular medical treatment. Hawthorn, for instance, is no substitute for established heart-disease therapy.

Chamomile Used for indigestion. The tea, from tiny flower-heads, may suppress muscle spasms and cut inflammation in the digestive tract; it's used for menstrual cramps as well. (Topically, chamomile oil or ointment may be applied as an anti-inflammatory, for skin and mucous membrane problems.) A volatile oil is mainly responsible, so the tea must be made from fresh herb—fresh smells like apples; old, like hay—and steeped long enough to release the oil. Peo-

ple allergic to ragweed or flowers in the daisy family could suffer reactions.

Echinacea Used as an immunity booster. Also in the daisy family, this herb was sold as a drug before antibiotics existed. A few controlled trials suggest it can increase resistance to upper respiratory infections, perhaps by stimulating certain white blood cells. Benefits may be lost with continued use, however. May cause reactions among people allergic to the sunflower family.

Feverfew Used for migraine headache. Chewing the leaves is a folk remedy, but may cause mouth sores. A double-blind British study has suggested that feverfew taken daily can cut the occurrence of attacks by one-fourth.

Garlic Used for high cholesterol. Considering only the best-designed of numerous studies, a 1993 analysis showed that the equivalent of one-half to one clove daily could lower cholesterol an average of 9 percent; a similar 1994 "meta-analysis" gave stronger results. It might not work for all people, however. Enteric-coated pills, which dissolve in the intestine, cut odor and improve the absorption of allicin, apparently a key ingredient. Too much garlic can hinder blood clotting, so people on anticoagulants should be wary.

Ginger Used for nausea. Double-blind research shows that taking ginger before traveling can prevent motion sickness. This root can quell other nausea as well. Crystallized ginger, a confection sold in Oriental food markets, works too. No side effects have been noted with therapeutic dosages, but there's potential to inhibit clotting.

Ginkgo biloba Used for circulation. Enhances blood flow to the brain, according to a review of several published studies. For the elderly, that supposedly can improve concentration and memory, absent-mindedness, headaches, and tinnitus, a ringing in the ears. May also aid circulation to legs, to relieve painful cramps.

Hawthorn Used for heart disease. Substances in the fruit, leaves, and flowers dilate blood vessels and lower blood pressure. It relaxes smooth muscle in coronary vessels and thus may help avoid angina. Should not be used without consulting a doctor.

Milk thistle Used for liver damage. This plant's small, hard fruits have been shown to protect the liver against a variety of toxins. Human trials called "encouraging" for hepatitis, cirrhosis. Standardized extracts concentrate silymarin, a substance that apparently prevents the membrane of undamaged liver cells from letting toxins enter. Should not be used without consulting a doctor.

Saw palmetto Used for enlarged prostate. Was prescribed for a variety of urogenital ailments until 1950. Several studies suggest the extract can improve urinary flow in men with benign prostate enlargement. Also shows anti-inflammatory effects. Slows conversion of testosterone into a more active form that enlarges the gland.

Valerian Used for sleep problems. May have mild sedating and tranquilizing effects. Probably depresses brain centers and relaxes smooth muscle directly. May be used as tea, tincture (alcohol-based solution), or extract in capsules. The most unpleasant aspect may be its odor, like old socks or sharp cheese.

HERBS THAT CAN HARM

The U.S. Food and Drug Administration has identified a number of herbs that can cause serious harm. Some, including these five, are still being sold under various brand names.

Chaparral Sold as tea, tablet, and capsule and promoted as a blood purifier, cancer cure, acne treatment, and natural antioxidant. Has caused at least six cases of acute nonviral hepatitis (rapidly developing liver damage) in North America; one patient required a transplant. Sometimes an ingredient in combination-herb formulas.

Comfrey Sold as tea, tablet, capsule, tincture, poultice, and lotion. In the past decade, comfrey taken orally has been linked to at least seven cases of obstructed blood flow from the liver, with potential for cirrhosis (scarring); one person died. A woman's drinking comfrey tea when pregnant is suspected in her newborn's liver disease. Animal studies show lung, kidney, and

gastrointestinal problems are also possible. Four countries (Australia, Canada, Germany, and Great Britain) restrict comfrey's availability.

Ephedra Also called ma huang and sometimes epitonin. Contains the stimulants ephedrine and pseudoephedrine, found in asthma drugs and in decongestants. Promoted for weight-control and in energy-boosting formulas, sometimes with caffeine, which can augment the adverse effects. Can raise blood pressure and cause palpitations, nerve damage, muscle injury, psychosis, stroke, and memory loss. Several states limit sales, for instance by putting it behind pharmacists' counters. Last year, Ohio restricted all ephedrine products, including ma huang, after the death of a high-school student who'd taken an over-the-counter ephedrine product. Texas is moving in that direction, after the death of a woman who'd used an ephedra-and-caffeine herbal supplement. In August, a coalition of state drug regulators wrote to the FDA asking the agency to limit ma huang to prescription use only.

Lobelia This "Indian tobacco" acts like nicotine, though it's less potent. It can both stimulate and depress the autonomic nervous system. In low doses, lobelia dilates the lungs' bronchi and steps up breathing. As little as 50 milligrams of dried lobelia (less than a capsule) can bring on these reactions. Larger amounts could reduce breathing, drop blood pressure, induce sweating and a rapid heart beat, and cause coma and death.

Yohimbe From the bark of an African tree. Sold as a men's aphrodisiac. Its active compound, yohimbine, is a prescription drug sometimes used to treat impotence but probably is ineffective. (One medical review calls the evidence for yohimbine's efficacy "sparce and inconclusive.") An overdose can cause serious problems: weakness and nervous stimulation, followed by paralysis, fatigue, stomach disorders, and ultimately death. Georgia has branded yohimbine a "dangerous drug" and forbids selling even yohimbe herb without prescription.

them, that have the desired therapeutic effect. The result is a hodgepodge of products that consumers cannot sensibly compare.

Several studies have demonstrated the chaos that results from a lack of industry standards.

☐ Our tests of 10 ginseng supplements found wide variations in composition; the details are on page 699.

☐ Other tests of the ginseng content of 50 products, published last year in The Lancet, a British medical journal, found a few "ginseng" supplements that contained no ginseng at all.

☐ The Center for Science in the Public Interest, a consumer group, reported this year on its tests of several brands of garlic pills. Allicin, a compound purported to be the active cholesterol-lowering ingredient, varied more than 40-fold among brands. And the cost of a clove's worth of allicin varied from $2 down to 6 cents (for a garlic powder off the spice rack).

☐ The National Organization for Rare Disorders tested 12 brands of L-carnitine, a supplement crucial for people with a deadly metabolic disease. Carnitine is also sold to bodybuilders, supposedly to help them add muscle. Two brands offered no detectable carnitine, and another's pills varied, containing from 20 percent to 85 percent of the labeled quantity. A few other brands also showed wide pill-to-pill discrepancies—or their pills didn't disintegrate in a test simulating what occurs in the stomach.

"If there were standards for each herb," says Varro Tyler of Purdue, "it would put a lot of companies out of business."

Eventually, according to the new supplement act, the FDA must specify minimal quality controls. Standards will likely include protections from filth, methods for determining potency, and overall quality assurance—pills must contain what's listed on the label. Rules may also cover packaging, expiration dates, and lot numbers, to trace a product if something goes wrong. But those standards won't exist for at least two years.

You may see supplements labeled "USP"—for the United States Pharmacopeial Convention, the nonprofit group that sets standards for all prescription and over-the-counter drugs sold in the U.S. But at least for the next few years, any USP logo simply means that the ordinary vitamins and minerals in the pills—not

the herbal or exotic ingredients—meet the group's standards. The group is considering writing standards for some herbal supplements but has not yet decided whether it will do so.

Is it safe?

You might reasonably assume that a "natural" product, won't harm you. "People are often surprised by herbs—they equate 'natural' with 'safe,'" says Rossanne Philen, an epidemiologist at the Centers for Disease Control and Prevention (CDC) who handles reports of herbs' adverse effects. But her work has shown these pills can be dangerous.

Among the problems Philen sees are poisonings caused by misidentifications. The workers who pick the plants—often hired hands in developing countries—"are not Ph.D.

botanists," she says. They may collect a poisonous part of the plant they're after, or the wrong plant entirely.

For instance, she told us, last year seven New Yorkers fell ill after drinking an herbal tea contaminated with a poisonous plant in the belladonna family. Three of the people were rushed to hospitals for emergency treatment. Symptoms included rapid heartbeat, fever, dilated pupils, and flushed skin.

Earlier this year, the shrub chaparral—touted as a cancer cure and blood purifier—was found to be a potential cause of serious liver damage. One woman needed a transplant after taking the herb for 10 months, according to an article in the Journal of the American Medical Association.

A Journal editorial speculated that

BEYOND THE HYPE

THREE HOT SELLERS

While most of the new dietary supplements are herbs, several are not—including these three, which appear to be among the hottest-selling pills in health-food stores. Here is what is known about their properties.

Melatonin. This year's craze. Synthetic versions of this human hormone are said, by the more conservative promoters, to fight insomnia and jet lag. The more daring proponents also claim that it can slow aging, fight disease, and enhance one's sex life. The authors of several new books are spreading the word.

The hormone is produced during the night by the pineal gland at the base of the brain. Studies have found that taking a fraction of a milligram can, in fact, hasten sleep; the evidence for the other claims is weak, however. Several pharmaceutical companies are hoping to turn melatonin into a prescription drug, but you can already buy melatonin in the store. The drawbacks: No one knows the right dosage, the interactions with other drugs, or the long-term effects. One brand lists extensive cautions, including warnings addressed to people with diabetes, depression, leukemia, epilepsy or autoimmune diseases, and to women who are pregnant or nursing.

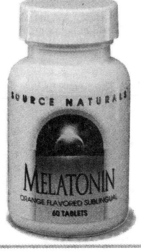

· **Chromium picolinate.** This patented form of chromium, a trace metal, is promoted for weight loss—it's claimed to target fat, spare muscle, and increase strength. Chromium helps bind insulin to cell membranes and thus may play a role in how the body uses carbohydrates. Much of the research has been done by the patent's holder; independent research does not support the claims. Picolinate's promoters say that most Americans don't get enough chromium in their diet. But documented cases of chromium deficiency are rare. In fact, animal experiments suggest that too much chromium can be harmful. And some picolinate pills, if taken as directed, would deliver several times the daily limit of chromium—200 micrograms—considered safe for people. The FDA says it has "safety concerns" and that it has received reports of adverse effects, including irregular heart beat.

Coenzyme Q10. Sellers claim the supplement can "strengthen the heart" and "inhibit the aging process." Produced in virtually every cell of the body, this substance helps convert food into energy; it's also an antioxidant. But there's disagreement over whether it works when it's swallowed.

liver damage of unknown origin might stem from herbs more often than doctors realize—and urged doctors to question their patients more carefully about the use of supplements.

Illness and death have also been tied to kombucha "mushrooms." Kombucha is really a fermenting colony of yeasts and bacteria, sold in health-food stores and passed among users, who start new colonies. The liquid is said to have tonic properties. But one Iowa woman died this spring, and another was hospitalized, after taking kombucha tea. Investigators could not definitely pin down the cause; one theory is that the tea may have reacted with a drug the dead woman took. FDA officials say there's always a risk that harmful microorganisms can taint home-grown kombucha, and they warn people with suppressed immunity to be cautious.

Perhaps the most famous outbreak of deaths from supplements was traced to the once-popular L-tryptophan. Pills containing this amino acid, which was marketed for insomnia, were linked to a painful ailment of the connective tissue and blood, eosinophilia-myalgia syndrome. Eventually, more than 1500 cases surfaced, and at least 38 people died. It's not clear if contamination at a factory or the supplement itself was to blame, but tryptophan pills are off the market.

Some supplements' contaminants are added deliberately, says the CDC's Philen. Herbal remedies may be adulterated with real drugs for extra punch—arthritis products spiked with pain killers, tranquilizers, or steroids, for example.

Patrolling the market

Even if a product has harmed someone, there's no way to be sure that it will be yanked from your local store shelves. No one is systematically tracking bad reactions.

The FDA's system for catching bad supplements is "passive surveillance," says an official at the agency's Office of Special Nutritionals. The FDA waits until reports roll in from doctors, hospitals, health agencies, or individuals. Problems can take a month or more to wend their way from district offices to Washington. It often takes even longer before a pattern reveals itself. "It's a very small office in a very big area," the official told us. "Only nine people—and not all are doing adverse-effects monitoring. We tend to see only the tip of the iceberg."

FDA staffers often don't know what to make of the problems they do notice. There's no way for them to tell just how many people have suffered similar illnesses, and no way to tell how many Americans in all have been using a particular supplement. (Reports of adverse reactions to prescription drugs are sent to the FDA by the same route, but in those cases investigators begin with much more information: They know what's in the drug, who makes it, how much is prescribed, the safe dosage, and what sorts of side effects turned up during years of testing.) What's more, neither the CDC nor the American Association of Poison Control Centers have systematic mechanisms to track problems with herbs or other supplements.

The industry's attempts to regulate itself have been incomplete. The American Herbal Products Association has recommended detailed warnings on bottles of ma huang—also called ephedra—which contains amphetamine-like chemicals and can cause serious side effects. For a time the association had also asked its members to stop selling chaparral; then it suggested only that the labels on chaparral bottles include detailed cautions and a phone number to report adverse

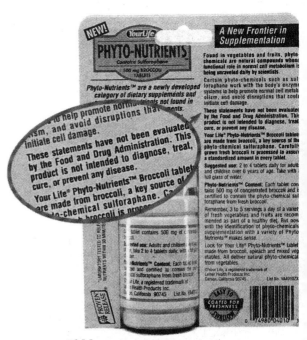

Hidden message Manufacturers now are required to tell consumers that their health claims have not been reviewed by the U.S. Food and Drug Administration. But there is no requirement that they make that message stand out.

effects. The group has also recommended that a third dangerous herb, comfrey, be recommended for external use only, and not on abraded skin.

We checked a few stores to see the recommendations' effects; the results were inconsistent. We found ephedra carrying a stern warning. We found chaparral capsules, carrying a lukewarm warning and no hotline number. We also found comfrey—in capsules, for internal use.

Some states have attempted to step in. Georgia bans nonprescription sale of yohimbe, an herb carried elsewhere in health-food stores and sold as an aphrodisiac; Georgia classifies it a "dangerous drug." Several states have already restricted, or are moving to restrict, the sale of

Unchecked claims Consumers typically get much of their information about supplements from pamphlets and books whose accuracy gets little official scrutiny. That is unlikely to change under the new law.

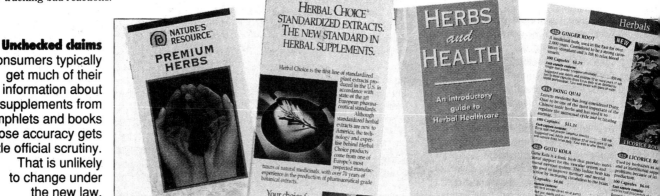

BUZZWORDS ON BOTTLES

Supplement bottles abound with impressive terms. Many turn out to be elaborate ways of describing the commonplace.

Antioxidants Compounds—such as vitamin C, vitamin E, and beta carotene—presently taking much of the credit for the apparent protective effects of fruits and vegetables. Antioxidants control "free radicals," which damage cells through oxidation. Some marketers suggest all antioxidants can prevent cancer and heart disease, but the evidence from controlled clinical trials is mixed and suggests that different antioxidants have different effects.

Energy Sometimes a euphemism for stimulants like caffeine and ephedra. In other cases, a perfectly safe throwaway word, since all digestible plant products provide chemical energy, measured in calories.

Enzymes Proteins that work as catalysts to enhance chemical reactions. (We've seen products containing cytochrome C, involved in cells' energy production, and papain, a papaya enzyme.) But enzymes taken orally usually are broken down by digestion, like other protein, and are thus of no special use to the body.

Phytonutrients From "phyto," Greek for plant, these botanical substances are a new supplement category. Some are extracted from vegetables such as broccoli. It's too early to say whether the manufacturers have picked the right active ingredients (there may be thousands to choose from), or whether the amount packed into a pill is meaningful.

RNA and DNA Genetic material said to rejuvenate cells, enhance memory, prevent wrinkling. Already present in many foods anyway. Often destroyed by digestion.

---

ephedra, following deaths linked to the herb or its active ingredient, ephedrine.

But there is an effort in Congress to block such local safety regulations on supplements, and to further limit Federal authority over their safety. The bill, H.R. 1951, was introduced in June; its outcome is uncertain at this writing.

Recommendations

Herbal supplements have become serious business—and pose serious problems. They're sometimes expensive, they may mislead you with false promises, and they offer no assurances that what's on the label is what's inside.

We'd like to see Congress clean up the mess it's made of supplement regulations. These products should at least carry much clearer disclaimers, in large type, saying that any claims of safety and efficacy are strictly the opinions of the manufacturer and have not been confirmed by the FDA or other medical authorities. Consistent manufacturing standards should be established swiftly. Clearly dangerous supplements, like chaparral and ephedra (ma huang), should be banned immediately.

In the long run, we would like to see the United States emulate the German system for regulating herbs. There, druggists may sell herbs if there's some evidence they work, and no evidence that they are unsafe. And a national commission compiles monographs discussing each herb's pros and cons, which are then published.

If you want to try a supplement despite the uncertainties, don't rely on what's printed on the packages or in pamphlets. Do your best to seek out independent sources of information about what the herbs and other supplements are supposed to do. We recommend two books, both by Varro Tyler, an expert in the medicinal use of plants: *The Honest Herbal—A Sensible Guide to the Use of Herbs and Related Remedies* (third edition, 1993); and *Herbs of Choice—The Therapeutic Use of Phytomedicinals* (1994). Both are published by Pharmaceutical Products Press (Haworth); the first book is organized by herb, the second by disease.

Here are several other suggestions for playing it safe:

☐ Before trying a supplement, consider changes to your diet or lifestyle that might accomplish your goals. If you have high cholesterol, for example, cut your intake of saturated fat and begin an exercise program before you consider taking garlic pills.

☐ Check with your doctor before taking an herb or other supplement. Many people don't, for fear of looking silly or getting a lecture. But it's worth the risk of embarrassment. A supplement may interact with a drug you take or pose a serious side effect. And the doctor may know of an effective conventional treatment you should try first.

☐ Pregnant and nursing women and anyone with chronic and serious health problems should not take herbal supplements, unless their doctor gives the green light.

☐ Check the warnings on packages and on related material. Start with small doses.

☐ Buy herbs that at least claim to be "standardized"—so you have a fighting chance of consistent contents from pill to pill.

☐ Stick to single-herb products, not combinations, whose actions might be hard to sort out.

☐ Be alert to the herb's effects—positive and negative. If you can track progress objectively—with cholesterol tests, say, or by keeping tabs on your urinary flow if you're taking a prostate remedy—you'll be less susceptible to the power of suggestion.

☐ Stop immediately if there's a problem, and call the doctor. For instance, abdominal pain, darkened urine, and jaundice can signal liver complications that an herb may have brought on.

☐ If you think a product made you sick or otherwise harmed you, the FDA advises you to contact your doctor, who should then call the agency's MedWatch hotline for professionals to report adverse effects. The agency also suggests contacting your state and local health departments and consumer protection agency.

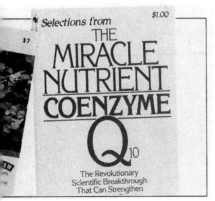

$1.00

Selections from
THE
MIRACLE
NUTRIENT
COENZYME
Q10

The Revolutionary
Scientific Breakthrough
That Can Strengthen

Herbal Warning

Health-food stores have built a new natural-drug culture.
How safe are their wares?

GEOFFREY COWLEY

THE CALL CAME AT 6 A.M. ON MARCH 7, just as Tom and Karen Schlendorf were getting up for work in suburban Long Island. The local police department was on the line, and an officer said he'd be right over because he had something to tell them. "For two or three minutes I didn't think anything of it," Karen recalls. "Then my blood just went cold as ice and I said, 'Oh, my God, I hope it's not Pete'." The Schlendorfs had spoken a few days earlier with their 20-year-old son, a junior studying history and theater at the University of Albany. He was in Panama City, Fla., enjoying spring break with several buddies. Now, as she feared, her life was changing. "I'm sorry to have to tell you this," the officer said after greeting them at the door. "Your son is dead."

If the fact of his death was hard to accept, so was the cause. From talking to her son's friends, Karen has surmised that they spent the day of March 6 wandering in and out of the beach town's novelty shops, where they were inundated by flashy signs and posters touting herbal supplements with names like Cloud 9, Herbal Ecstacy (sic) and Ultimate Xphoria. According to the promotions, these little packets of pills would deliver increased energy, "inner visions," "sexual sensations" and "cosmic consciousness." Best of all, they were natural, legal and cheap. That night, by Karen's account, the kids settled on Ultimate Xphoria. The package suggested a dose of four tablets, but most of them followed a store clerk's advice and took 12 to 15. Pete took just eight, but they hit him hard. Complaining of tingling sensations and a headache, he decided

to stay behind at the motel while his pals went out for the evening. They found him dead on the floor when they returned. According to the local medical examiner's report, he died from the "synergistic effect of ephedrine, pseudoephedrine, phenylpropanolamine and caffeine," the active ingredients in Ultimate Xphoria.

The product's distributor, Alternative Health Research Inc. of Tempe, Ariz., isn't commenting on the incident. But just about everyone else is. Peter Schlendorf's death was just the latest of several linked to ephedrine-containing compounds. It has alarmed parents and health officials and it raises new questions about the safety of the largely unregulated nutritional-supplements industry. States and localities are rushing to clamp down on the new herbal stimulants—the state of Florida announced last week that it is banning them altogether—and the Food and Drug Administration is voicing official outrage. "When a 20-year-old dies from taking a product like this, something is very wrong," says FDA Commissioner David Kessler. "We need to be sure it doesn't happen again."

THE QUESTION IS, HOW? IF THE SUPPLEments craze were confined to a few twenty-somethings looking to get high, the issue would be straightforward. But they're just a small part of the picture. Whether they want to lose weight, gain muscle, soothe nerves or stave off the AIDS virus, Americans are taking up natural remedies as never before. We spend some $6 billion annually on nutritional supplements—everything from vitamins and minerals to herbs,

seeds, pollens, oils and enzymes—and the market is growing by 20 percent every year. Critics say this burgeoning industry has run amok and needs regulation. Herb lovers say most natural nostrums are harmless if used sensibly, and they bristle at the prospect of having the government tell them what they can put in their bodies. In the wake of the Florida incident, each camp is accusing the other of bad faith. Unfortunately, they're both right.

Critics of the industry say the trouble started in 1994, when Congress passed the Dietary Supplement Health and Education Act (DSHEA), cosponsored by Sens. Orrin Hatch and Ted Kennedy. By classifying vitamins, minerals and herbs as food supplements rather than drugs, the bill reduced the FDA's control over them. Now marketers can't make explicit health claims for a supplement ("cures cancer"), but they can promote its known effects on the "structure and function" of the body ("protects against cell damage"), and they can give it any name they like ("Tumor Be Gone!"). Unless the FDA can show that the product is dangerous, it can't restrict sales.

The catch is that many herbs are, in effect, drugs. Ephedra, the key ingredient in Ultimate Xphoria and its kin, is a plant that Chinese physicians have used for 2,000 years to treat upper-respiratory ailments. Its active chemical, ephedrine, is in many decongestants and bronchodilators. But what interested some supplement makers in ephedrine was its stimulant effect. By combining it with caffeine, another natural upper, they created nonprescription speed. For the past couple of years, 80 or so com-

'We're Squeaky Clean'

And, says Mr. Herbal Ecstacy, there's more in store

Sean Shayan is not given to understatement. The 20-year-old CEO's company, Global World Media Corp., has a name only Rupert Murdoch could love. His headquarters, a cramped warren of offices a few blocks off the beach in Los Angeles, are New Age baroque: purple and green walls, low-slung crescent-shaped desks and a black triangular conference table. Pillows on the floor serve as chairs, and shoes are strictly optional. It's all a bit much. But then what would you expect from an outfit whose chief product, Herbal Ecstacy (unaccountably misspelled), is hyped as "synergistically blended to insure visionary vibrations"?

'We'd like to thank the FDA': The Herbal Ecstacy CEO says sales are up 25% since the agency threatened action

---

Sounds far out. In reality, Shayan and his colleagues are more P. T. Barnum than Timothy Leary. As Shayan acknowledges, Herbal Ecstacy's effects are much subtler than its packaging—and far less dramatic than those if its illicit namesake. "We're selling the concept of ecstacy," he explains. Shayan claims his company controls 90 percent

of the market, having peddled more than 150 million pills—which retail for $2 to $3 apiece—in four years. *His brand has never been linked to death, Shayan says—a claim that apparently is true. Nevertheless,* Newsweek has learned that California health regulators began investigating the company, and others like it, several months ago. Not that controversy fazes Shayan. "We're squeaky clean," he insists. The pleasant, long-locked CEO has been entertaining a media parade since the FDA began threatening action against ephedra-based pseudodrugs like Herbal Ecstacy. Shayan claims sales are up by 25 percent since the saber rattling started. "We'd like to thank the FDA," he says, smiling.

Born in Tehran and raised in Los Angeles, Shayan says he left school and home at 15, cutting his marketing teeth as a promoter on L.A.'s club scene. Noticing that club hoppers were fueling all-night dancefests with the designer drug Ecstasy, he and some pals had an idea. "We thought, God, if we could come up with an alternative product like that that was safe, legal and natural, there would be a huge market for it," he recalls. They ran across a group of herbalists who had been experimenting with mildly psychoactive herbs. "These were brilliant guys scientifically, but they didn't have it as far as marketing," he says. Enter Shayan. Ads in High Times magazine and elsewhere helped sell a purported

500,000 10-pill packages in the company's first weeks.

Now Shayan and his company drive mainstream herbalists nuts. "I don't consider them part of the industry," says Michael Q. Ford, executive director of the National Nutritional Foods Association, a trade group for supplement makers. "God knows we'd like to see this company out of business." Shayan calls it sour grapes. "We've got a dynamic idea. We've got intense marketing," he says. "They can only get $5.95 for 10 pills. We get $3 per pill." Shayan says his pills, made somewhere "in the United States," cost him less than 60 cents apiece. "We're way overpriced," he volunteers, then rethinks, "I take that back. We're the best, and it costs more to buy us."

Shayan insists ephedra is safe if taken in recommended doses. Nonetheless, Global has released a reformulated "Herbal Ecstacy 2" that substitutes kavakava root, described in one textbook as "a mild narcotic, a soporific, a diuretic and a major muscle relaxant." Shayan's excited. "Kavakava is the next big thing," he says. "We think it can be as big as coffee." What's more, he promises, Global will release "40 new products within 60 days." As P. T. Barnum might have figured it, Shayan should have at least 86,400 new customers by then.

Kendall Hamilton and
Andrew Murr

---

panies have promoted the blend as a safe way to lose weight, boost energy, stay alert or get high. Though hard figures are unavailable, the makers of Herbal Ecstacy say they alone have sold 150 million pills. "Consumers may not realize it," says Norman Farnsworth, a phar-

macognosist (herb expert) at the University of Illinois in Chicago, "but what they're dealing with here is a medicine."

And a potent one. Within 20 minutes of taking an ephedrine-based stimulant, users experience a jump in heart rate and blood pressure. In some people, says

Purdue University pharmacognosist Varro Tyler, that surge can lead to seizures, heart attacks and strokes. Police Sgt. Charles Nanney of Miami was 28 and in peak physical condition when he started taking an ephedrine-based sports-training formula two years ago. After a

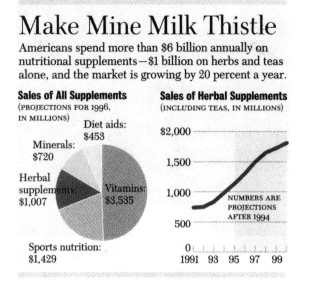

Make Mine Milk Thistle

Americans spend more than $6 billion annually on nutritional supplements—$1 billion on herbs and teas alone, and the market is growing by 20 percent a year.

Sales of All Supplements
(PROJECTIONS FOR 1996, IN MILLIONS)

Diet aids: $453
Minerals: $720
Herbal supplements: $1,007
Vitamins: $3,535
Sports nutrition: $1,429

Sales of Herbal Supplements
(INCLUDING TEAS, IN MILLIONS)

NUMBERS ARE PROJECTIONS AFTER 1994

tive-medicine enthusiasts tout the extract as a natural way to induce abortion. That's what 24-year-old Kristina Humphrey had in mind two years ago. Humphrey, a sociology student at San Jose State University, didn't like the thought of ending her unwanted pregnancy in a cold, impersonal surgical suite, her parents recall. So she bought a container labeled FRESH PENNYROYAL HERB and followed directions that said, "Add 20-40 drops of extract to a small amount of warm water and take 3 times daily as needed" (to avoid "medical claims," most labels don't mention what a supplement might be used for).

few months of popping one or two tablets before his daily workout, one morning he suffered a stroke, which he says caused him permanent brain damage (for which he's suing the maker and the distributor). His experience, like Peter Schlendorf's, suggests the new stimulants have an extremely narrow safety margin. But there's no reason to think that every user is equally vulnerable. Though the products have become staples among truckers, dieters and nightclub kids, the FDA has recorded only 400 health complaints and 15 possible deaths.

No other supplement has caused as much trouble as ephedrine—and for many other widely used remedies, the risks appear negligible. There's no evidence, for example, that the millions of Americans who take echinacea to prevent colds and flu are in danger. And though countless aging baby boomers now end the day with a few milligrams of melatonin—a naturally occurring hormone touted as an antidote to afflictions from insomnia to the aging process—no one has documented any toxic effects. But several other commonly used herbs are giving health experts the jitters.

Some herb lovers take an extract from the leaves and twigs of chaparral, an evergreen desert shrub, in the hope of preventing cancer, preserving youth or alleviating arthritis. Several medical reports suggest it can damage the liver. One, published last year, involved a 60-year-old woman who'd been taking one

or two capsules a day to boost energy. When she upped her dose to six capsules, she developed such severe hepatitis that she required a liver transplant. Many pharmaceuticals—even over-the-counter analgesics—can cause liver damage in susceptible people. But because they're tested and prescribed at specific doses, risks and benefits are well known. "We don't have any idea about the magnitude of the risk in chaparral," says University of Chicago hepatologist Alfred Baker.

Even dicier is comfrey, a coarse, hairy perennial whose leaves and roots have been used in folk medicine for everything from wound healing to blood cleansing. There's little danger in using a comfrey tincture topically, says Tyler, but taken orally, it's "definitely hazardous." Comfrey contains chemicals called PAs (pyrrolizidine alkaloids), which can gum up the vessels in the liver, starving it of blood. Canada has banned it, and most European countries regulate the concentrations in which it's sold. But comfrey is unregulated in the United States, and readily available in most health-food stores. Says Tyler: "It shouldn't even be on the market."

You could also say that about pennyroyal, a member of the mint family whose concentrated extract can cause liver damage, coma, convulsions and death—in amounts of less than a teaspoon. Native Americans once used the leaves (which are far less noxious) for coughs and menstrual cramps. Alterna-

ONE NIGHT, HER PARENTS SAY, SHE broke into a cold sweat and crawled into a bathtub hoping to ease a stabbing abdominal pain. When her boyfriend found her unconscious he called paramedics, who rushed her to San Jose Hospital. There, emergency physicians surgically removed what turned out to be an ectopic pregnancy. The fetus hadn't ruptured her fallopian tube, yet she bled so profusely that she lapsed into a fatal coma. "The cardiac arrest occurred because of shock," the emergency physician's report said. "The shock occurred because of abnormal blood clotting ability due to liver damage. The liver damage was caused by pennyroyal." In a lawsuit against the herb's packager, Humphrey's parents are seeking not only money but a clear warning on every bottle sold: "Pennyroyal in tincture form has been known to cause liver damage and should not be used as a substitute for medical abortion under any circumstances."

Active ingredients aren't the only ones that can make a supplement dangerous. With no regulation, contamination is always possible. In the late 1980s, 1,500 people got a painful connective-tissue disease called EMS (eosinophilia-myalgia syndrome) after taking the amino acid L-tryptophan as a sleep aid. The illness, which claimed at least 38 lives, was linked to contaminants in a single Japanese brand (the FDA responded by banning L-tryptophan entirely). Contaminants have also turned up in herbal teas. Two years ago officials traced several New York City poisonings, none fatal, to Paraguayan tea that contained belladonna leaves. And even when a supplement is harmless by itself, it can interact with other foods or medications in unexpected ways (chart).

For all the fear they inspire, herbal horror stories are rare. According to the American Association of Poison Control Centers, pharmaceutical products kill roughly 500 people for every person killed by an herb. And while plants cause about 50 nonfatal poisonings each year (that's if you count all the jade, holly and poinsettia that kids eat by mistake), pharmaceuticals cause about 7,000. "The data just doesn't support the view that these products cause widespread harm," says Loren Israelsen, executive director of the Utah Natural Products Alliance.

The FDA hasn't exactly discouraged that view in recent weeks. No one faults the agency for the consumer alert it issued on April 10, urging people to avoid ephedrine-based stimulants (Kessler calls them "street drugs masquerading as dietary supplements"). But supplement makers were outraged two weeks later, when The New York Times portrayed agency officials as complaining that DSHEA, the 1994 congressional act, had left them powerless to police even known poisons such as hemlock "until the bodies piled up." In fact, the agency can ban any product for which it can show "substantial or unreasonable

risk"—not a hard standard to meet where hemlock is concerned. It can also mandate warnings. Last fall, after reviewing the safety of ephedrine, an ad-

---

Bad Bedfellows

Herbal remedies that are safe by themselves can have bad effects when combined with other food or drugs. Some examples:

• Long-term use of stimulant herbal laxatives such as **cascara** and **senna** can increase the potency of the heart medicine digoxin, placing stress on the heart.

• When mixed with lithium, a diuretic herb such as **birch leaf, dandelion leaf** or **juniper** may increase the drug's concentration in the bloodstream.

• **Yohimbe,** an herb used as an aphrodisiac and for energy, can cause skin rashes when mixed with a tyramine-rich food such as liver, cheese or red wine. Yohimbe can also cross-react with over-the-counter products containing phenylpropanolamine, such as nasal decongestants and diet aids.

---

visory committee suggested mandatory warning labels for products like Ultimate Xphoria and Herbal Ecstacy—labels describing side effects, drug interactions and the risk of overdose. The agency has done nothing about that recommendation because, says a spokesman, the committee wasn't specific about how the label should be worded. Kessler says the Schlendorf death "will now allow us to go into court and take regulatory action."

If the FDA has dropped the ball, so have the supplement makers. In early 1994, the American Herbal Products Association urged its members to suspend sales of chaparral and to place clear warnings on products containing ephedrine. But it later withdrew the chaparral recommendation. And though some ephedrine products do include cautions and dosing instructions, the warnings are vague, inconsistent and voluntary. "We need either self-regulation or government regulation," says Joseph Pizzorno, the naturopath who heads Seattle's Bastyr University. For now, it seems we'll have to settle for mutual finger-pointing.

With MARY HAGER *in Washington,* KAREN SPRINGEN *in Chicago,* PATRICIA KING *in San Francisco and* SUSAN MILLER *and* BRAD STONE *in New York*

Hunger and Global Issues

You cannot reason with a hungry belly; it has no ears.
—Greek Proverb

Hunger respects no geographical boundaries. Although it is most common in Africa, it is known on every continent and in every country. The absolute number of hungry people has dropped in recent years in spite of world population growth, but it is said that 800 million face persistent hunger. Even larger numbers face temporary hunger and malnutrition. Thirty-five thousand of them die every day.

Famines have been frequent throughout history, and they always bring an acute focus to hunger. One of the most famous is the Irish potato famine of 1845–1850, which resulted in thousands of deaths and huge numbers of immigrants to the United States. A decade ago two million Ethiopians died, but even more had died a few years earlier. The same can be said for the Sahel, East Africa, and the Sudan. Periodic famines have faced China throughout the nineteenth and twentieth centuries, affecting millions each time. India's repeated famines were substantially reduced once the nation became independent, and it now claims to be self-sufficient in food production; but government leaders have not solved the problem of chronic hunger.

The causes of hunger are multiple, and experts acknowledge that their complexity is difficult to analyze and define: natural disasters, such as periodic cycles of droughts and

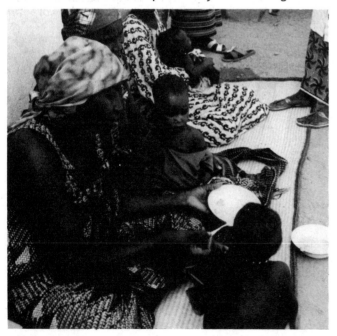

floods, which are particularly devastating in vulnerable economies; overpopulation and environmental degradation; social upheaval and wars; and an absence of commitment on the part of local governments. But the lack of purchasing power is ultimately behind the failure to secure food. Most of the world's poor are in semisubsistence agriculture and unable to produce cash crops. They will spend half or more of their small incomes to feed themselves and may still eat less than dietary requirements. For example, the average person in Afghanistan consumes only 72 percent of the estimated daily caloric requirements; the percentage is 84 in Bolivia. Paradoxically, those of us in the United States receive 138 percent.

Malnutrition accompanies hunger in many cases. It may be too few calories or too little protein. It may be the absence of essential vitamins or minerals. Many of those affected are children. The extent of the harm depends upon the length and severity of the malnutrition and upon when it occurs in the growth period. The effects can be evidenced in behavior, physical growth, and mental development. It is impossible to determine the extent to which a child's recovery might be accomplished or permanent problems avoided with appropriate intervention.

A mother's nutritional status before and during pregnancy dramatically affects the outcome of that pregnancy. One good indicator of this is the infant mortality rate (IMR). High IMRs are said to show that hunger exists as a chronic, society-wide condition. Worldwide, in 1996, the IMR is 62, but in Afghanistan it is 163. In Africa, where the average IMR is 91, only 6 of the 55 countries have infant mortality rates under 50. By contrast, the rate in the United States has dropped to 7.5, while in Japan it is only 4.2.

Pragmatic leaders realize that future food disasters must be headed off now and are trying to find innovative and acceptable ways to accomplish this formidable task. "Averting a Global Food Crisis" portrays some of the crucial problems that must be addressed and some of the possible solutions. In particular, the critical role of China is discussed. In recent years China has dramatically increased purchasing power and moved toward being a meat-consuming culture. Within the past year, China has become an importer of rice and corn; it was already the largest wheat importer. The magnitude of China's population, together with these shifts, raises large questions about the world's response.

The second article, "Nibbling at Famine's Edge," is a portrayal of the situation in bordering North Korea, where a second year of major flooding has increased food shortages once again. This situation is representative of other areas of the world, many of them in Africa. In Liberia, for example, food and medicine were recently rushed to a town of 35,000, where 60 percent of the population was said to be suffering from extreme hunger and hundreds of children were on the verge of death. In this case, the cause was internal war. They had been cut off from aid for seven months.

Hunger is also visible at home. Experts say that U.S. hunger differs from hunger in developing countries in that its cause is poverty uncomplicated by natural disasters, war, or an undeveloped economy. More people go to bed hungry now than did in the mid-1980s, and millions in our country are said to have food insecurity. While they may not be hungry every day, the food available will not stretch over an entire month. They may skip meals, scavenge, or rely on soup kitchens. Quality and ethnic appropriateness of foods are also concerns. Minorities represent a disproportionate number of the poor, with one-third of all African American families and one-quarter of Hispanics living in poverty. Nor has hunger remained within class boundaries. People from all social levels have lost jobs, and there is ample evidence that hunger and malnutrition have spread to the middle class as well.

Patricia Splett, in "Federal Food Assistance Programs: A Step to Food Security for Many," reports on the many efforts being made by the federal government to feed the needy. Food programs that are intended to supplement the family's food budget sometimes become the primary source of food. Even these have been under political attack in an election year when both parties have been jockeying for position and welfare programs have been targeted for revision. WIC (an aid program for women, infants, and children) in particular has been documented to be extremely cost-effective, saving three dollars in potential medical costs for every dollar spent, according to the General Accounting Office.

Even these programs do not reach all of the needy. Since 1980, private sector emergency feeding programs such as soup kitchens, food pantries, and homeless shelters have multiplied all over the country. Many of them report turning people away or closing temporarily due to increased demand and dwindling resources.

But hunger is more than a physical phenomenon. It has significance beyond its capacity to feed the body. "Thunder in the Distance" is included in this book because, in our zeal to learn facts and to be scientific, we must not forget the damage to one's psyche from the hunger experience. The science of nutrition is applied to people, and people are the grand sum of social, mental, emotional, and spiritual dimensions, as well as the physical dimension. Food, or the lack of it, nourishes and shapes the soul as well as the body and influences our response to the world.

Nobody really knows what the carrying capacity of the world, or even an individual country, is. Over the past century estimates have ranged from fewer than one billion to more than one trillion people. The actual number does, of course, depend upon the standard of living one is willing

to accept. Headlines tend to be pessimistic: "Africa will need to produce 300% more food by 2050," or "Once a breadbasket, Ukraine expecting poor grain harvest." There is much evidence to support this pessimism. Per capita food production since 1960 has decreased in 75 of the poorest countries. In fact, over the past few years world grain harvests have shrunk, and the carryover grain stocks have been reduced to 48 days of consumption. As supplies dwindle, prices rise. Many believe that grain expansion has neared its limits. The significant contributions of the "green revolution" have been absorbed, additional fertilizer is having little impact on yields, and vast areas of rangeland are overgrazed and converting to wasteland. Furthermore, irrigation demands are pressing the limits of the hydrological cycle, reducing aquifers to below normal levels. Ongoing deforestation is causing more soil erosion. The Food and Agriculture Organization reports that all major oceanic fishing areas are being fished beyond capacity. Total fish harvests have been increasing since 1993, but some of this is due to expanded aquaculture. While grain is more efficiently used in producing fish than red meat or poultry, it still represents choices about how grain will be used. Yet the world's population keeps growing at the rate of 90 million per year.

Not everybody agrees with this pessimistic outlook, however. Dennis Avery, in an opinion commentary, claims that those with doomsday predictions have been wrong in the recent past. He believes that science can and will rise to the occasion and will find ways to increase crop yields so that several billion more people can be fed on the same amount of productive land. Perhaps so. There will still be the problems of cooperation, purchasing power, and distribution to be solved.

Mark Twain said that hunger is the handmaid of genius. This aphorism notwithstanding, hunger felt or vicariously experienced by millions has certainly aroused intense emotions of survival and compassion. Experts and ordinary citizens have been challenged to find solutions. Their tireless courage and successful efforts will provide the energy from which future victories will come.

Looking Ahead: Challenge Questions

Should more be done about hunger in the United States? Whose responsibility is it, that of the government or of the private sector? How could you help?

What should be the roles of the United States and other developed countries in solving world hunger? To what extent should countries be expected to solve their own problems?

What criteria would you use to decide when to help another country and how much?

Some argue that we should all become vegetarians. Would this solve the hunger problem at home or abroad? What are the implications of changing the Western diet to one based on plants?

Averting a Global Food Crisis

Lester Brown

LESTER BROWN is president of the Worldwatch Institute, a private, nonprofit environmental-research organization in Washington, D.C., and author of Who Will Feed China? Wake-Up Call for a Small Planet *(W.W. Norton, September 1995), on which this article is based. Before founding Worldwatch, he was administrator of the U.S. Department of Agriculture's International Agricultural Development Service and Advisor to the Secretary. He started his career as a farmer, growing tomatoes in New Jersey.*

[In] February [1995], while giving a speech in Oslo, Norway, at a conference on sustainable development, I illustrated some of the global dilemmas that lay ahead as a result of China's headlong dash toward industrialization. I suggested that when countries become densely populated before they begin to industrialize, as is the case with China, they inevitably suffer a heavy loss in grainland as farms are devoured by factories, roads, and parking lots. If industrialization is rapid, land losses quickly outstrip rises in agricultural productivity, which leads to a decline in grain production.

*I*ronically, the same industrialization that shrinks grain harvests also raises income and with it the demand for grain. Indeed, given the opportunity, people will quickly shift from a monotonous fare—in which a staple such as rice supplies the bulk of calories—to one that includes a substantial portion of pork, beef, poultry, milk, eggs, and other livestock products. Unfortunately, these items require more grain than would otherwise be consumed in a starchy diet. For example, 4 kilograms of grain are needed to produce 1 kilogram of pork, and 7 kilograms of grain are needed for 1 kilogram of beef.

I pointed out that before China, only three countries—Japan, South Korea, and Taiwan—were densely populated before they industrialized. Within 30 years, each had lost more than 40 percent of its grainland. And since the huge losses could not be offset by productivity gains, grain output fell in Japan by 32 percent and in both South Korea and Taiwan by 24 percent. Add to this equation the widespread demand by the suddenly affluent populations for greater diversity in their diets, and the three countries went from being largely self-sufficient to collectively importing 71 percent of their grain needs. In no case was the heavy dependence on imports a conscious policy goal, but rather it was the result of industrialization in a region of land scarcity.

While the problem was severe for these three smaller countries, I showed that it will be overwhelming in China, with its immense and rapidly growing population—which at nearly 1.2 billion is 10 times larger than that of Japan and amounts to more than one-fifth of the world's population. Meanwhile, the country is on track for adding some 490 million people between 1990 and 2030—the equivalent of four Japans—swelling its population to more than 1.6 billion. Moreover, in China's increasingly industrial society, incomes are rising faster for more people than ever before in history. If the country's economy continues growing at its breakneck pace—it has expanded by a phenomenal 56 percent in just four years—China could overtake the United States as the world's largest economy by 2010 and will accelerate its demand for more food at a record rate.

China could thus become such a massive importer of grain that the United States and all the rest of the exporting countries combined will not be able to meet the need. For the first time in history, the collision between expanding human demand for food and the earth's natural limits will produce devastating effects worldwide. Because of China's effect on our global economy, its land scarcity will become everyone's land scarcity, its grain shortages will become everyone's grain shortages, and its rising food prices will spread throughout the world.

In short, I proposed that China's emergence as a massive grain importer will serve as the "wake-up call" signaling trouble in the relationship between ourselves and the natural systems and resources on which we depend. It will force governments everywhere to address long-neglected issues such as the need to stabilize population, to rethink agricultural priorities, and to redefine security in terms of food scarcity rather than military aggression.

CHINA'S REBUTTAL, AND ADMISSION

Following the presentation, which was well received, I had to leave after the coffee break for the airport. Later I learned that when the session reconvened, the Chinese ambassador to Norway, Xie Zhenhua, asked for the floor even though he was not a scheduled speaker. According to the *Times of India*, one of the papers covering the conference, the ambassador claimed that my analysis was off-base and misleading. "We are giving priority to agricultural productivity," he said. "Our family-planning program has been very successful. Science and technology and economic growth will see us through." In concluding, he repeated the question I had asked—"Who will feed China?"—and solemnly proclaimed to the audience that "the Chinese people will feed themselves." The following day, Xie held a news conference, and contended "unequivocally that China does not want to rely on others to feed its people and that it relies on itself to solve its own problems."

Although I was aware that the Chinese were sensitive to the notion that they might need to import large amounts of grain, I had not realized just how politically charged the issue is. All the leaders of China today are survivors of the massive famine that occurred from 1959 to 1961 in the aftermath of the "Great Leap Forward." This misguided effort under Mao Tse-tung to employ millions of farmers in large construction projects—including roads, huge earthen dams, and backyard steel furnaces—sharply reduced food production, claiming a staggering 30 million lives and driving perhaps a few hundred million more to the edge of starvation. The national psyche of China has been so deeply affected by this devastating event that the prospect of depending on the outside world for a substantial share of the country's food supply is both psychologically difficult to accept and politically anathema.

If China's croplands shrink and its population swells at present rates, the total amount of grainland per person will dwindle to about one-tenth the present U.S. figure in the next three decades, creating an import deficit in China that may be twice the current level of world exports.

As it happened, however, during the time when my indirect dialogue with Chinese officialdom was taking place, the food situation was already tightening within China. In late February, a Reuters story referred to the "sounding of alarm bells" by Communist Party chief and President Jiang Zemin and by Premier Li Peng regarding the state of the country's agriculture. Premier Li talked about 1995 being "significant for the increase of grain output, and the task is a very hard one." President Jiang warned that "lagging agricultural growth could spawn problems that would threaten inflation, stability, and national economic development." He indicated that some developed coastal areas where industrialization was particularly rapid had suffered a precipitous drop in the amount of acreage under cultivation, saying that this is "a trend that must be reversed . . . this year."

Accounts of the National People's Congress meeting in mid-March said officials acknowledged that "China is facing a looming grain crisis, with a hike in imports the only apparent solution to the demands of a growing population on a shrinking farmland." Experts cited "a series of vicious circles that threatened to lock grain production into a downward spiral." Such extensive consideration of the matter at the Congress suggests that feeding China is indeed now a pressing matter of official concern.

EBBING WAVES OF GRAIN

China's cropland crisis can be blamed partly on the country's geography. Although China covers essentially the same land area as the United States, much of the country is desert and mountain. In fact, only one-tenth of the land—most of it a 1,000 mile-wide strip along the eastern and southern coasts—is cultivable. Given that China has the largest population on the planet, this relatively meager allotment means that China ranks among nations with the smallest amount of grainland per person. In fact, in 1990, grainland per person was 0.08 hectares, less than one-third that of the United States.

Since 1990, however, harvested grainland area dropped from 90.8 million hectares to 85.7 million. This decline of 5.6 percent in four years, combined with a 4.9 percent population growth totaling 59 million people, reduced the harvested area per person by just over 10 percent. If the trend continues, grainland per person will dwindle to 0.03 hectares by 2030. By the time Japan reached this point, it was importing two-thirds of its grain.

The major factor contributing to such losses is the conversion of cropland to nonfarm uses. Today China's labor force totals nearly 800 million people, most of whom work in agriculture. A shift of only 100 million workers from the farm labor force to the industrial sector over the next decade or so—assuming roughly 100 workers per factory (about par for China's private sector)—would require construction of 1 million factories.

These factories will consume valuable cropland, since they will be constructed where the people are and the people are concentrated where the cropland is. (Wastelands in the western half of the country contain so little water that they can't support even dry-land crops much less cities and industries—and the cost of transporting water from the southeast would be prohibitive.) The factories also need access roads and parking lots as well as warehouses to store raw materials and finished products.

Residential demands are also claiming cropland. The 490 million people added to China's population between 1990 and 2030 will have to be housed. If each family consists of five individuals—a married couple, one child, and one set of in-laws—the additional people will require 98 million more housing units. Whether this need is satisfied with apartments or freestanding homes, it will consume a vast area of land, much of it cropland.

A consequence of rising affluence is an increase in the living space per person. In many cases, villagers are expanding their homes, adding a room or two. Others are simply building new, much larger homes. In Japan, by way of comparison, floor space per person expanded from 20.5 square meters in 1970 to 28.6 square meters in 1990, an increase of more than one-third. Given China's nationwide housing shortage and the extent of its crowding, this trend set in Japan will likely be followed in China as incomes rise.

Automobiles, too, are "consuming" cropland. In an industrial policy announced in July 1994, Beijing indicated that automobiles are to become one of the major growth industries during the next two decades. Ironically, even as the Ministry of Agriculture is calling for new measures to protect cropland, the Ministry for Machinery Building is pressing for a massive expansion of the automobile fleet and planning incentives that will encourage people to trade their trusty bicycles for cars.

Annual sales of cars, vans, trucks, and buses, which totaled 1.2 million in 1992, are expected to approach 3 million by decade's end. By 2010, ministry projections show production of automobiles above 3.5 million per year. Meanwhile, the car fleet is projected to grow from 1.85 million in 1994 to 22 million by 2010. A fleet of this size will require millions of hectares of land for a network of roads, highways, service stations, and parking lots. And as with factories, these will have to be built where the people are.

Finally, farmland is being claimed by shopping centers, tennis courts, golf courses, and private villas. In rapidly industrializing Guangdong province, for example, some 40 golf courses have been built in the newly affluent Pearl River Delta region alone. Concern about this wholesale loss of cropland has led the Guangdong Land Bureau to cancel construction of all golf courses planned but not yet completed.

Chinese political leaders may be tempted to think that they can somehow avoid a massive loss of cropland to nonfarm uses. But if they look at the experience in Japan, they will see how difficult protecting cropland can be. Few governments have worked as strenuously at this as Japan did with its system of

---

Though as many as 300 Chinese cities face severe water shortages, demand will more than double in the next 30 years. Thus many of China's farmers—who now rely on irrigated fields for four-fifths of the country's harvest—will soon be forced to revert to lower-output rain-fed crops.

---

zoning. For example, some 13,000 Japanese families grow rice within the Tokyo city limits; if this land were released for sale, it might be worth easily 100 times its value as farmland. But even with such concentrated efforts, Japan lost half its grainland during the last four decades. If China maintains its present course, the country will likely lose at least as much of its grainland to industrialization in the same span of time.

SPREADING WATER SCARCITY

Along with the continuing disappearance of farmland, China faces another threat to food production—one that its trio of neighbors did not: water scarcity from an extensive diversion of irrigation water to nonfarm uses. This is an acute concern in a country where nearly four-fifths of the harvest comes from irrigated land.

As recently as mid-century, water supplies in China were abundant relative to demand. Surface and underground sources together could more than satisfy the needs of the country's 500 million people. Since then, however, the water supply-demand ratio has decreased as water use has increased sixfold as a result of population growth, expanding irrigation, rising affluence, and industrialization. Water scarcity became extreme enough in 1993 for that Minister of Water Resources Niu Mao Sheng to observe that "in rural areas, more than 82 million people find it difficult to procure water. In urban areas, the shortages are even worse: more than 300 Chinese cities are short of water and 100 of them are very short."

The most severe water shortages are being felt in the northern half of China. That's largely because the area north of the Yangtze River encompasses nearly two-thirds of the country's cropland, yet it holds only one-fifth of the total surface water. In contrast, more than four-fifths of the surface water in China is found in the Yangtze and other river basins in the south, which has only 37 percent of the country's cropland.

The situation is most acute in the northern province. In Shanxi, where one-tenth of the peasants face chronic shortages of drinking water, farmers are limited to using far less water for irrigation than they need. In fact, one-quarter of the province's irrigated fields cannot be guaranteed water during the growing season. Likewise, burgeoning water demand in Beijing, also located in the north, has produced such severe water shortages that farmers in the region immediately around the city were recently banned from the reservoirs from which they traditionally draw irrigation water. With 300 cities in China already short of water, it is likely that in the years ahead farmers near many other urban areas will be forced to join those around Beijing who have reverted to less intensive rain-fed farming.

Meanwhile, water needs in China are expected to continue growing at a rapid pace in all sectors. Industry's use of water, now growing by more than 11 percent a year, could easily double within seven years. In agriculture, the combination of a population reaching 1.6 billion by 2030 and the continuing rise of individual consumption of livestock products, could nearly double the demand for water over today's levels. And in the residential sector, though families often share sanitary facilities and use only 10 gallons of water per person daily, millions more every year are moving into homes with indoor plumbing, where they can easily double or triple their consumption.

DON'T COUNT ON BOOSTING PRODUCTIVITY

In a country where the land area devoted to crops is no longer expanding, as in China, future growth in food output can come only from raising land productivity. The central question, therefore, is whether Chinese Ambassador Xie Zhenhua's proclamation—that China's farmers can raise grain yield per hectare fast enough to offset any loss of cropland—will come true. Alas, data for the four years since 1990 indicate that they are losing the race, just as farmers in Japan, South Korean, and Taiwan did two or three decades earlier.

Since mid-century, changes in China's grain productivity break down into four distinct periods. In the first, from 1950 to 1977, productivity per hectare doubled. One of the keys to this gain was an expansion of irrigated areas along with the adoption of higher-yielding varieties of wheat and rice, developments that paralleled those in other Asian countries participating in the Green Revolution.

The most dynamic period in China's recent agricultural history occurred from 1977 to 1984, when the nation led the world by raising grain yield per hectare by 62 percent, posting a phenomenal annual rate of nearly 7.1 percent. The 1978 economic reforms, which broke up farm production teams and returned farmers to family farm units, triggered the Agricultural Revolution and with it a dramatic rise in the use of fertilizer, which was primarily responsible for the phenomenal growth. After 1984, however, raising productivity proved more difficult. As gains from irrigation and fertilizer use peaked, yields slowed, growing less than 2 percent a year through 1990. Then from 1990 to 1994, yield per

Hopes have faded that biotechnology will provide the necessary doubling or tripling in the production of rice, wheat, and corn—the crops that occupy most of China's farmland. The science has failed to produce a single dramatic gain in the yield of any grain in more than 20 years.

hectare rose even more slowly, edging up only 0.7 percent per year.

Improving productivity further will require raising yields of the three crops that occupy most of China's farmland: rice, wheat, and corn, each of which accounts for roughly 100 million tons of the 340 million-ton annual grain harvest. Rice and wheat, of course, are the two national staples, with rice dominating in the south and wheat in the north. Some corn is also consumed as food but most of that harvest is now fed to livestock.

Of these grains, rice appears to hold the greatest promise for productivity gains. In fact, in the fall of 1994 the International Rice Research Institute in the Philippines, the world's leading center for rice breeding, announced that it had designed a rice variety that would lift yields 20 to 25 percent above the highest-yielding varieties now available in Asia (see "A Job for Super Rice," TR August/September 1995, page 20). By cross-breeding the highest-yielding varieties created during the Green Revolution, scientists essentially designed a plant that boosts the share of metabolic energy it devotes to the formation of seeds, thus raising the amount of grain produced per hectare. But even if the so-called super rice is successful and boosts yields by the maximum 25 percent, it would add only about 30 million tons to the country's harvest—just one-tenth of the projected growth in demand for grain between now and 2030.

As with rice, China can boast of an impressive history in boosting wheat production: from 1975 to 1984, yields climbed 81 percent, a remarkable gain for such a large country. But here, too, growth has since slowed considerably: during the past 10 years, productivity has risen only 17 percent. And with water scarcity reducing irrigation application rates in the north where wheat is grown, achieving greater yields may become progressively more difficult.

China has made similarly impressive progress with corn, but production per hectare is still scarcely 60 percent of that in the United States. This gap could narrow somewhat, but few countries can approach the yields achieved in the U.S. Corn Belt, which has an ideal combination of deep soils, temperatures, day length, and rainfall, the latter near-optimal in both annual amount and seasonal distribution.

At one time, there was high hope that biotechnology would create another generation of high-yielding strains that would greatly increase yields, much like the earlier generation of varieties produced by conventional plant breeding. Unfortunately, this hope has faded as biotechnology has failed to produce a single dramatic yield gain for any grain in more than 20 years. The prudent assumption, therefore, is that there is not likely to be another generation of grains that will double or triple the yield of existing varieties. Yet production improvements of that scale will be required.

A Growing Deficit

Even allowing for some boosts in rice yields from research such as the super rice prototype, the long-term prospect for large additional rice yield increases in China is not bright. The plateauing in grain production during the last four years suggests that the loss of cropland is already offsetting modest gains in land productivity. Indeed, as harvested grain area shrank by 5.6 percent between 1990 and 1994, grain yield per hectare rose by 2.8 percent, which translates into a total decline in grain harvest of 2.8 percent, or 0.7 percent a year.

This suggests that the long-term decline in grain output that accompanied industrialization in Japan, South Korea, and Taiwan may now have begun in China. Indeed, once the decline in Japan's grain production got under way after 1960, output fell by roughly 1 percent a year for more than 30 years, accounting for some 32 percent in total. In looking ahead to 2030, a conservative assumption would be that China's grain production would fall by at least 20 percent. If this happens, the 1990 harvest of 340 million tons would fall to 272 million tons by 2030.

In projecting China's potential grain demand, two scenarios can be considered. Under the first, demand increases only as a result of population growth and there are no further rises in per capita consumption of meat, milk, eggs, or other food products dependent on the use of grain. The second scenario assumes that the Chinese people continue their recent move up the food chain, albeit at a much slower rate than that of Japan. It suggests that the current annual consumption of just under 300 kilograms of grain per person, including that consumed directly as well as that consumed indirectly in the form of livestock products and alcoholic beverages, will increase to 400 kilograms by the year 2030, roughly the same as Taiwan today and half the U.S. per capita grain consumption of more than 800 kilograms per year.

Under both scenarios, the resulting grain deficit is huge, many times that of Japan—currently the world's largest grain importer. In 1990, China produced 340 million tons of grain and consumed 346 million tons. In the first scenario, allowing only for the projected population increase, China's demand for grain would increase to 479 million tons in 2030. Given a projected 20 percent drop in grain production to 272 million tons, as explained earlier, this would leave a shortfall of 207 million tons—roughly equal to the world's entire 1994 grain exports.

But China's newly affluent millions will not likely be content to forgo further increases in consumption of livestock products. If per capita grain consumption climbs to 400 kilograms in the year 2030, total demand for grain will reach a staggering 641 million tons. Under this scenario, the import deficit would reach 369 million tons, nearly double current world grain exports.

While China's political leaders are reluctant to recognize the possibility of so large a grain deficit, at least one Chinese scientist has made calculations similar to these. **Professor Zhou Guangzhao, head of the Chinese**

Academy of Sciences, observes that if consumption per person nationwide reaches the level of the most affluent coastal provinces (about the same level as Taiwan) and if the nation continues to squander its farmland and water resources in an all-out effort to industrialize, "then China will have to import 400 million tons of grain per year from the world market."

WHO WILL FEED CHINA?

In confronting such a deficit, two key questions arise: Will China have enough foreign exchange to import the grain it needs? And will the grain be available? On the first count, if the premise underlying this demand is a continuation of the economic boom, there would likely be ample income from industrial exports to pay for the needed grain imports at current prices. Since China's economic reforms were launched in 1978, nonagricultural exports have been growing at a prodigious rate, surpassing $100 billion for the first time last year. Moreover, record levels of foreign investment by global corporations—designed largely to capitalize on China's vast pool of low-wage labor—will help ensure competitiveness in world market and increase exports.

Filling a 100-million-ton import deficit, which is equal to nearly half of current world grain exports, by bringing in wheat or corn at 1994 prices of roughly $150 a ton would require $15 billion. But given its trade surplus with the United States alone, which in 1994 reached nearly $30 billion, China could buy all U.S. grain exports—grain that now goes to more than 120 grain-deficit countries—even if grain prices doubled. Given the likely continuing growth in China's nonagricultural exports, importing 200 million or even 300 million tons of grain at current prices would be within economic range if the country's leaders were willing to use a share of export earnings for this purpose.

The more difficult question is, who could supply grain on this scale? The answer: no one. No single exporting country nor even all of them together can likely expand exports enough to cover more than a small part of this huge additional claim on the world's exportable grain surplus.

The handful of countries that traditionally produce an exportable grain surplus—including the United States, Canada, Australia, Argentina, and Thailand—face a number of similar constraints to raising yields. For example, in the United States, which accounts for half the world grain exports, the diversion of irrigation water to satisfy the demands of Sun Belt cities—such as Los Angeles, Phoenix, Tucson, Las Vegas, El Paso, and Denver—will reduce the water available to farmers in the southern Great Plains and the Southwest during the next four decades. Also, as the U.S. population swells by some 95 million in this period, the country's cropland will shrink as these new Amer-

icans will need the space to build approximately 30 million houses and apartments and a proportionate number of factories, schools, churches, shopping malls, golf courses, cars, roads, and parking lots. Finally, this growing population will demand some 75 million tons of additional grain for its own consumption.

FOOD: THE NEW THREAT TO SECURITY

Even as China is facing the potential need for massive imports of grain, many other countries are in a similar situation. For example, six of the world's more populous developing countries—Iran, Nigeria, Ethiopia, Pakistan, Bangladesh, and Egypt—are expected to double or triple in population over the next four decades. These and other growing countries—including India, Brazil, Mexico, and Eritrea—face huge grain deficits. In 1990, this group of 10 nations imported 32 million tons of grain, roughly one-sixth of the world total. By 2030—assuming no change in diet—they will need to import 190 million tons, six times the amount they import today and nearly equal to total world grain exports in 1994.

The point of these projections is that competition for grain imports in the years ahead is likely to intensify dramatically even without China's emergence as a massive importer. This suggests that the world grain market soon will be converted from a buyer's to a seller's market. From mid-century through the early nineties, strong competition among exporting countries substantially lowered the real price of grain. This created an ideal environment for alleviating hunger as even low-income countries with limited foreign exchange enjoyed gradually declining outlays for grain imports. But in a seller's market, importing countries will soon find themselves competing vigorously for supplies of grain that never seem adequate, and at ever-increasing prices.

Thus, as the world contemplates the prospect of scarcity, it must face the issue of distribution. As long as the economic pie was expanding more rapidly than population was growing, political leaders could always urge the poor to be patient because eventually their share would also increase. But if the food supply is expanding much more slowly than population, the question of how the pie is divided becomes a much more immediate political issue.

One way of distributing scarce resources is to let the market do its job. Indeed, given the economic reforms in the former Soviet Union and China, reliance on the market to distribute food is now nearly worldwide. Whenever demand outruns supply, the price rises, reducing demand while encouraging additional supply.

From a purely economic standpoint, the market does a good job of balancing demand and supply and distributing food. But from a social point of view, rising food prices can quickly produce a life-threatening situation for the world's poorest. For the Third World's rural landless and its shantytown residents who already may spend 70 percent of their income on food, even a modest rise in food prices can threaten survival. In a global economy, rising food prices could jeopardize security in food-importing countries worldwide, leading to potentially unmanageable inflation, abrupt shifts in currency exchange rates, widespread political unrest, and even swelling flows of hungry migrants across national borders.

SETTING PRIORITIES

Clearly, the most urgent need is to stabilize world population, and thus the demand for food, as soon as possible. China's leaders took a step in the right direction in 1979 when, faced with a trade-off between smaller families in the present or deteriorating living conditions in the future, they instituted a "one-couple, one-child" policy. As a result, China's population growth rate has dropped from 2.7 percent to 1.1 percent, and is now roughly the same as that of the United States. Still, implementing the one-child-per-family policy has become more difficult in recent years, as some families are becoming so affluent that they can readily pay the stiff penalty for having more children.

Meanwhile, the goals of the World Population Plan of Action—adopted at the United Nations Conference on Population and Development in Cairo in September 1994—may not be ambitious enough. The plan calls for achieving universal, primary-level education for all young women, which by itself is expected to reduce birth rates, and to implement family-planning practices more widely. But some densely populated developing countries may have to choose between quickly reducing family size to "replacement level," that is, no more than two children per family, or accept a decline in food consumption per person in the decades ahead.

Another top priority is to expand food production by conserving water. For example, water marketing—pricing water at full cost—would reduce wasteful use and encourage investment in water-efficient technologies and practices in agriculture, industry, and cities. Avoiding acute water scarcity depends on investing in water efficiency on a scale comparable to the investment in energy efficiency in the mid-seventies, and thus buying more time to stabilize population.

Many countries also need to take steps to actively protect cropland from nonfarm uses. One of the principal threats to the world's cropland is the trend toward automobile-centered transportation systems: the evolution of such systems not only leads to the extensive paving of cropland, but it also encourages land-consuming urban sprawl. The alternative is a combination of public transport and bicycles.

With world grain stocks at their lowest level in 20 years and with the prospect of spreading food scarcity, we need an inventory of the various reserves that can be tapped to alleviate scarcity and buy time to stabilize population, now growing by 90 million per year. The most easily tapped reserve is the cropland in the United States and Europe that is idled under supply management programs that are designed to avoid surpluses. If this land were returned to production in 1996, it could boost the world grain harvest by an estimated 34 million tons, enough to cover the demand stemming from world population growth for 15 months.

Another source of land for food production is the fields used to grow nonfood products such as tobacco. If the 5 million hectares of cropland now devoted to tobacco growing were switched to grain, assuming the average world yield of 2.4 tons per hectare, the production would provide enough grain to support the growth in world population for nearly six months.

Almost as large a potential source of food is the 1.4 million hectares of highly productive U.S. cornland that now produces the 11 million tons of corn annually used to make roughly 1 billion gallons of ethanol for use as an automotive fuel. Making this grain available for human consumption could cover four months of world population growth.

The area now growing cotton could also be reduced. If consumers could be persuaded to replace half of the cotton clothing they buy with clothes made from synthetic fibers, some 9 million hectares of land worldwide would be freed up, providing enough grain for 11 months of world population growth. China, the world's leading cotton consumer, is already investing heavily in the manufacture of synthetic fibers on a scale that could eventually lower demand for cotton.

A tax on the consumption of beef, pork, poultry, eggs, and other livestock products—which require far more grain to produce than would otherwise be consumed in a starchy diet—would be unpopular but could be one means of ensuring global stability in an era of scarcity.

By far the largest food reserve is the 37 percent of the world grain harvest, some 630 million tons in 1994, used to produce livestock and poultry products for human consumption. To some degree, rising grain prices will push up prices of livestock products and reduce their consumption. But the price level at which a substantial reduction occurs is so high that it could force food consumption among millions of the world's poor below the survival level. Rationing the consumption of livestock products in the more affluent societies would free up grain without leading to dramatic price rises.

The same reduction in consumption could be achieved by imposing a tax on consumption of livestock products, one that would be similar to those that governments put on alcoholic beverages and cigarettes. Such a tax could affect eating habits not only in industrial countries but in developing ones as well, as China is now the world's largest consumer of red meat. Reducing the 630 million tons of grain used for feed by 10 percent would free up 63 million tons of grain for direct consumption—enough to cover world population growth for 28 months. Unprecedented and unpopular though a livestock-products tax would be, it could be the price of global stability in an era of scarcity.

Beyond this, an international food-reserve organization is urgently needed—one that would acquire stocks when prices are low in order to release them when they are higher, thus helping to stabilize food prices.

Finally, there is a need for much greater global investment in agricultural research. Although the likelihood of another breakthrough like the development of hybrid corn or the discovery of chemical fertilizer is low, in a world of food scarcity every technological advance that helps expand production, however small, is important.

Effectively addressing the threat of food scarcity to our future will take a massive mobilization of resources, both financial and political. But if we really care, we have no choice but to launch such an effort. For our generation, the overriding issue is whether we can reestablish a stable relationship between our numbers and aspirations on the one hand and the earth's natural support systems on the other. Unless we act quickly and decisively, neither history nor our children will judge us kindly.

Nibbling at famine's edge

N. Korea: *Economic mismanagement and floods that wiped out the rice crop have left North Korea desperate for food. The government radio is offering recipes for grass.*

SUN FOREIGN STAFF

TUMEN, China—Returning to China, Tian Jijun told of his frustrating business trip to North Korea. "They have nothing to sell," he said.

North Korea is desperate for food. Chinese traders have food to sell. But 50 years of economic mismanagement have left North Korea with little cash and nothing to sell other than scrap metal, smuggled cars and the few remaining trees on its mountains.

North Korea remains off limits to most foreigners, but its problems are evident even from the periphery.

Here, in northeastern China's Yanbian district, 40 percent of the population is ethnically Korean, with hundreds of Chinese-Koreans a day crossing into North Korea carrying rice for impoverished relatives.

After months of gathering intelligence, U.S. officials say they now agree with international relief agencies that famine could occur and formally announced yesterday that they will offer North Korea food worth $6.2 million.

The country's food shortage comes after floods devastated much of the countryside in August. Some areas received 80 percent of their annual rainfall in just 24 hours, leading to flood waters that carried away

homes and crops. Paddies were buried under mud and rock, making it impossible in many areas to plant new crops.

North Korea claimed it had suffered $15 billion in damages, a figure that other countries thought was exaggerated to mask long-term economic mismanagement. But it became apparent that even though the country's economic policies of self-reliance and collectivization had ruined agriculture, a genuine disaster had taken place and aid was needed.

Recently, for example, North Korean radio has broadcast recipes for using grass to make the national staple, kim chee, which is usually made of pickled cabbage. Visitors say people can be seen scrounging along roadsides for edible plants.

"It's not at the famine stage but the initial signs of malnutrition are appearing slowly and consistently," said Robert Hauser, head of the U.N. World Food Program office in Pyongyang.

Besides its failed economic policies, many observers blame North Korea's leadership for allowing part of its population to go hungry while preserving privileges for others, such as urban residents and the army.

"The leadership has decided to write off the rural population," said a Western diplomat in Beijing.

"I would not underestimate the ability of the North Korean people to endure," the diplomat said. "But sometime in the future [the system] will collapse. Their economic system is a failure on the most basic level: the ability to provide food for its people."

North Korea is making use of its reputation for unpredictability. With a huge army facing South Korean and U.S. troops, the thought of starvation and a desperate leadership makes outsiders doubly willing to offer aid.

Cui Shunjin, an ethnic Korean who is general manager of Taoyuan Co. Ltd., said that during a recent business trip to the North the country's fuel shortage meant that buses did not run and cars were few. Restaurants served cold noodles, while tourist sites were empty.

"At this time of the year, all the hotels should have been full," said Cui, "but they were almost empty"— for lack of fuel for buses and lack of electricity for the hotels.

Residents of the capital, she said, had to spend a day a week working in the fields, while food was so severely rationed—700 grams of rice a day—that people went hungry. Relief agencies estimate that North Koreans are receiving 900 calories of food a day, 1,400 calories less than an average manual laborer needs for survival.

But Cui and other visitors inevitably point out that North Korea is tightly disciplined and not imploding. Food is distributed, people go to work, government agencies function.

Still, the signs of a failed economy are visible.

Cui, whose company carries out barter trade, said she imports from North Korea handicrafts, cars that were stolen from Japan and steel. Other traders say the steel is scrap from dismantled factories and railroads. Seafood also is for sale— when North Korean fishermen have enough fuel to leave port.

She and other Chinese exporters sell the North only food, primarily flour and sugar. China, which imports grain itself to feed its huge population, discourages the export of grain. Nevertheless, Cui and others say they could export more food products if North Korea had products worth buying.

Recently, a Chinese government official said, North Korea was buying grain on credit, promising bartered products when they are available. But with North Korea's economic situation worsening, the Chinese government stepped in to forbid state-run firms from selling grain on credit.

With trade falling, most contacts are personal. Cui makes regular trips to bring help in the form of rice for her relatives. Although her family and the other city people she visits are surviving, Cui is unsure about conditions in the countryside.

So are the relief agencies.

North Korea allows the United Nation's World Food Program, for example, to monitor food distribution to make sure that donated food is given to the needy. But relief workers are not allowed free access to rural areas for a true assessment of the country's needs.

The higher standard of living in Pyongyang—where grain rations may be double those in the countryside—makes it clear that the government is pacifying the potentially volatile urban residents at the expense of people in the countryside.

Few ethnic Koreans are willing to talk openly about the situation, out of embarrassment at their people's suffering or fear of North Korea's security apparatus. One elderly lady named Kim, however, said her family was in need of food.

Standing next to half a dozen 110-pound bags of rice, Kim said she was planning to smuggle the rice past Chinese customs officials—who turn a blind eye out of humanitarianism or for a small bribe—and over the border.

Privation is nothing new to North Koreans. Ethnic Koreans in China have been carrying grain over to hungry relatives for years, while the Red Cross estimates that grain harvests started falling after 1985, the last time North Korea published statistics on grain production.

Federal Food Assistance Programs

A Step to Food Security for Many

Food Assistance Programs supported by the Federal government in the United States and currently funded to a level of over $37 billion are designed to either enhance the buying power of participants by issuing vouchers or stamps for the purchase of food in the marketplace or to provide food directly to supplement or spare family food supplies. The scope, goals, successes and limitations of current programs in enhancing the food security of targeted populations are discussed.

PATRICIA L. SPLETT, M.P.H., Ph.D.

Dr. Splett is Assistant Professor in the School of Public Health at the University of Minnesota. Her research focuses on the cost and effectiveness of nutrition and health programs and services.

Many citizens of the United States do not have access to sufficient food on a regular basis. Federal food assistance programs are an important means of assuring that all Americans have access to an adequate, safe, nutritious and reliable food supply at reasonable cost. The food programs of the United States represent a range of goals, services, delivery models and eligibility criteria. They are intended to improve the nutrition and health status of the targeted beneficiaries by improved access to food. . . .

The current levels of participation and 1993 federal appropriations for the major food assistance programs are shown in Table 1. Federal government expenditures for food assistance help subsidize the distribution of over 100 million meals a day. Together, the food assistance programs play an important role in reducing food insecurity in U.S. households.

Food insecurity has been described to include four components. First is the *quantitative* aspect, which addresses whether the household has access to a sufficient quantity of food—enough to eat, not going to bed hungry. Second is a *qualitative* component, which is concerned with the nutritional adequacy of the available food as well as its suitability for the family. Suitability includes consideration of cultural factors and capacity for food storage and preparation, which may be affected by skills and access to usable cooking utensils and appliances. To sustain health, available food must be nutritionally

> **All food assistance programs extend the quantity of food available.**

balanced, and it must be acceptable and usable. The third component of food security is *psychological*. This has to do with anxiety, lack of choice and feelings of deprivation when hunger and food insecurity are experienced. A *social* component completes the definition of food insecurity. When food security for an individual or household is threatened, food acquisition methods and eating patterns may deviate

From *Nutrition Today*, March/April 1994, pp. 6-13. © 1994 by Williams & Wilkins. Reprinted by permission.

from what is generally considered socially acceptable—stealing, gathering food from dumpsters and eating pet food are examples of this. Understanding these components is crucial to appropriate steps to addressing the food security needs of individuals and families. . . .

SCHOOL-BASED FOOD PROGRAMS

The school-based Child Nutrition Programs include school lunch, school breakfast, special milk, and summer feeding programs. These began with the school lunch program in 1947.

School Lunch Program. The National School Lunch Program is the nation's widest scale effort to support the nutrition of children. It was created to safeguard the health of American children by encouraging consumption of nutritious foods and to provide an outlet for surplus agricultural commodities. It operates through federal reimbursements as cash and commodity foods to schools for lunches that meet federally defined meal pattern requirements. The lunch with five prescribed meal components is intended to provide approximately one-third of the Recommended Dietary Allowance (RDA) for children.

Almost all primary and secondary public schools in the United States offer school lunch to students. In fiscal year 1992, 42.7 million students (58% of school enrollment) participated in the School Lunch Program, which was supported with federal funds of $3.8 billion distributed to 92,300 schools. Nearly half of the lunches are provided free or at a reduced price to children from low-income families. For example, in 1992 children in a family of four with an annual income of $18,135 or less qualified for free lunch. . . .

The School Lunch Program has been the subject of numerous evaluations over the years. Many benefits of participation in the program have been documented. A recent study found that low-income children participating in school lunch consume more protein, calcium, riboflavin, phosphorus, vitamin A and vitamin B_6, but less magnesium and vitamin C than nonparticipants of similar income. In addition, children not eating school lunch have significantly greater polyunsaturated fat, carbohydrate and sucrose intake. Older school lunch participants (aged 12 to 18 years) consume an average of 728 calories more per day than nonparticipants.

The last comprehensive national study was completed in 1983. At

that time, school lunch participants were found to have an overall higher quality of diet than nonparticipants. Participants also weighed more for their age than nonparticipants. A second comprehensive evaluation of the school lunch program is now under way. This study will help determine the degree to which school lunch is safeguarding the health of American children taking into account our new understanding of diet as it is related to the risk of future chronic disease.

Because school lunch reaches a large proportion of the nation's children, it is an excellent channel for influencing the nutritional intake and health of children. The School Lunch Program is also an important means to influencing food preferences and food choices in childhood and for a lifetime. With the help of the Nutrition Education and Training Program (NET) and the initiative and creativity of many school food service directors, teachers and university, industry and other collaborators, many schools have built exciting and effective nutrition education into their School Lunch Program.

School Breakfast Program. Congress passed the School Breakfast Program in 1966. Its aim is to offer a meal to children who would oth-

Table 1
Federal Food Assistance Programs, 1992 Participation and 1993 Appropriations*

Program	No. of Participants	Government Appropriation (million dollars)†
Food Stamps	25.4 million	27,000
Child Nutrition		
National School Lunch	25.0 million/day	4,100
School Breakfast	5.3 million/day	891
Special Milk	175 million ½ pints	14.9
Summer Food Service Program	2 million	230.4
Child and Adult Care Food Program		1,300
Children	1.9 million/day	
Adults	32,000/day	
Supplemental Food		
Commodity Supplemental Food	342,000/mo	94.5
Women, Infants and Children (WIC)	5.4 million/mo	2,860
Food Distribution		
Nutrition Program for Elderly (congregate dining and home delivered meals)	929,000 meals/day	142.9
Emergency Food Assistance (TEFAP)		163

* *Source:* Food Program Facts: The Food and Nutrition Service, USDA, May 1993.
† Excludes administrative costs except for WIC.

COMPONENTS OF FOOD SECURITY

Quantitative—Is there access to a sufficient quantity of food?

Qualitative—Is food nutritionally adequate?

Suitability—Is food culturally acceptable and the capacity for storage and preparation appropriate?

Psychological—Does it alleviate anxiety, lack of choice and feelings of deprivation?

Social—Does food gathering involve socially acceptable methods?

erwise not eat breakfast. School Breakfast Program resources are earmarked for schools enrolling low-income children and schools in locations that require children to travel long distances.

In 1990, over 4.4 million school breakfasts were served daily. Breakfast is primarily used by low-income children evidenced by the fact that over 86% are provided to children who qualify for free or reduced-price meals.

Research has shown that the availability of a school breakfast is a factor in determining whether or not children eat any breakfast, and eating a breakfast is significantly related to attention span and school performance. School breakfast was found to contribute positively to the 1987 comprehensive test of basic skills battery total score and negatively to 1987 tardiness and absence rates. Studies have shown significant improvements in academic functioning among low-income elementary school breakfast participants.

Special Milk Program. The Special Milk Program provides half pints of fluid milk to children in schools and child care. After the widespread availability of school lunch, the milk program is now used primarily to provide a milk break to kindergarten students.

Summer Food Program. The Summer Food Program extends the benefits of school lunch by providing nutritious meals to needy children during the summer months. The Summer Food Program is delivered through park and recreation departments, community centers, camps and schools. The Summer Food Program plays an important role in extending food resources for low-income families during the summer months when, compared to the school year, the family is responsible for two more meals each day for school-aged children. Summer food programs often become a component of summer recreational and educational programs. This offers the opportunity to merge nutritional benefits with physical exercise, education and socialization in a supervised setting

where positive role models are available.

FOOD STAMP PROGRAM

The Food Stamp Program was created in 1964 to help low-income households obtain a more nutritious diet by using government issued stamps to purchase foods in the marketplace. The program increases the food-buying power of participating families and stimulates demand for agricultural commodities.

In fiscal 1991, government spending for the program was $18.8 billion for 22.6 million participants. The households receiving food stamps had an average monthly income of $472. The additional income represented by food stamps averaged $162 per month. In 1992, the federal expenditure for food stamps rose to $22.4 billion. This was distributed to 25.4 million individuals and provided a larger benefit for each participating household.

Like Social Security, the Food Stamp Program is an *entitlement* program. That means that all who meet eligibility criteria have the right to receive benefits. Unfortunately, only about half of eligible families participate. The most common participating household is a family with children. Low-income elderly have the lowest participation rates.

The Food Stamp Program is an entitlement program with all who meet eligibility requirements having the right to receive benefits.

Participation numbers and total program costs are controlled through adjustments in eligibility standards. Periodic changes include redefining net income calculations by modifying allowable deductions and exemptions, requiring participation in employment and training programs, or raising or lowering the level of benefits to eligible households. Changes to limit eligibility (and therefore the number "entitled") and to control fraud and abuse have caused application and

verification procedures to be complicated and burdensome. Reports suggest that administrative hassles, as well as poor outreach and a welfare stigma associated with using stamps, are barriers to participation. USDA and advocacy groups are attempting to reduce these and other barriers.

Food stamp participation fosters a more nutritious diet by designating that a specific amount of the household's resources be spent on food. Participants are free to exercise their preferences for types of food and ways to meet nutritional needs using food stamps. Studies have shown that food stamp families purchase more nutrient-dense foods and have higher nutrient intakes than nonparticipating low-income families.

Evaluations have found that Food Stamp Program participation does increase household food expenditures, and participants have higher levels of 12 key nutrients relative to the RDA. Food stamp participation has been found to significantly increase the consumption of calcium, vitamin C and iron and eight other nutrients.

The monetary value of food stamps allocated to a household is based on the Thrifty Food Plan, one of four USDA food plans. USDA food plans are national standards of costs for nutritious diets at four levels of food expenditure. They are based on food consumption patterns and food costs of U.S. households as identified by the 1977–78 U.S. Nationwide Food Consumption Survey and a supplemental survey of food stamp-eligible households. The plans take into account current knowledge of nutritional needs (i.e., Dietary Guidelines and RDAs) and nutrient content of foods. The lowest cost plan, the Thrifty Food Plan, is used as a basis to determine benefits in the Food Stamp Program, even though it results in a diet below the RDA for calcium, zinc, iron, magnesium and folacin. These nutrient shortfalls are of special concern for young children, teenaged girls and women who are highly represented among food stamp recipients.

The cost of the Thrifty Food Plan is updated monthly based on the

Bureau of Labor Statistics market-basket survey of actual food costs. Food stamp benefits are adjusted annually; thus, food stamp allot-

---

Monetary value of food stamps is based on family size and income adjusted annually to reflect the cost of the USDA Thrifty Food Plan.

---

ments are behind the actual cost of the Thrifty Food Plan by 3 to 15 months.

Food stamp benefits are calculated on the assumption that 30% of net household income will be spent on food in addition to food stamps. Evidence indicates that this is a faulty assumption. In 1988, the average grant to families receiving Aid to Families with Dependent Children was 47% of the federal poverty level in 39 states; and food stamp plus Aid to Families with Dependent Children benefits together raised the families' income to only 75% of the poverty level.

Thus, even with food stamps families are likely to experience food insecurity. In a Boston study, food assistance benefits (food stamps plus school lunch) covered only 33.8 to 66.3% of estimated household food costs in 1987. The investigators showed that high housing costs dramatically limited resources available for food. When food stamp families participated in one to five additional food assistance programs (e.g., school lunch, WIC, etc.) 71% of families in Cleveland still did not meet the Thrifty Food Plan's nutritional recommendations. Consumption of breads and cereals and fruits and vegetables was commonly lacking for all family members. Female adolescents and adults were at the greatest nutritional risk with low intakes of milk and fruits and vegetables. . . .

WIC

WIC is targeted to low-income pregnant or lactating women and infants and children up to age 5 who are certified as having health or nutritional risks. The program was created to supplement diets in specific nutrients by providing milk or cheese, iron-fortified cereal, vitamin C juice, eggs and peanut butter or dry beans. Iron-fortified formula is also provided to infants who are not breast-fed. Participants receive an average of $35 worth of nutritious food each month. In addition to the specified package of supplemental foods, the program provides nutrition education and facilitates contact with the health care system.

WIC has strong congressional and public support. Funding from the Federal government for WIC has grown from $20 million in 1974 to over $2.5 billion in 1992. In some states, WIC receives an additional state appropriation, which funds the expansion of services to more women, infants and children. About 4.9 million participants receive monthly WIC benefits. This is estimated to be approximately 60% of those eligible. Legislative efforts are underway to get "full funding" for WIC in future years. The goal is to bring the federal allocation to a level that makes WIC available to all who are eligible.

WIC is the most thoroughly evaluated food assistance program and is probably the most highly evaluated human service program. Such evaluations are important to assuring that the program operates efficiently and achieves its stated purpose. Early management studies compared using vouchers (like bank checks) at local grocers with warehousing and direct distribution of food. More recently, innovations are being studied, such as the use of vouchers at farmers' markets and a computerized "credit card" (e.g., automatic benefits transfer) in place of food vouchers. States have initiated steps to control food costs and thereby increase the number served. Contracting with one formula company as a "single source" provider of formula for the state has greatly reduced food costs and enabled expansion of the number served by WIC.

Studies of the nutrition and health effects of WIC have found that participation in WIC has positive effects on iron nutriture and growth and development of infants and children. WIC participation during pregnancy has been found to decrease the risk of delivering a

---

WIC participants have longer gestation periods, fewer preterm deliveries, and fewer low and very low birth weight infants. Infants and children have better growth and development and iron nutriture.

---

low birth weight (less than 2500 g) infant or a very low birth weight (less than 1500 g) infant by 25 and 44%, respectively.

A comprehensive, national evaluation of WIC was completed in 1985. Major findings included the following. Pregnant WIC participants were more likely to register for prenatal care in the first trimester and were less likely to have inadequate prenatal care compared to nonparticipants. WIC children were more likely to have a regular source of medical care and were better immunized compared to nonparticipating children.

Women's dietary intake improved for protein, iron, calcium and vitamin C (key WIC nutrients), as well as for energy, magnesium, phosphorus, thiamin, riboflavin, niacin, vitamin B_6 and vitamin B_{12}.

Women who participated in WIC during pregnancy had a longer length of gestation by 1.4 days compared with nonparticipants. The rate of preterm deliveries was significantly reduced among less educated white and black mothers. Birth weight differences appeared to be related to the quality of the local program operation and were greater among women who were members of racial/ethnic minority population groups or who had less education. Infants of women who participated during pregnancy had larger head circumferences.

The 1985 National WIC Evaluation did not find differences in pregnant women's intention to breast feed or on actual breast-feeding rates. Since then, breast-feeding promotion within WIC has been greatly expanded and an increase in breast-feeding rates has been observed.

WIC has been the subject of several cost-benefit studies. These studies have focused on cost savings resulting from heavier infants with longer periods of gestation and fewer infants requiring intensive care in the immediate postnatal period. The most comprehensive study involved five states and found positive benefit-cost ratios ranging from $1.77 to $3.13 for WIC services to pregnant women. A study is underway that will assess the cost benefit of WIC services provided to children. The government's General Accounting Office estimated that each dollar invested in WIC saves $2.89 in Medicaid, SSI, and special education and other health care within the first year after birth, and saves $3.50 over 18 years.

The positive effects of WIC are due, in part, to the nutrition education that all participants get as a part of WIC benefits. Every woman, infant and child has a nutrition assessment and receives nutrition education and counseling tailored to his or her needs and problems that are identified. Monthly contacts at WIC sites allow for reinforcement of education and recommendations.

WIC dietitians/nutritionists have information on child nutrition and nutrition in pregnancy and lactation. These nutrition professionals are excellent resources for others who are working with individuals and families to promote good nutrition and good health.

WIC is widely recognized as an important and effective program that successfully reaches large numbers of low-income women and their children. Because of this, several special activities have been piggybacked onto the responsibilities of WIC staff (e.g., immunization outreach, drug and alcohol screening, cholesterol screening, food stamp and Medicaid eligibility determination). These requests and mandates are in response to a recent emphasis on one-stop social services. While this appears to make good sense, it is possible that the advantages of program integration will be outweighed by the disadvantages stemming from a diffusion of effort and reduced focus on the nutrition education aspects of WIC. Many WIC programs are working to make service delivery procedures and education approaches and materials appropriate to the diverse cultures served. This remains an important challenge for WIC and for other food assistance programs.

WIC, through the provision of selected foods, nutrition education, counseling and support and referral to or coordination with health care, has become an extremely important program for fostering food security and increasing access to health services for the youngest and most vulnerable members of our society.

ELDERLY NUTRITION PROGRAM

The elderly are vulnerable to the risk of poor nutritional status because of the physiologic changes, psychological, sociological and economic factors, and chronic disease that accompany aging. They also experience major difficulties related to buying groceries, cooking and chewing. It is estimated that half of the nation's elderly population suffer from poor nutrition. Deteriorating nutritional status contributes to the greater utilization of health care services by this age group and to greater institutionalization. There is great interest in identifying effective community-based services that enable elderly persons to maintain health status and stay active in their communities.

Congregate Dining and Home Delivered Meals. Congregate dining and home delivered meal programs, funded by Title III of the Older Americans Act and operated through local Area Agencies on Aging, provide some food security while bringing elderly persons in regular contact with others. . . .

Congregate dining was created in 1965. It was the first federal nutrition program specifically targeted to older adults. The purpose of congregate dining is:

to provide older Americans, particularly those with low income, low cost, nutritionally sound meals served in strategically located centers. . .where they can obtain better social and rehabilitative services. Besides promoting better health among the older segment of the population through improved nutrition, such a program is aimed at reducing the isolation of old age, offering older Americans an opportunity to live their remaining years in dignity (*Federal Register*, 1972, p. 16845).

The home delivered meals program was added later for the frail and homebound elderly. Participation in home delivered meals can bridge a period after discharge from the hospital or recovery from illness, or it can be a permanent service that is crucial for allowing elderly persons to stay in their own homes.

Approximately 929,000 meals are served per day to older Americans who participate: 60% at congregate dining sites and 40% through home delivered meals. USDA support for the Nutrition Programs for the Elderly, as cash and commodity foods, was almost $143 millon in 1993. In addition, more than $617 million dollars (in 1990) were allocated for operation of Title III nutrition services by the Department of Health and Human Services.

Almost one million meals are served daily to older Americans—60% at congregate meal sites and 40% home delivered.

Because resources are limited, programs strive to target higher risk elderly persons. A past evaluation found that approximately 75% of delivered meals and congregate dining participants had one or more priority traits defined as advanced age, low-income, social isolation, minority status, mobility impairment or limited ability to speak English. Many participants have a high level of risk for nutritional deficiency. A study of the nutritional status of meals on wheels participants using weight and biochemical values by Lipschitz found a high prevalence of nutritional deficiencies; 36% were identified as at risk of protein-calorie malnutrition.

Local contributions are important to the operation of nutrition programs for the elderly. A study in the early 1980s found that federal funds supported 64% of costs of providing congregate meals and 60% of the cost of home delivered meals. In addition to this, hospitals, churches and other organizations in some communities offer meals on wheels programs that are independent from the federal nutrition programs for the elderly.

According to federal regulations congregate dining and home delivered meals must provide a minimum of one-third of the RDA. Studies have shown great variation in the nutritional quality of congregate meals. The levels of nutrients provided ranged from 24 to 133% of the RDA. Nutrients frequently found lacking include vitamin D, vitamin E, vitamin B₆, folacin, magnesium and zinc. Nutrient analysis of home delivered meals found that protein, iron, phosphorus, vitamin A and niacin were higher than 33% of the RDA, while energy, thiamin, riboflavin and vitamin C were below 33% of the RDA.

There is concern about the nutritional needs of homebound elderly persons on weekends. Those who receive home delivered meals 5 days per week generally have insufficient intakes of protein, thiamin, riboflavin, calcium, iron and phosphorus on weekends com-

pared to weekdays. Weekend meal services for the elderly are being explored and implemented in some areas. Some programs deliver frozen meal for weekends on Friday. This arrangement saves delivery costs and assures the the elderly person will not go hungry.

Evaluation Findings. Several studies have examined the association of Title III nutrition program participation with biochemical and anthropometric measures. In Mississippi, meals program participants were more likely to consume two-thirds of the RDA for calcium, vitamin A and ascorbic acid compared to nonparticipants. No differences in blood values were found.

Missouri investigators reported anthropometric, biochemical and dietary data from elderly women and men, 75 years and older. Men who participated in congregate dining once per week had significantly lower hemoglobin and hematocrit levels than men who participated regularly. Mean hematocrit levels for men who never participated or infrequently participated were in the unacceptable range. Serum vitamin A concentrations were lower for those who had never participated; this was statistically significant for women. Serum total protein and albumin were significantly lower for women who never participated.

The dietary intakes of homebound elderly who were recipients

of home delivered meals were compared with dietary intakes of a group of elderly on a waiting list. Waiting clients had significantly higher intakes of carbohydrate, thiamin and iron than meals recipients. Energy intake did not exceed the RDA for any one. More than 50% of both groups consumed less than the RDA for vitamin A, riboflavin, thiamin, calcium, phosphorus and iron. Calcium consumption was the nutrient most likely to be deficient. Sixty-three percent of waiting clients and 88% of recipients had daily intakes of less than 66% of the RDA for one or more

APPLICATION

Dietitians and other health professionals in various settings interact with patients/clients and community members who are living in poverty. Many of these people could be eligible for food stamps or other food assistance programs. Health professionals need to be attuned to food security needs. They need to recognize signs of food insecurity and refer patients/clients to programs when appropriate. Table 2 outlines targeted beneficiaries of the federal assistance programs and suggests indicators that could cue providers to identify individuals who would likely be eligible for and could benefit from specific programs. Through sensitivity and awareness, health and social serv-

Table 2
Referral Guide for Food Assistance

Program	Targeted Beneficiaries	Indicators of Need	Where to Call
School Lunch	Nation's school children	Poor nutritional status	Local school district
School Breakfast	Children who would be unlikely to eat before school	Harried household, low-income, poor nutrition status	Local school district
Summer Food Program	Children in low-income neighborhoods	Economic stress, poor nutritional status	State department of education
Food Stamps	Low-income households	Economic stress, low quantity/quality of available food	County social services office
WIC	Low-income pregnant and lactating women, infants and children up to age 5	Risk of or existing health or nutrition problem	City or county health department or community action agency
Congregate Dining	Elderly, especially low-income, minority and frail	Few social contacts, poor quality or quantity of diet	Area Agency on Aging
Home Delivered Meals	Frail, homebound elderly	Unable to shop or prepare food, no available caretaker	Area Agency on Aging or local hospital

ices providers can take appropriate action and extend the benefits of federal food assistance programs to those in need.

SUGGESTED READINGS

Emmons L. Relationship of participation in food assistance programs to the nutritional quality of diets. *Am J Public Health* 1987;77:856–8.

Farris RP, Nicklas TA, Webber LS, Berenson GS. Nutrient contribution of the School Lunch Program: implications for Healthy People 2000. *Sch Health* 1992;62:180–4.

Hunger in the '80s and '90s. *J Nutr Educ* 1992; 24(suppl).

Kohrs MB. Evaluation of nutrition programs for the elderly. *Am J Clin Nutr* 1982;36:812–8.

Kohrs MB. Effectiveness of nutrition intervention programs for the elderly. In Hutchinson ML, Munro HN. *Nutrition and aging.* Orlando, FL: Academic Press, 1986.

Lipschitz DA, Mitchell CO, Steel RW, Milton KY. Nutritional evaluation and supplementation of elderly subjects participating in a "Meals on Wheels" program. *JPEN* 1985;9:343–7.

Lopez L, Berce M. Food stamp use and the nutrition practices of participants in the Colorado Expanded Food and Nutrition Education Program. *J Am Diet Assoc* 1989;89:1312–3.

Mathematica Policy Research, Inc. *The savings in Medicaid costs for newborns and their mothers from prenatal participation in the WIC program.* Volume I. Washington, DC: U.S. Department of Agriculture, Food and Nutrition Service, 1990.

Matsumoto M. Recent trends in domestic food programs. *Natl Food Rev* 1990;13:31–3.

Meyers A. School Breakfast Program and school performance. *Am J Dis Child* 1989;143:1234–9.

Public Policy and Legislative Committee. *Universal vision: America's children ready to learn.* Legislative Issue Paper. Alexandria, VA: American School Food Service Association, February 1992.

Radzikowski J, Gale S. The national evaluation of school nutrition programs: conclusions. *Am J Clin Nutr* 1984;40:454–61.

Snyder MP, Story M, Lytle T, Renkner L. Reducing fat and sodium in School Lunch Program: The Lunchpower! Intervention Study. *J Am Diet Assoc* 1992;92:1087–91.

Tak J. Commercial frozen meals: a cost effective alternative for home-delivery in feeding programs for the elderly. *J Nutr Elderly* 1993;12:15–25.

United States Department of Agriculture Research Service. Effects of food stamps on food consumption: a review of literature. *Fam Econ Rev* 1991;4:28.

Wiecha JL, Palombo R. Multiple program participation: comparison of nutrition and food assistance program benefits with food costs in Boston, Massachusetts. *Am J Public Health* 1989; 79:591–4.

Thunder in the Distance

A University of California study on poverty estimates that two million California children are hungry. What happens when that hunger turns to anger, and those children grow up?

Al Martinez

Al Martinez is an award-winning columnist for the Los Angeles Times *and the author of several books, including a collection of essays published under the title "Ashes in the Rain."*

The year was 1936. I was in the second grade and we were living in a shack on a hillside in East Oakland. It was Thanksgiving. I remember the feelings of festivity in the air, and the good smells that seemed to emanate from the kitchens of others. It didn't come from ours. We were poor, and lived like we were poor. Our shack had no gas and no electricity. It hovered precariously over a steep slope, partially propped up by a single board wedged against a tree. We cooked on a wood stove and lighted the house with kerosene lanterns.

It was the time of the Great Depression, and my angry old stepfather had been out of work for God knows how long, and it gnawed at his soul like a hound of heaven. I remember we were on "relief" and were given occasional handouts of food and clothing by abrupt and harried people at long tables in cold and cavernous buildings.

I hated the grayness of the buildings, the attitudes of the workers and the terrible oppressiveness of those who stood in lines that wound out the door, waiting their turn for food and clothing. Even at age seven, I disliked being there. I could feel the resentment of a relief worker who jammed new shoes on my feet to see if they fit, handling me as though I were less than human, a job he hated that had to be done.

I suppose, in a way, I could have taken all that had it not been for Thanksgiving. I mentioned the smells and the warmth of other households in the neighborhood. No one was rich on Burr Street, but they had somehow managed to put together a holiday dinner. In our house, it was bread and a homemade meatless soup. Even in our terrible poverty, I had somehow expected there would be a Thanksgiving, but there wasn't. The shock of the meager dinner remains etched on my memory. And I think of all the children, in this Golden Age and this Golden State, who are today what I was back then: hungry, angry and terribly sad.

I was reminded of it recently by a report from the University of California, Berkeley, that said there are five million hungry people in California, and two million of them are children—enough to create a city more than twice the size of San Francisco. They comprise about 25 percent of all the children in the state up to age 18, a figure that, according to the U.S. Census Bureau, almost doubled in the decade of the 1980s. More children have entered poverty in the past five years than in the previous 20.

We don't always recognize them as poor by their outward appearance. They go to school, play outside and then disappear. Some go to houses, some to trailers and some to the cars or trucks or vans they call home. What awaits them are the kinds of meals that awaited me back then, or possibly less. They're what John Steinbeck called the children of fury, pushing at the thin line between hunger and anger.

We are coming full circle in my lifetime from an era of intense privation, through war and full bellies, to a period in which children wonder once more what became of Thanksgiving. The poor, the unseen people, have always been with us, and no doubt always will be, but their ranks, like armies of despair, are steadily growing. The number of Californians living below poverty level rose from 11 percent in 1980 to

18.2 percent in 1993. What makes their existence more painful than ever is a widening gap between the haves and have-nots, bringing into sharper contrast those who sign multimillion dollar contracts for hitting balls and sinking baskets and those with no place to go and nothing to eat.

Social scientist Michael Harrington, acknowledging the invisibility of the poor, observed that "They are not simply neglected and forgotten as in the old rhetoric of reform; what is much worse, they are not seen." And yet, evidence of their existence surfaces occasionally with such poignancy that we can't deny their pain.

I wrote once in my column for the *Los Angeles Times* of my search for a homeless family I had heard of living in a small cluster of trees near a freeway off-ramp. There are about 80,000 homeless people living in Los Angeles County, and I, like most everyone else, had tended to ignore their existence. They were like passing traffic, or leaves carried on a stray breeze, sensed briefly and gone quickly. I wanted to correct my own dispassion by writing about a family I'd been told lived in an encampment at the northern terminus of the Long Beach Freeway. So I went looking.

Neighbors told me they'd been there but had been chased off by the police. I searched the abandoned encamp-

ment and found the debris of their existence: a barbecue grill, a paper cup, a few cans, a ragged shirt . . . and a note. It was written in black crayon on a piece of lined notebook paper by a child who might have been seven or eight years old. On one side was a picture of a house in rough outline, without doors or windows, standing bleakly alone. On the other, printed with determined care, were the words, "I love you mom."

I looked at that note for a long time, drawn into it by the terrible sadness of its circumstances. I could picture a little girl, the age of my own granddaughters, sitting in that vacant lot, carefully printing the words, and just as meticulously drawing a picture of a home that might have existed in a small corner of her memory. It was a house without her in it, a place beyond the horizons of her reach, cold and distant and empty.

When I think of that child, and of all the children in California whose dreams are trampled by poverty, I wince at the dogged efforts of those who would deny them assistance in order to drive them away. The passage of Proposition 187 and attacks on welfare, affirmative action and free food programs burn with acrimony bordering on hatred toward the kinds of people who need help the most. Frustrated by

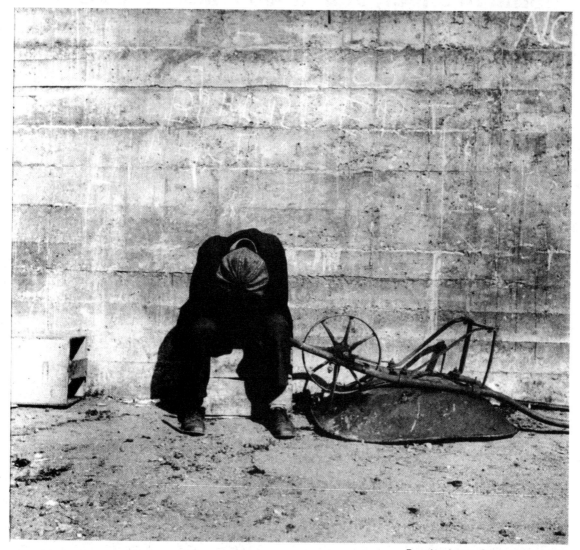

Man Beside Wheelbarrow

Dorothea Lange, San Francisco, 1934,
Courtesy of the Oakland Museum

growing tax burdens and crushing unemployment, we look around for someone to blame and place it on the shoulders of the poor, whether they are immigrants, the mentally ill we dumped into the streets when we stopped "warehousing" them, or those who forever wander in search of existence.

overty isn't always a choice we make by reasons of indolence or the absence of skill. Sometimes it is thrust upon its victims when wars end, government contracts dry up and huge industries move away. We've seen the aerospace plants

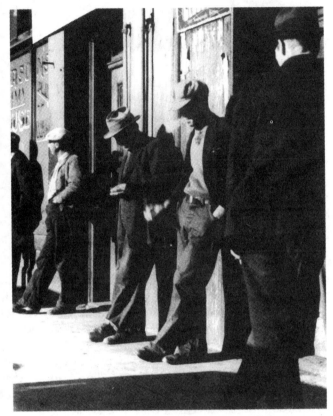

"Thirteen million unemployed fill the cities in the early '30's"

**Dorothea Lange, San Francisco, 1934,
Courtesy of the Oakland Museum**

shut down and General Motors move and a recession-rooted downsizing of businesses from Yreka to San Diego. It all happened for reasons so complex that only a small percentage of the population even begins to understand them. We didn't deliberately add to the problem of poverty, and if you sat down with the guy next door you'd find he hates the idea of people being out of work and kids going hungry.

But poverty in the abstract is something else, and politicians can easily transform the homeless into bums and welfare recipients into leeches as they play upon the fears of a vast middle class to enhance their own positions on the political spectrum. We're going broke, they say, because bums refuse to work; we're going broke because Mexicans are taking our jobs; we're going broke because illegals are burdening our social systems and driving our taxes upward.

They find ready listeners, because many Californians stand a paycheck away from poverty themselves. The same University of California report that found five million Californians hungry found another 8.4 million at risk of being hungry. They're the working poor, to whom a layoff can mean disaster. I saw it happen when the General Motors plant shut down in Van Nuys and 26,000 employees were suddenly out of work. Unexpected illness can similarly wipe out a lifetime of building. I've seen that happen too among those who least expected it.

One of them was Liz McVey.

She was a successful woman in her mid-40s, a restaurateur and the owner of two private detective agencies. A graduate of Bryn Mawr, she was raised in a gray stone mansion in a wealthy section of Chester, Pennsylvania, and numbered the DuPonts among her schoolmates. She came to California in the mid-1950s as an Air Force comptroller, then, intrigued by detective work, earned a private investigator's license. By 1970, she owned two agencies. Such was the success of the agencies that within 10 years she had opened a pair of restaurants. Then the roof fell in.

Business setbacks were followed by a bad fall, followed by a series of illness that kept her hospitalized for seven months. Without medical insurance, her savings disappeared. Lacking the ability to function, her businesses failed. If it is true we are all fate's children, she was selected for punishment beyond reason.

Once out of the hospital, she remained on medication for asthma and diabetes. When I saw her, she was still on oxygen and bedbound. She had no money for food or rent and was about to be evicted from the small Hollywood apartment she occupied alone. "I always wondered why homeless people couldn't just pull themselves up by the bootstraps," she said to me. "I guess I'll find out."

As it turned out, McVey was helped by friends and ultimately gained enough public assistance to get her back on her feet. But this was a university graduate who finally could figure out how to work her way through a maze of bureaucracies to get the help she needed to keep her off the streets. This was a woman with friends.

The five million people in California who live below the poverty level lack the mental resources McVey had. There are damned few university graduates among them, and no friends to extend helping hands. We are their friends. We are their resources. If the California Dream, already blurred, is not to end up as a nightmare, we've got to stop ignoring the armies of despair that occupy our state, and, even more urgently, stop attempting to deprive them of the little they receive from us.

I keep coming back to that Thanksgiving almost 60 years ago and the feelings of hopelessness and despair that poverty created; they are an indelible part of my soul. And I keep coming back to the children of poverty, because by the year 2000 they will be one-third of all the children in California. I grew up in an age relatively free of an inclination toward street violence and found avenues for my rage that were socially acceptable. But this is a different world, a different state, a place that bristles with new armaments and new hatreds, and I can't help but wonder how the anger in the bellies of the children, the sad and hungry kids in the shadows, will react when they're grown up enough to let us know how they feel. I hear thunder in the distance, and wonder when the storm will arrive.

Modern farming yields bountiful fields of dreams

Dennis T. Avery

Dennis T. Avery is editor of Global Food Quarterly *and was formerly the State Department's senior agriculture analyst.*

CHURCHVILLE, va.—A new report from the World Resources Institute invites us to expect a world with "storm-battered islands of biological diversity" in the sea of humans, as wildlands give way to farm, pasture and settlements.

The environmentalists are right that food production is the biggest danger to our wildlife.

The world's cities take up only 1.4 percent of the global land area. Nine billion people in 2040 will occupy only about 3.5 percent of the land area. One-third of the land on this planet is used for farming.

To avoid plowing up more wildlife, we will need to triple today's yields on the world's existing farmland. Can that be done?

Paul Ehrlich and Lester Brown say "No." But they said it could not be done in 1965 and we have already done it.

In fact, the world is full of people who do not know how modern farming has already tripled the world output, but who are firmly convinced we cannot do it again.

The pessimists' favorite argument is that agriculture is up against the law of diminishing returns. But history says the law of diminishing returns may not apply to farming—yet.

When man first started growing crops, he had to find a way to keep weeds from drowning out the wheat and millet.

The first real answer was a method known as "clean fallow." The farmer left half of his field unplanted for a whole season and pulled out any weeds that sprouted. Then he planted. But that wasted half the cropland.

By the early 20th century, American farmers controlled their weeds with horse-drawn "cultivators," which had pointed steel shoes that tore out the weeds between the crop rows. Corn was "check-planted," enabling the horse to pull the cultivator both between and across the rows. This let the farmer get most of his weeds—but he could plant only about 5,000 plants per acre.

Growing crops takes nutrients out of the soil. In the old days, the only ways to put them back (and keep the farm from "wearing out") were

crop rotation and adding manure. Rotation crops such as clover and alfalfa added nitrogen and organic matter to the soil; but a field growing clover was not growing grain.

Nor did crop rotation and manure put back very high levels of nutrients into the soil. Crop yields were limited to between 25 and 30 bushels per year.

Crop rotation was also the only insect control. The better the farmer's corn crop, the more insects he could expect to attract.

With these constraints, a Corn Belt field in the 1920s could grow only two corn crops and a wheat crop every seven years. That made for an average year's yield of perhaps 13 bushels of grain per acre.

Today, a farmer does not need to check-plant his field when he can control his weeds with chemical weedkillers.

Nor do the corn rows have to be wide enough for a horse. Many farmers are planting 25,000 corn plants per acre. A seed company in Michigan says it is testing a variety that can thrive even if crowded in at 50,000 plants per acre.

High levels of plant nutrients result from using available manure with chemical fertilizers. The chemicals provide more soil nutrients per acre than farmers ever got from green manure crops.

The fields have plenty of organic matter because a corn crop that is producing 175 bushels of corn also produces lots of stalks to till back into the soil.

Integrated pest management uses crop rotation, timing and a variety of chemical pest-killers to keep insect damage down to tolerable levels.

Today's Corn Belt farmer can grow big crops of corn, wheat and soybeans almost every year. In seven years, he might grow three 175-bushel corn crops, two hefty soybean crops and one crop of 80-bushel wheat. That is equal to 109 bushels of grain per acre per year—*eight times* the yield of the 1920s.

What about the future? What if these high-yield plant populations are protected with supplemental irrigation systems for the occasional dry spell? And with inbred pest-control from genetic engineering? The farmer could well produce 300-bushel corn yields!

Maximum yields

A Dutch researcher calculated 30 years ago that the maximum edible crop yield per acre was between 6 tons and 9 tons (depending on distance from the equator). The world's current average corn yield is only about 2.5 tons, and the average rice yield is 3.5 tons.

The American Corn Belt farmer (at 4.5 tons) has reached only half this theoretical maximum.

We cannot, of course, repeal the law of diminishing returns. But there seems to be quite a bit of room within the statute to feed a projected peak human population of 9 billion to 10 billion people.

We need to increase investments in high-yield agricultural research, and encourage chemical companies to develop new pesticides, with new methods to prevent buildup of resistant pests.

We need free trade in farm products, to use the world's best farmland wherever it lies.

If we do, the global future should feature islands of high-yield farming and high-rise human habitation amid virtually the same wildlands we have today.

Glossary

Absorption The process by which digestive products pass from the gastrointestinal tract into the blood or lymphatic systems.

Acid/base balance The relationship between acidity and alkalinity in the body fluids.

Amino acids The structural units that make up proteins.

Amylopectin A component of starch, consisting of many glucose units joined in branching patterns.

Amylase An enzyme that breaks down starches; a component of saliva.

Amylose A component of starch, consisting of many glucose units joined in a straight chain, without branching.

Anabolism The synthesis of new materials for cellular growth, maintenance, or repair in the body.

Anemia A deficiency of oxygen-carrying material in the blood.

Anorexia nervosa A disorder in which a person refuses food and loses weight to the point of emaciation and even death.

Antioxidant A substance that prevents or delays the breakdown of other substances by oxygen; often added to food to retard deterioration and rancidity.

Arachidonic acid An essential polyunsaturated fatty acid.

Arteriosclerosis Condition characterized by a thickening and hardening of the walls of the arteries and a resultant loss of elasticity.

Ascorbic Acid Vitamin C.

Atherosclerosis A type of arteriosclerosis in which lipids, especially cholesterol, accumulate in the arteries and obstruct blood flow.

Avidin A substance in raw egg white that acts as an antagonist of biotin, one of the B vitamins.

Basal metabolic rate (BMR) The rate at which the body uses energy for maintaining involuntary functions such as cellular activity, respiration, and heartbeat when at rest.

Basic Four The food plan outlining the milk, meat, fruits and vegetables, and breads and cereals needed in the daily diet to provide the necessary nutrients.

Beriberi A disease resulting from inadequate thiamin in the diet.

Betacarotene Yellow pigment that is converted to vitamin A in the body.

Biotin One of the B vitamins.

Bomb calorimeter An instrument that oxidizes food samples to measure their energy content.

Buffer A substance that can neutralize both acids and bases to minimize change in the pH of a solution.

Calorie The energy required to raise the temperature of one gram of water one degree Celsius.

Carbohydrate An organic compound composed of carbon, hydrogen, and oxygen in a ratio of 1: 2: 1.

Carcinogen A cancer-causing substance.

Catabolism The breakdown of complex substances into simpler ones.

Celiac disease A syndrome resulting from intestinal sensitivity to gluten, a protein in some cereals.

Cellulose An indigestible polysaccharide made of many glucose molecules.

Cheilosis Cracks at the corners of the mouth, due primarily to a deficiency of riboflavin in the diet.

Cholesterol A fatlike alcohol found only in animal products; important in many body functions but also implicated in heart disease.

Choline A substance that prevents the development of a fatty liver; frequently considered one of the B-complex vitamins.

Chylomicron A very small emulsified lipoprotein that transports fat in the blood.

Cobalamin One of the B vitamins (B_{12}).

Coenzyme A component of an enzyme system that facilitates the working of the enzyme.

Collagen Principal protein of connective tissue.

Colostrum The yellowish fluid that precedes breast milk, produced in the first few days of lactation.

Cretinism The physical and mental retardation of a child resulting from severe iodine or thyroid deficiency in the mother during pregnancy.

Dehydration Excessive loss of water from the body.

Dextrin Any of various small soluble polysaccharides found in the leaves of starch-forming plants and in the human alimentary canal as a product of starch digestion.

Diabetes (diabetes mellitus) A metabolic disorder characterized by excess blood sugar and urine sugar.

Digestion The breakdown of ingested foods into particles of a size and chemical composition that can be absorbed by the body.

Diglyceride A lipid containing glycerol and two fatty acids.

Disaccharide A sugar made up of two chemically combined monosaccharides, or simple sugars.

Diuretics Substances that stimulate urination.

Diverticulosis A condition in which the wall of the large intestine weakens and balloons out, forming pouches where fecal matter can be entrapped.

Edema The presence of an abnormally high amount of fluid in the tissues.

Emulsifier A substance that promotes the mixing of foods, such as oil and water in a salad dressing.

Enrichment The addition of nutrients to foods, often to restore what has been lost in processing.

Enzyme A protein that speeds up chemical reactions in the cell.

Epidemiology The study of the factors which contribute to the occurrence of a disease in a population.

Essential amino acid Any of the nine amino acids that the human body cannot manufacture and that must be supplied by the diet, as they are necessary for growth and maintenance.

Essential fatty acid A fatty acid that the human body cannot manufacture and that must be supplied by the diet, as it is necessary for growth and maintenance.

Fat An organic compound whose molecules contain glycerol and fatty acids; fat insulates the body, protects organs, carries fat-soluble vitamins, is a constituent of cell membranes, and makes food taste good.

Fatty acid A simple lipid—containing only carbon, hydrogen, and oxygen—that is a constituent of fat.

Ferritin A substance in which iron, in combination with protein, is stored in the liver, spleen, and bone marrow.

Fiber Indigestible carbohydrate found primarily in plant foods; high fiber intake is useful in regulating bowel movements, and may lower the incidence of certain types of cancer and other diseases.

Flavoprotein Protein containing riboflavin.

Folic acid (folacin) One of the B vitamins.

Fortification The addition of nutrients to foods to enhance their nutritional values.

Fructose A six-carbon monosaccharide found in many fruits as well as honey and plant saps; one of two monosaccharides forming sucrose, or table sugar.

Galactose A six-carbon monosaccharide, one of the two that make up lactose, or milk sugar.

Gallstones An abnormal formation of gravel or stones, composed of cholesterol and bile salts and sometimes bile pigments, in the gallbladder; result when substances that normally dissolve in bile precipitate out.

Gastritis Inflammation of the stomach.

Glucagon A hormone produced by the pancreas that works to increase blood glucose concentration.

Glucose A six-carbon monosaccharide found in sucrose, honey, and many fruits and vegetables; the major carbohydrate found in the body.

Glucose tolerance factor (GTF) A hormonelike substance containing chromium, niacin, and protein that helps the body use glucose.

Glyceride A simple lipid composed of fatty acids and glycerol.

Glycogen The storage form of carbohydrates in the body; composed of glucose molecules.

Goiter Enlargement of the thyroid gland as a result of iodine deficiency.

Goitrogens Substances that induce goiter, often by interfering with the body's utilization of iodine.

Heme A complex iron-containing compound that is a component of hemoglobin.

Hemicellulose Any of various indigestible plant polysaccharides.

Hemochromatosis A disorder of iron metabolism.

Hemoglobin The iron-containing protein in red blood cells which carries oxygen to the tissues.

High-density lipoprotein (HDL) A lipoprotein that acts as a cholesterol carrier in the blood; referred to as "good" cholesterol because relatively high levels of it appear to protect against atherosclerosis.

Hormones Compounds secreted by the endocrine glands that influence the functioning of various organs.

Humectants Substances added to foods to help them maintain moistness.

Hydrogenation The chemical process by which hydrogen is added to unsaturated fatty acids, which saturates them and converts them from a liquid to a solid form.

Hydrolyze To split a chemical compound into smaller molecules by adding water.

Hydroxyapatite The hard mineral portion (the major constituent) of bone, composed of calcium and phosphate.

Hypercalcemia A high level of calcium in the blood.

Hyperglycemia A high level of "sugar" (glucose) in the blood.

Hypocalcemia A low level of calcium in the blood.

Hypoglycemia A low level of "sugar" (glucose) in the blood.

Incomplete protein A protein lacking or deficient in one or more of the essential amino acids.

Inorganic Describes a substance not containing carbon.

Insensible loss Fluid loss, through the skin and from the lungs, that an individual is unaware of.

Insulin A hormone produced by the pancreas that regulates the body's use of glucose.

Intrinsic factor A protein produced by the stomach that makes absorption of B_{12} possible; lack of this protein results in pernicious anemia.

Joule A unit of energy preferred by some professionals over the heat energy measurements of the calorie system for calculating food energy; sometimes referred to as "kilojoule."

Keratinization Formation of a protein called keratin which, in vitamin A deficiency, occurs instead of mucus formation; leads to a drying and hardening of epithelial tissue.

Ketogenic Describes substances that can be converted to ketone bodies during metabolism, such as fatty acids and some amino acids.

Ketone bodies The three chemicals—acetone, acetoacetic acid, and beta-hydroxybutyrie—which are normally involved in lipid metabolism and accumulate in blood and urine in abnormal amounts in conditions of impaired metabolism (such as diabetes).

Ketosis A condition resulting when fats are the major source of energy and are incompletely oxidized, causing ketone bodies to build up in the bloodstream.

Kilocalorie One thousand calories, or the energy required to raise the temperature of one kilogram of water one degree Celsius; the preferred unit of measurement for food energy.

Kilojoule *See* Joule.

Kwashiorkor A form of malnutrition resulting from a severe protein deficiency and a mild to moderate lack of other essential nutrients but an adequate or even excessive calorie intake.

Lactase A digestive enzyme produced by the small intestine that breaks down lactose.

Lactation Milk production/secretion.

Lacto-ovo-vegetarian A person who does not eat meat, poultry, or fish but does eat milk products and eggs.

Lactose A disaccharide composed of glucose and galactose and found in milk.

Lactose intolerance The inability to digest lactose, due to a lack of the enzyme lactase in the intestine.

Lacto-vegetarian A person who does not eat meat, poultry, fish, or eggs but does drink milk and eat milk products.

Laxatives Food or drugs that stimulate bowel movements.

Lignins Certain forms of indigestible carbohydrate in plant foods.

Linoleic acid An essential polyunsaturated fatty acid.

Lipase An enzyme that digests fats.

Lipid Any of various substances in the body or in food that are insoluble in water; a fat or fatlike substance.

Lipoprotein Compound composed of a lipid (fat) and a protein that transports both in the bloodstream.

Low-density lipoprotein (LDL) A lipoprotein that acts as a cholesterol carrier in the blood; referred to as "bad" cholesterol because relatively high levels of it appear to enhance atherosclerosis.

Macrocytic anemia A form of anemia characterized by the presence of abnormally large blood cells.

Macroelements (also macronutrient elements) Those elements present in the body in amounts exceeding 0.005 percent of body weight and required in the diet in amounts exceeding 100 mg/day; include sodium, potassium, calcium, and phosphorus.

Malnutrition A poor state of health resulting from a lack, excess, or imbalance of the nutrients needed by the body.

Maltose A disaccharide whose units are each composed of two glucose molecules, produced by the digestion of starch.

Marasmus Condition resulting from a deficiency of calories and nearly all essential nutrients.

Melanin A dark pigment in the skin, hair, and eyes.

Metabolism The sum of all chemical reactions that take place within the body.

Microelements (also micronutrient elements; trace elements) Those elements present in the body in amounts under 0.005 percent of body weight and required in the diet in amounts under 100 mg/day.

Monoglyceride A lipid containing glycerol and only one fatty acid.

Monosaccharide A single sugar molecule, the simplest form of carbohydrate; examples are glucose, fructose, and galactose.

Monosodium glutamate (MSG) An amino acid used in flavoring foods; causes allergic reactions in some people.

Monounsaturated fatty acid A fatty acid containing one double bond.

Mutagen A mutation-causing agent.

Negative nitrogen balance Nitrogen output exceeds nitrogen intake.

Niacin (nicotinic acid) One of the B vitamins.

Nitrogen equilibrium (zero nitrogen balance) Nitrogen output equals nitrogen intake.

Nonessential amino acid Any of the 13 amino acids that the body can manufacture in adequate amounts, but which are nonetheless required in the diet in an amount relative to the amount of essential amino acids.

Nutrients Nourishing substances in food that can be digested, absorbed, and metabolized by the body; needed for growth, maintenance, and reproduction.

Nutrition (1) The sum of the processes by which an organism obtains, assimilates, and utilizes food. (2) The scientific study of these processes.

Obesity Condition of being 15 to 20 percent above one's ideal body weight.

Oleic acid A monounsaturated fatty acid.

Organic foods Those foods, especially fruits and vegetables, grown without the use of pesticides, synthetic fertilizers, etc.

Osmosis Passage of a solvent through a semipermeable membrane from an area of higher concentration to an area of lower concentration until the concentration is equal on both sides of the membrane.

Osteomalacia Condition in which a loss of bone mineral leads to a softening of the bones; adult counterpart of rickets.

Osteoporosis Disorder in which the bones degenerate due to a loss of bone mineral, producing porosity and fragility; normally found in older women.

Overweight Body weight exceeding an accepted norm by 10 or 15 percent.

Ovo-vegetarian A person who does not eat meat, poultry, fish, milk, or milk products but does eat eggs.

Oxidation The process by which a substrate takes up oxygen or loses hydrogen; the loss of electrons.

Palmitic acid A saturated fatty acid.

Pantothenic acid One of the B vitamins.

Pellagra The niacin deficiency syndrome, characterized by dementia, diarrhea, and dermatitis.

Pepsin A protein-digesting enzyme produced by the stomach.

Peptic ulcer An open sore or erosion in the lining of the digestive tract, especially in the stomach and duodenum.

Peptide A compound composed of amino acids joined together.

Peristalsis Motions of the digestive tract that propel food through the tract.

Pernicious anemia One form of anemia caused by an inability to absorb vitamin B_{12}, owing to a lack of intrinsic factor.

pH A measure of the acidity of a solution, based on a scale from 0 to 14: a pH of 7 is neutral; greater than 7 is alkaline; less than 7 is acidic.

Phenylketonuria (PKU) A genetic disease in which phenylalanine, an essential amino acid, is not properly metabolized, thus accumulating in the blood and causing early brain damage.

Phospholipid A fat containing phosphorus, glycerol, two fatty acids, and any of several other chemical substances.

Polypeptide A molecular chain of amino acids.

Polysaccharide A carbohydrate containing many monosaccharide subunits.

Polyunsaturated fatty acids A fatty acid in which two or more carbon atoms have formed double bonds, with each holding only one hydrogen atom.

Positive nitrogen balance Condition in which nitrogen intake exceeds nitrogen output in the body.

Protein Any of the organic compounds composed of amino acids and containing nitrogen; found in the cells of all living organisms.

Provitamins Precursors of vitamins that can be converted to vitamins in the body (e.g., betacarotene, from which the body can make vitamin A).

Pyridoxine One of the B vitamins (B_6).

Pull date Date after which food should no longer be sold but still may be edible for several days.

Recommended Daily Allowances (RDAs) Standards for daily intake of specific nutrients established by the Food and Nutrition Board of the National Academy of Sciences; they are the levels thought to be adequate to maintain the good health of most people.

Rhodopsin The visual pigment in the retinal rods of the eyes which allows one to see at night; its formation requires vitamin A.

Riboflavin One of the B vitamins (B_2).

Ribosome The cellular structure in which protein synthesis occurs.

Rickets The vitamin D deficiency disease in children characterized by bone softening and deformities.

Saliva Juices, produced in the mouth, that help digest foods.

Salmonella A bacterium that can cause food poisoning.

Saturated fatty acid A fatty acid in which carbon is joined with four other atoms; i.e., all carbon atoms are bound to the maximum possible number of hydrogen atoms.

Scurvy The vitamin C (ascorbic acid) deficiency disease characterized by bleeding gums, pain in joints, lethargy, and other problems.

Standard of identity A list of specifications for the manufacture of certain foods, stipulating their required contents.

Starch A polysaccharide composed of glucose molecules; the major form in which energy is stored in plants.

Stearic acid A saturated fatty acid.

Sucrose A disaccharide composed of glucose and fructose, often called "table sugar."

Sulfites Agents used as preservatives in foods, to eliminate bacteria, preserve freshness, prevent browning, and increase storage life; can cause acute asthma attacks, and even death, in people who are sensitive to them.

Teratogen An agent with the potential of causing birth defects.

Thiamin One of the B vitamins (B_1).

Thyroxine Hormone containing iodine that is secreted by the thyroid gland.

Toxemia A complication of pregnancy characterized by high blood pressure, edema, vomiting, presence of protein in the urine, and other symptoms.

Transferrin Protein compound, the form in which iron is transported in the blood.

Triglyceride A lipid containing glycerol and three fatty acids.

Trypsin A digestive enzyme, produced in the pancreas, that breaks down protein.

Underweight Body weight below an accepted norm by more than 10 percent.

United States Recommended Daily Allowance (USRDA) The highest level of recommended intakes for population groups (except pregnant and lactating women); derived from the RDAs and used in food labeling.

Urea The main nitrogenous component of urine, resulting from the breakdown of amino acids.

Uremia A disease in which urea accumulates in the blood.

Vegan A person who eats nothing derived from an animal; the strictest type of vegetarian.

Vitamin Organic substance required by the body in small amounts to perform numerous functions.

Vitamin B complex All known water-soluble vitamins except C; includes thiamin (B_1), riboflavin (B_2), pyridoxine (B_6), niacin, folic acid, cobalamin (B_{12}), pantothenic acid, and biotin.

Xerophthalmia A disease of the eye resulting from vitamin A deficiency.

Credits/Acknowledgments

Cover design by Charles Vitelli

1. Trends Today and Tomorrow
Facing overview—Dushkin/McGraw·Hill illustration by Mike Eagle.

2. Nutrients
Facing overview—United States Department of Agriculture photo.

3. Through the Life Span
Facing overview—Dushkin/McGraw·Hill photo by Pamela Carley.

4. Fat and Weight Control
Facing overview—New York State Department of Commerce photo.
132—Illustrations by Scott Williams.

5. Food Safety
Facing overview—Dushkin/McGraw·Hill photo by Frank Tarsitano.
164, 166—University of Illinois Archives photos.

6. Health Claims
Facing overview—Dushkin/McGraw·Hill photo by Nick Zavalishin.

7. Hunger and Global Issues
Facing overview—WHO photo by M. Jacot.

ANNUAL EDITIONS ARTICLE REVIEW FORM

■ NAME: _____ DATE: _____

■ TITLE AND NUMBER OF ARTICLE: _____

■ BRIEFLY STATE THE MAIN IDEA OF THIS ARTICLE: _____

_____

■ LIST THREE IMPORTANT FACTS THAT THE AUTHOR USES TO SUPPORT THE MAIN IDEA:

_____

_____

_____

_____

_____

■ WHAT INFORMATION OR IDEAS DISCUSSED IN THIS ARTICLE ARE ALSO DISCUSSED IN YOUR
TEXTBOOK OR OTHER READINGS THAT YOU HAVE DONE? LIST THE TEXTBOOK CHAPTERS AND
PAGE NUMBERS:

_____

_____

_____

_____

_____

■ LIST ANY EXAMPLES OF BIAS OR FAULTY REASONING THAT YOU FOUND IN THE ARTICLE:

_____

_____

_____

_____

■ LIST ANY NEW TERMS/CONCEPTS THAT WERE DISCUSSED IN THE ARTICLE, AND WRITE A SHORT
DEFINITION:

_____

_____

_____

_____

*Your instructor may require you to use this ANNUAL EDITIONS Article Review Form in any
number of ways: for articles that are assigned, for extra credit, as a tool to assist in developing
assigned papers, or simply for your own reference. Even if it is not required, we encourage
you to photocopy and use this page; you will find that reflecting on the articles will greatly
enhance the information from your text.

We Want Your Advice

ANNUAL EDITIONS revisions depend on two major opinion sources: one is our Advisory Board, listed in the front of this volume, which works with us in scanning the thousands of articles published in the public press each year; the other is you—the person actually using the book. Please help us and the users of the next edition by completing the prepaid article rating form on this page and returning it to us. Thank you for your help!

ANNUAL EDITIONS: NUTRITION 97/98
Article Rating Form

Here is an opportunity for you to have direct input into the next revision of this volume. We would like you to rate each of the 59 articles listed below, using the following scale:

1. **Excellent: should definitely be retained**
2. **Above average: should probably be retained**
3. **Below average: should probably be deleted**
4. **Poor: should definitely be deleted**

Your ratings will play a vital part in the next revision. So please mail this prepaid form to us just as soon as you complete it.
Thanks for your help!

Rating	Article	Rating	Article
	1. Consumer Nutrition and Food Safety Trends 1996		32. Dieting and Weight Loss Increase Osteoporosis Risk
	2. The 1995 Dietary Guidelines: Changes and Implications		33. Losing Weight Safely
			34. Surgery for Obesity
	3. The Food Pyramid: How to Make It Work for You		35. The New Paradigm of Trust
	4. The Not-So-Great Mediterranean Diet Pyramid		36. Foodborne Illness: Role of Home Food Handling Practices
	5. Phytochemicals: Drugstore in a Salad?		37. New Risks in Ground Beef Revealed
	6. Taking Soy to Heart		38. Botulinum Toxin
	7. Taking the Fat Out of Food		39. Mad Cow Madness
	8. Fast Food: Fatter than Ever		40. How Much Are Pesticides Hurting Your Health?
	9. Genetic Engineering: Fast Forwarding to Future Foods		41. New Scientific Review Reaffirms Safety of MSG
	10. Genetically Altered States		42. After the Glow
	11. Alcohol: Spirit of Health?		43. Naturally Occurring Toxins: Part of a Balanced Diet?
	12. Should You Be Eating More Protein—or Less?		44. How Quackery Sells
	13. What's Wrong with Sugar?		45. Changing Channels
	14. The Facts about Fats		46. Confessions of a Former Women's Magazine Writer
	15. Food for Thought about Dietary Supplements		47. Food for Thought: Can You Trust Your Favorite Magazine to Tell You What to Eat?
	16. Vitamin A: Pregnancy Hazard?		48. Why Do Those #&*?@! "Experts" Keep Changing Their Minds?
	17. The Trials of Beta-Carotene: Is the Verdict In?		
	18. Vitamin E		49. Vitamin Pushers and Food Quacks
	19. Vitamin C: Is Anyone Right on Dose?		50. Supplement Bill Passes
	20. Special Report: Iron Overkill		51. Supplements Are Unnecessary to Enhance Athletic Performance
	21. Fiber		52. Nutrition Shortcut in a Can?
	22. Nutritional Implications of Ethnic and Cultural Diversity		53. Herbal Roulette
			54. Herbal Warning
	23. Breast-Feeding Best Bet for Babies		55. Averting a Global Food Crisis
	24. Kids Just Want to Have Fun		56. Nibbling at Famine's Edge
	25. Teens at Risk: Nutrition Issues for the '90s		57. Federal Food Assistance Programs: A Step to Food Security for Many
	26. Boning Up on Osteoporosis		
	27. Is Butter Really Better for Me?		58. Thunder in the Distance
	28. Health Implications of Vegetarian Diets		59. Modern Farming Yields Bountiful Fields of Dreams
	29. Obesity: No Miracle Cure Yet		
	30. New Study Questions Weight Guidelines		
	31. New Study Finds Higher Weight Protects Elderly		

(Continued on next page)

ABOUT YOU

Name _____ Date _____

Are you a teacher? ❑ Or a student? ❑

Your school name _____

Department _____

Address _____

City _____ State _____ Zip _____

School telephone # _____

YOUR COMMENTS ARE IMPORTANT TO US !

Please fill in the following information:

For which course did you use this book? _____

Did you use a text with this *ANNUAL EDITION*? ❑ yes ❑ no

What was the title of the text? _____

What are your general reactions to the *Annual Editions* concept?

Have you read any particular articles recently that you think should be included in the next edition?

Are there any articles you feel should be replaced in the next edition? Why?

Are there other areas of study that you feel would utilize an *ANNUAL EDITION?*

May we contact you for editorial input?

May we quote your comments?

ANNUAL EDITIONS: NUTRITION 97/98

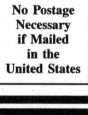
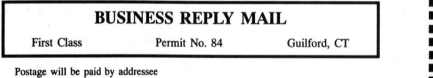